Cyberbullying Across the Globe

Raúl Navarro • Santiago Yubero • Elisa Larrañaga
Editors

Cyberbullying Across the Globe

Gender, Family, and Mental Health

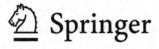
Springer

Editors
Raúl Navarro
Santiago Yubero
Elisa Larrañaga

Department of Psychology
University of Castilla-La Mancha
Cuenca
Spain

ISBN 978-3-319-25550-7   ISBN 978-3-319-25552-1 (eBook)
DOI 10.1007/978-3-319-25552-1

Library of Congress Control Number: 2015956037

Printed on acid-free paper

Springer International Publishing AG Switzerland is part of Science+Business Media (www.springer.com)

Foreword: An International Perspective on Cyberbullying

Over the past 30 years, a revolution has occurred in how we understand and deal with bullying in schools. No doubt bullying has occurred ever since schools came into being; but for many decades it was ignored or denied. Since the 1980s however, social scientists, educators, teachers, and parents have combined efforts to raise awareness of the negative effects that school bullying can have, and to find ways to reduce and prevent it. In fact, a very considerable research program on school bullying has developed over this period. I have argued (Smith 2014) that this has gone through four phases. The first, origins (from 1970s to 1988), occurred in western cultures in Scandinavia, notably through the work of Dan Olweus, including the beginning of measurement techniques and intervention procedures; however, separate origins in eastern cultures such as Japan should be noted. The second (1989–mid-1990s) involved the spread of these ideas to many other countries, and a bringing together of western and eastern studies into one international endeavor. The third (1990s–2004), saw a well-established international research program on bullying which by now commanded considerable attention in academic circles and which had resulted in many publications, but also resources for anti-bullying programs, which have been shown to have some degree of success (Ttofi and Farrington 2011).

The fourth phase has been the advent of cyberbullying. This will have been present more or less since mobile phones and the Internet were invented; but the spread of these devices and the awareness of cyberbullying have happened this century. Press reports and academic publications on cyberbullying took off rapidly from around 2004. This has had ramifications for both academic research and for anti-bullying practice.

So far as academic research is concerned, cyberbullying has both revitalized the bullying research program and challenged it. It has revitalized it in part by bringing in a new mix of disciplines and researchers, from for example, media, communication, and legal studies, to complement the work of (mainly) psychologists and (sometimes) sociologists up to that time. Publications on cyberbullying have rocketed in the past decade as this influx of research and researchers has borne fruit. It has also challenged the research program in several ways. One is definitional—can we apply the usual criteria for school bullying, namely repetition and imbalance of power, to the cyber domain? Another is in terms of scope. The school bullying research stuck rather narrowly to peer–peer bullying in school (with, for example, workplace bullying as a largely separate research area). Such a narrow focus is difficult to sustain when studying cyberbullying, much of which is instigated outside school, and a great deal of which may involve adults as well as children or young people as victims or perpetrators. There are also challenges for practitioners, and for academics seeking to make their research relevant, to ensure that useful resources for coping with cyberbullying become available and disseminated.

The available research on school bullying, including findings from regular surveys such as Health Behavior of School-Aged Children (HBSC), indicate that rates have been in decline in a majority of countries surveyed, over the past 10–15 years. It is plausible that the school bullying research program and its practical applications has been a major contributor to this. But the evidence regarding cyberbullying, although much more limited, does not show any clear decrease and indeed sometimes shows an increase in recent years. Developing awareness and resources to cope with cyberbullying is a work in progress. It may be a work in progress for some time, as modes of use of mobile phones and the Internet change rapidly and is measured in years rather than decades.

This book brings together contributions from seven countries across the globe, to focus on a range of issues around cyberbullying. It includes issues around family and gender; research perspectives from different countries; and practical contributions on prevention and intervention. The authors are experts in their respective areas, and this will surely be a most useful book for researchers and practitioners concerned about understanding cyberbullying and ameliorating or preventing the negative and sometimes devastating consequences it can have.

Goldsmiths College, University of London, UK   Peter K. Smith

References

Smith, P. K. (2014). *Understanding school bullying*. Sage Publications.
Ttofi, M. M., & Farrington, D. P. (2011). Effectiveness of school-based programs to reduce bullying: A systematic and meta-analytic review. *Journal of Experimental Criminology, 7,* 27–56.

Acknowledgements

No one makes the road without help. Apart from the names appearing on the cover of this volume, we would like to express our gratitude to all who have walked and walk with us in our academic and personal life. Particularly, we are indebted to all contributors involved in this project. The volume presented here is the result of the close collaboration of an interdisciplinary group of distinguished scholars whose own knowledge, time, and interest have contributed to the formation of this book. Finally, we offer our thanks to the Springer editorial team, especially to Garth Haller for his assistance, supervision, and much-needed encouragement during the entire process.

Acknowledgements

Contents

About the Editors

Raúl Navarro Ph.D. is a lecturer in the Department of Psychology at the University of Castilla-la Mancha, Spain. He received his bachelor's degree in education and psychology from the University of Castilla-la Mancha, a master's degree in social education from the University Pablo Olavide and his Ph.D. in psychology from the University of Castilla-La Mancha. Dr. Navarro's research has focused on relationships among bullying behaviors and gender, aggression and school adjustment, online communication, antecedent factors of cyberbullying, and parental mediation and Internet victimization. He has coauthored several book chapters on gender socialization and bullying, and has written articles about cyberbullying, which have been published in international journals. Dr. Navarro has given conferences and seminars with adolescents, teachers, and parents about how to deal with bullying. He has been on research stays in Goldsmith College, London, with Peter K. Smith, Ph.D., and at the University of Massachusetts, Boston, with Martha Montero, Ph.D., to analyze bullying behaviors. He is currently teaching courses about social psychology, gender development and psychology values in the Social Education Degree and the Master of Psychology.

Santigo Yubero Ph.D. is the dean of the Faculty of Education and Humanities at the University of Castilla-La Mancha, Spain. He obtained his bachelor's degree and his doctorate degree in psychology from the Complutense University in Madrid. In the past few years, he has been teaching courses about social psychology, social intervention, and intergroup relations in the Social Work and Social Education Degree as a member of the Department of Psychology at the University of Castilla-la Mancha. His research interests include group conflict, workplace aggression, bullying and socialization processes. He has edited several books about social education, intergroup conflict, violence and bullying with Professor Peter K. Smith, Ph.D., at Goldsmith College, London, Professor Anastasio Ovejero, Ph.D., at the University of Valladolid, and Professor Francisco Morales, Ph.D., at the National University of Distance Education. He is also the deputy director of the Centre of Studies for the Promotion of Reading and Children's Literature at the University of Castilla-

La Mancha. He has given conferences about reading promotion in diverse Latin-American countries like Argentina, Mexico, Colombia, or Brazil. Dr. Yubero has worked in a private practice as a counseling psychologist.

Elisa Larrañaga Ph.D.   is the dean of the Faculty of Social Work at the University of Castilla-La Mancha, Spain. She obtained her bachelor's degree in psychology at the Complutense University in Madrid, and her doctorate degree from the University of Castilla-La Mancha. She has been teaching courses about developmental psychology, psychopathology, and language acquisition in the Social Work and Education Degrees as a member of the Department of Psychology at University of Castilla-La Mancha. Her research interests include reading practices, sexism, behavioral problems, gender, and cyberbullying. She has edited several books on violence and social exclusion working with Amalio Blanco, Ph.D., at the Complutense University in Madrid. She has coauthored several book chapters on reading promotion, violence and traditional bullying. She collaborates with the Centre of Studies for the Promotion of Reading and Children's Literature at the University of Castilla-La Mancha. She has been working with teachers and parents about promotion of reading as a tool to prevent and intervene in sexist attitudes, violence behavior, and resilience. Dr. Larrañaga has also worked in a private practice as a counseling and clinical psychologist focusing on language problems.

Contributors

Sofía Buelga Department of Social Psychology, University of Valencia, Valencia, Spain

Fabiola Cabra Torres Facultad de Educación, Pontificia Universidad Javeriana, Bogotá, Colombia

Cristina Cañamares Department of Philology, University of Castilla-La Mancha, Cuenca, Spain

Wanda Cassidy Faculty of Education, Simon Fraser University, Burnaby, BC, Canada

Lucie Corcoran School of Arts, Dublin Business School, Dublin 2, Ireland

Susan Hanley Duncan University of Louisville, Louisville, KY, USA

Steven Eggermont School for Mass Communication Research, University of Leuven, Leuven, Belgium

Chantal Faucher Centre for Education, Law and Society, Simon Fraser University, Surrey, BC, Canada

Gary W. Giumetti Department of Psychology, Quinnipiac University, Hamden, CT, USA

Wannes Heirman Department of Communication Studies, University of Antwerp, Antwerp, Belgium

Margaret Jackson School of Criminology, Simon Fraser University, Burnaby, BC, Canada

Robin M. Kowalski Department of Psychology, Clemson University, Clemson, SC, USA

María de la V. Moral Department of Social Psychology, Universtiy of Oviedo, Oviedo, Spain

Elisa Larrañaga Department of Psychology, Faculty of Social Work, University of Castilla-La Mancha, Cuenca, Spain

Seung-Ha Lee Department of Early Childhood Education, Yeungnam University, Gyeongsan-si, Gyeongsangbuk-do, South Korea

Gloria Marciales Vivas Department of Psychology, Pontificia Universidad Javeriana, Bogotá, Colombia

Belén Martínez-Ferrer Department of Education and Social Psychology. Pablo de Olavide University, Seville, Spain

Conor Mc Guckin School of Education, Trinity College Dublin, Dublin 2, Ireland

Gonzalo Musitu Department of Psychology, Pablo de Olavide University, Seville, Spain

Raúl Navarro Department of Psychology, Faculty of Education and Humanities, University of Castilla-La Mancha, Cuenca, Spain

Anastasio Ovejero Department of Psychology, University of Valladolid, Valladolid, Spain

Sara Pabian Department of Communication Studies, University of Antwerp, Antwerp, Belgium

Sandra Sánchez-García Department of Philology, University of Castilla-La Mancha, Cuenca, Spain

Cristina Serna Department of Psychology, University of Castilla-La Mancha, Faculty of Social Work, Cuenca, Spain

Heidi Vandebosch Department of Communication Studies, University of Antwerp, Antwerp, Belgium

Michel Walrave Department of Communication Studies, University of Antwerp, Antwerp, Belgium

Denis Wegge Department of Communication Studies, University of Antwerp, Antwerp, Belgium

Santiago Yubero Department of Psychology, Faculty of Education and Humanities, University of Castilla-La Mancha, Cuenca, Spain

Chapter 1
Cyberbullying: Definitions and Facts from a Psychosocial Perspective

Anastasio Ovejero, Santiago Yubero, Elisa Larrañaga
and María de la V. Moral

School coexistence is one of the main objectives that schools must pursue in at least two ways: (1) an objective on school coexistence must be formulated to allow good interpersonal relationships among all members of schools and (2) in parallel, the objective must make achieving all other scholarly objectives possible. Consequently, we must make every necessary effort to face all the obstacles and problems that make a suitable and positive school life difficult. These obstacles include violent conduct, which also causes much harm and suffering to many young and adolescent students, among which bullying and cyberbullying stand out. This chapter centers on analyzing cyberbullying as an extremely harmful psychosocial phenomenon for not only children and adolescents but also for positive school life. The reason why we face this phenomenon is because numerous adolescents have committed suicide in several countries worldwide. So, we must systematically study it if we want psychology to become a real solution to social problems and to alleviate people's pain and suffering. The gravest aspect is that victims, who have committed suicide, have made us aware of the seriousness of this matter. This was the case of a 13-year-old boy called Ryan who committed suicide in the USA on October 7, 2003. It was not by chance that considering conducting research into cyberbullying began systematically since 2004 (Smith 2013), which became the fourth phase of studies on school bullying (Smith 2013). Since then, we have studied the reasons why some

A. Ovejero (✉)
Department of Psychology, University of Valladolid,
Valladolid, Spain
e-mail: tasio@psi.uva.es

S. Yubero
Department of Psychology, Faculty of Education and Humanities,
University of Castilla-La Mancha, 16071 Cuenca, Spain

E. Larrañaga
Department of Psychology, Faculty of Social Work, University of Castilla-La Mancha,
Camino del Pozuelo s/n., 16071 Cuenca, Spain

M. de la V. Moral
Department of Social Psychology, Universtiy of Oviedo, Oviedo, Spain

© Springer International Publishing Switzerland 2016
R. Navarro et al. (eds.), *Cyberbullying Across the Globe*,
DOI 10.1007/978-3-319-25552-1_1

schoolchildren get involved in cyberbullying, its negative effects, what it shares, or does not share, with traditional bullying, the prevalence of such harmful conduct or ways to prevent it. This chapter attempts to review the current situation of this particular matter.

It is quite surprising that although since 1992 violence at school has never stopped diminishing (Robers et al. 2014), there is increasing concern about bullying, and of both the traditional and online kinds (see Giumetti and Kowalski in this volume). This reflects an insecure and intimidated society. Let us not forget that the most important aspect is the suffering of thousands and thousands of victims, who are normally adolescents.

It is well known that many episodes of bullying, humiliation, and violence by students at school have appeared in the news in the past 10–12 years, and that these students employ new communication technologies to this end, above all the Internet and cell phones (Li 2006; Smith et al. 2006; Smith et al. 2008). Some of these episodes have even ended in the victim committing suicide. In fact, generalizing about the use of the two above-mentioned technologies has allowed a new phenomenon to emerge, cyberbullying (Belsey 2005), also known as electronic bullying (Raskauskas and Stoltz 2007) or digital bullying (Olin 2003).

Bullying already existed much earlier before the Internet and cell phones appeared. Young and adolescent students, and also more and more children, have used the new technologies to bully others, basically because these media provide them with this facility (or that is what they believe) to attack but remain anonymous (anonymity), which other cyberbullying aspects facilitate: not seeing the victim, nor his or her pain and suffering caused by bullying conduct. So, it is much easier for them to keep a moral distance from their victims. This means feeling less regret and having fewer scruples when harming someone else. So, it is not surprising that cyberbullying prevalence rates have never stopped rising.

Finally, we wish to add that a considerable number of chapters similar to the present one are available, but we wished to include a more psychosocial orientation that includes the reality that cyberbullying is a phenomenon that is understood only in a context that is group-like, family, school, community and cultural.

1.1   The Internet Galaxy and Cyberbullying

Although the Gutenberg Galaxy is still present, it is obvious that we now live in another era known as the Galaxy Internet (Castells 2001), which has completely changed our lives, to the point that we can un-mistakenly assert that a new era of humanity has commenced with the technology revolution, especially with the Internet. According to Manuel Castells (2001, p. 15), "The Internet is the fabric of our lives. If information technology is the historical equivalent of what electricity represented in the industrial era, in our era we can compare the Internet with the electric grid and the electric motor given its capacity to distribute the power of information to all areas of human activity." Therefore, it is for the right and wrong. More specifically, Castells adds (p. 20), "the elasticity of the Internet makes this means particularly suitable to stress our society's contradictory trends. The Internet is neither a utopia nor a dystopia, but a means we express ourselves in—by a specific communication code that we must understand if we intend to change our reality." So, in a violent society, people will use the Internet to attack and bully others, while a caring and altruistic society will use it to help others. So, right and wrong does not lie in the Internet, but in the way we use it.

However, the Internet is here to stay. So, we must do whatever we can to increase its positive effects, and there are many, and to cut its negative effects and risks to a minimum, of which there are also many, above all in the field of social interaction with young people and adolescents. Largely, they will depend on the cultural and ideological background in which they live. Nowadays, the dominant cultural pattern is none other than neoliberal capitalism, that is, "the neoliberal globalisation ideology" (see Ovejero 2014). This ideology shapes "neoliberal subjects" who consider that they can use all surroundings, including people, to consequently obtain some benefit as a result (Laval and Dardot 2010; Lazzarato 2011; Ovejero 2014). The features of this neoliberal ideology (selfishness, individualism, social Darwinism, fatalism, competition of everyone against everyone, internalization of the idea that benefit is all that matters), especially internalized by adolescents, are difficulting a suitable coexistence among people, even in the Internet, in at least two directions: it is quite likely that more and more people show less empathy to peers, which may promote cyberbullying; on the contrary, behaviors to defend and help victims may become less and less likely, which also may increase victim's pain. In this way, it is not surprising that cases of cyberbullying have increased so much. In only 10 years, the world of electronic communications has dramatically changed as we now find many other forms of electronic communication (chat, text messages, etc.), which makes the problem even worse, given the frequent diffusion of episodes that harm some people on web pages such as YouTube or MySpace, where thousands of people act as constant witnesses of the jokes or humiliation that victims are targets of. In the most serious cases, participation in such episodes has led a victim to commit suicide, and news items have a huge social repercussion which, at the end of the day, allows growing interest in this phenomenon.

Over the past 10–12 years, cyberbullying has appeared as a new form of violent conduct in the electronic communication context as the result of the vast communication possibilities that progress in electronics has enabled, especially among increasingly younger adolescents (Noret and Rivers 2006). Using a cell phone and the Internet has increased so much in recent years: in 2004, 68 % of Spanish students aged 10–15 years employed a computer, while 94.1 % did so only 4 years later (INE, 2008). The Internet and cell phone uses show a similar trend: 60.2 % in 2004 versus 82.2 % in 2008 and 45.7 % in 2004 versus 65.8 % in 2008, respectively. Since 2008, this trend has not stopped growing, to the point that current rates come close to 100 %. In Switzerland, 95 % of adolescents aged between 12 and 19 years have access to the Internet at home, 75 % do so in their own bedroom, and nearly all of them have and use a cell phone (Willemse et al. 2010). So, we can see that having access to these technologies has increased so much that they affect almost all students aged over 10 years in almost all countries worldwide. The extent is such that Talwar et al. (2014) state that electronic is now the most frequent communication type among adolescents and young people, and even among the under 14-year-olds (Print Measurement Bureau 2013), and even among small children (Monks et al. 2012). The Pew Internet Research Center (Pew 2009) reports that 93 % of adolescents in the USA use the Internet. In the same country, social networks, such as Facebook, are employed by around 70 million people, mostly young people. So, it is not strange to find that more and more teachers and education specialists worry about the effects of electronic communication. In fact, we can only understand cyberbullying if we frame it in this technological context where young people spend most of their time (Festl and Quandt 2013; Walrave and Heirman 2011; Ybarra and Mitchell 2008). We know that the more widespread the Internet is, the more frequent cyberbullying cases are (Erdur-Baker 2010; Floros et al. 2013; Kwan and Skoric 2013; Leung and Lee 2012; Staksrud et al. 2013). So, in the USA, between 20 and 40 % of young people who use the Internet have experienced cyberbullying at least once in their life (Tokunaga 2010), while 6 % of schoolchildren in Europe aged 9–12 years who use the Internet have been cyberbullied some time in the previous year (Livingstone et al. 2011). What is more, Kumazaki et al. (2011) discovered that a relationship exists in the first stage of adolescence between skills for using the Internet and cyberbullying conduct.

It is also a fact that adolescents increasingly employ social networks, such as Twitter or Facebook (Duggan and Smith 2014), where self-presentation plays an essential role (personal data, photos, etc.). However, it is quite likely that some people use such information and photos to harm others, either as a joke or for other purposes. Therefore, using the Internet not only has many unquestionable advantages but also severe risks (Carr 2010; Holfeld and Grabe 2012), among which cyberbullying stands out for its extent and serious consequences (Genta et al. 2013; Kowalski et al. 2012; Smith 2013).

1.2 Definition of Cyberbullying

Both bullying and cyberbullying are aggressive conducts whose objective is to harm another person, which most certainly refers to violent social conduct. This means that to study it, we must frame it within social psychology. Therefore, authors such as Bandura (1999) and his theory about moral disengagement, Milgram (1974) and his study on obeying authority, Zimbardo (2007) and his demonstration of power over the situation, or Baumeister and Leary (1995) and the consequences of not satisfying the need to belong, will be very helpful here. Social psychologists have demonstrated that it is not necessary to act aggressively to get involved in violent conducts because they depend, to a great extent, on situational variables, such as the group we belong to, or feeling satisfied or not with belonging, identity, or self-esteem (Aronson 2000; Putnam 2000). We face a general pattern of conduct that shows a clear relationship between social exclusion and/or social rejection and aggressive/violent behavior (Garbarino 1999; Garbarino and deLara 2003a, b). We also know that it is not a matter of a mere correlation, rejection and exclusion lead to aggressive behavior (Twenge et al. 2002, 2003) in such a way that exclusion even multiplies difficulties for self-regulation (Baumeister et al. 2005), which increases the likelihood of getting involved in aggressive and violent behavior. Its seriousness stems from the fact that ostracism and social exclusion in our societies today are becoming increasingly frequent (Putnam 2000; Williams 2007), which also lower the probability of prosocial behaviors (Twenge et al. 2007).

Another important factor responsible for online aggression is lack of inhibition and social disengagement. Online bullies do not have to deal with the inmediate emotional or psychological effects on their victims because they are separate by technology, which make it much easier to get involved in cyberbullying.

Although the definition of cyberbullying tends to be similar to that of bullying (see Ovejero et al. 2013 about bullying), there is still no consensus about its more specific characteristics (Olweus 2013; Smith et al. 2012; Ybarra et al. 2012). This is due to its intrinsic complexity and to the fact that many cyberbullying types exist depending on the means employed to practice them (e-mail, cell phone, text messages, web sites, chats, social networks, digital images, online games, etc.), and each one is used more in one age group than in another, or more by subjects depending on some characteristics or others (Juvonen and Gross 2008; Kowalski and Limber 2007).

Nevertheless, many definitions for cyberbullying resemble one another, and most repeat the bullying definition but require electronic means (Juvonen and Gross 2008; Menesini and Nocentini 2009; Smith et al. 2008; Tokunaga 2010). Smith et al. (2006) define cyberbullying as aggressive and intentional action that employs electronic forms of contact, repeatedly perpetrated by an individual or group, which remains constant over time with a victim who cannot easily defend oneself. Likewise, Belsey (2005) maintains that cyberbullying implies using electronic communication technologies as a platform of intentional, repeated, and hostile conduct applied to an individual or group to harm others. Yet some discussion continues as to whether it is necessary or not there being an intention to hurt someone, if it is necessary to repeat this conduct, if an imbalance of power must exist, etc. An example of such is, for victims, that the essential factor for talking about cyberbullying is not the intention but the real effects (Dredge et al. 2014a). As to whether repeating an attack with time is necessary, here things change with face-to-face bullying because, more often than not, only one harmful action presented to a large audience is sufficient to consider it cyberbullying.

1.3 Similarities and Differences Between Traditional Bullying and Cyberbullying

Cyberbullying shares some characteristics of traditional bullying (Almeida et al. 2012; Kowalski and Limber 2013; Kowalski et al. 2014; Menesini et al. 2012; Smith 2013), to the extent that some authors state that it is a continuation of bullying but occurs outside school and by electronic media (Giumetti and Kowalski in this volume; Kowalski et al. 2014; Mishna et al. 2010; Vandebosch and Van Cleemput 2009; Wegge et al. 2013), and they sometimes overlap (Modecki et al. 2014). In fact, the vast majority of adolescents involved in cases of bullying have been involved in both traditional and cyberbullying types as bullies and/or victims, while there are very few cases in which the people involved are either bullies or victims in only one of the bullying types (Landstedt and Persson 2014; Olweus 2012).

Nevertheless, cyberbullying has its own typical characteristics that clearly distinguish it from traditional bullying. This has led some authors, such as Dredge et al. 2014a, to doubt that the definition of traditional bullying can be applied to cyberbullying. It is true that traditional and electronic bullying considerably overlap, both positively relate to each other (Bauman 2009; Mitchell et al. 2011), and many traditional bullies are also cyberbullies (Smith and Slonje 2010). So, we can view cyberbullying as a new way of attacking people rather than a conceptually new phenomenon (Gradinger et al. 2010; Raskauskas and Stoltz 2007). Yet cyberbullying has its own different characteristics, which make it different to traditional bullying. Smith (2013, pp. 177–178) summarizes them as follows: (1) It requires a certain degree of technological specialization. Although it is quite easy to send emails and text messages, attacks are more sophisticated, such as forging one's identity, and require more technical skills; (2) it is a form of indirect aggression, which favors the bully's invisible and anonymous condition; (3) the bully does not normally witness the victims' reaction, which makes moral disengagement easier, and also favors cyberbullying because, as direct feedback is lacking, empathy or regret is less likely; (4) the variety of spectator's roles is more complex in cyberbullying than it is in bullying; (5) the bully tends to lose support, which increases the status that the traditional bully acquires before peers when exercising his or her power on the victim; (6) the size of the potential audience in cyberbullying is much larger; and (7) a cyberbully has access to his or her victims 24 h, 7 days a week, while a traditional bully only has access at school. So, cyberbullying victims "have nowhere to hide" and cannot avoid the bully, not even by changing school or moving to another city or town; the victims' fear of the bully can trigger genuine panic.

To these differences, we can add others. For example, cyberbullying tends to take place outside school, so it is difficult for teachers to control it (Kraft and Wang 2009; Stewart and Fritsch 2011). Being both a bully and a victim is more frequent than in traditional bullying (Kessel Schneider et al. 2012; Kowalski et al. 2012; Privitera and Campbell 2009; Smith et al. 2008; Walrave and Heirman 2011; Wong et al. 2014). In addition, bullies are either adolescents who feel isolated or have been rejected by classmates (Wright and Li 2013).

Basically, the relationships between both bullying types are more complex than they may appear at first sight. The new technologies have specific characteristics: anonymity, more likelihood of moral disengagement, more potential bystanders, difficulty to detect who the bully actually is, the duration of bullying episodes, this being 24 h/day in cyberbullying, etc., which make cyberbullying a distinct phenomenon and a more harmful one than face-to-face bullying (Campbell et al. 2013; Cassidy et al. 2013; Mishna et al. 2012; Park et al. 2014).

1.4   Measuring Cyberbullying and Prevalence Rates

Despite there being many studies on cyberbullying, serious measuring problems still exist (Mehari et al. 2014; Menesini and Nocentini 2009; Menesini et al. 2011; Rivers 2013), which relate mainly with these two factors: the nature of the items employed and the characteristics of the underlying definition (Kowalski et al. 2014):

(a) *Nature of the items employed*: Here, the two main problems are that the items employed do not well observe the phenomenon they say they measure. So each author uses items with different contents to measure cyberbullying. A complete, accurate definition agreed by all for both the above factors is necessary because, as previously mentioned, such a definition does not exist. Some authors measure cyberbullying with a single item, while others employ multi-item measures, which makes comparing the results difficult and gives rise to distinct prevalence rates. Clearly multi-item measures seem better than the single-item kind, but we need researchers to reach a consensus about the specific conducts to include, and also about the frequency with which these conducts must take place (e.g., "once a month", "at least 5 times in the two last 2 months", etc.) (Kowalski et al. 2014; Modecki et al. 2014).
(b) *Content of the definition used*: Despite the efforts made today to reach a consensus about a definition of cyberbullying (Gladden et al. 2014), we are still far from achieving this. So, while some authors do not include the term "bully" so they do not have to label students as "bullies" or "victims", others include it. Once again, we need to state that this makes comparing the results difficult and gives rise to distinct prevalence rates. For example, Ybarra et al. (2012) state that when we use the term "bully", we obtain lower prevalence rates (the following authors indicated a similar situation: Kann et al. 2014; Kowalski et al. 2014).

As for prevalence rates, the results of one of the first studies on this matter showed that 6% of North American adolescent students reported being bullied over the Internet (Finkelhor et al. 2000). Yet shortly afterward, in the work of Mnet (2001) this percentage rose to 25% for Canadian Internet users who received intimidating or aggressive messages about other people. However, nobody conducted specifically designed research to measure cyberbullying until 2004, and one of the first to do so were Ybarra and Mitchell (2004), who found that 19% of youngsters aged 10–17 years were involved in cyberbullying cases. This percentage rose to 38.3% in another study also conducted in the USA (Burgess-Proctor et al. 2006) and to 49% in another US study, with 21% as cyberbullies (Raskauskas and Stoltz 2007). In Australia, however, Campbell (2005) reported lower percentages: 14% of students indicated being a cyberbullying victim and 11% being cyberbullies. In the UK, victimization rates are 13% (MSN.uk, 2006), although Smith et al. (2006) reported a percentage of 22%. In Canada, Li (2006) speaks about 25% of cybervictims and 17% of cyberbullies. In Holland, Van den Eijnden et al. (2006) found that 17% of youngsters have been involved in cyberbullying situations at least on one occasion.

In Greece, Kapatzia and Syngollitou (2007) provided much lower percentages as they report 6% victims and 7% cyberbullies, and Slonje and Smith (2008) in Sweden found that 5.3% of students stated being cybervictims and 10.3% were cyberbullies. Finally in Turkey, Dilmaç (2009) found a 23% rate of cyberbullying, and one of 55% for cybervictims among university students. These data are similar to those indicated by Arıcak (2009) also for Turkish university students: 20% of cyberbullies and 54% of cybervictims.

As we can see, the variability in the prevalence of this phenomenon is very wide (Kowalski et al. 2014; Livingstone and Smith 2014; Sabella et al. 2013). Although Kowalski et al. (2014) stated that, in general, the prevalence of cyberbullying is approximately 10–14%, many studies have found much higher percentages; Carroll (2008) found that 69% of subjects were involved in cyberbullying as either bullies or victims. Some authors even indicate that 75% of youngsters at school have experienced cyberbullying at least once in the past year (Juvonen and Gross 2008; Katzer et al. 2009).

Therefore, the essential characteristic of cyberbullying prevalence rates is its huge variability. Patchin and Hinduja (2012) reviewed the data of 35 studies and concluded that victimization rates ranged from 5.5 to 72%, Cook et al. (2010) placed it between 5 and 44%, while Sabella et al. (2013) stated that it was between 6 and 30%.

By way of conclusion, existing data do not allow us to solve the matter of whether cyberbullying is rising or curbing because it is not easy to detect changes in this prevalence with such disperse data. What is clear, however, is that no matter how we measure, we will always find that this prevalence is worrying. If to this we add that its consequences for victims are more harmful than those of traditional bullying (Copeland et al. 2013; Vivolo-Kantor et al. 2014), it is obvious that both parents and teachers must be well informed about this field (Collier 2009; Juvonen and Gross 2008).

1.5   Effects of Cyberbullying

The effects of cyberbullying are similar to those preceded by traditional bullying (Cappadocia et al. 2013; Wade and Beran 2011), but are more harmful and last longer (Fredstrom et al. 2011; Machmutow et al. 2012; Menesini et al. 2012; Perren and Gutzwiller-Helfenfinger 2012; Sakellariou et al. 2012; Schneider et al. 2012; Ševčíková et al. 2012; Šléglová and Černá 2011; Smith et al. 2008; Sticca et al. 2013) given some of the aforementioned differential characteristics, to the extent that committing suicide is more likely in cyberbullying (Bonanno and Hymel 2013).

Results from the research that has been conducted to date in different countries are overwhelming. Avaliable evidences show that cyberbullying is a clear threat to adolescents health and well-being, physically (different somatic symptoms, such as sleeping disorders, headaches, loss of appetite, skin problems, etc.), psychologically (anxiety, anguish, depression, suicidal thoughts), and psychosocially (isolation, solitude, exclusion, etc.). Relations between cyberbullying and children's and adolescent's poor well-being have been found in Germany (Katzer et al. 2009), Australia (Hemphill et al. 2012), Spain (Estévez et al. 2010; Navarro et al. 2013; Navarro et al. 2012; Ortega et al. 2009), the USA (Wigderson and Lynch 2013), Finland (Sourander et al. 2010), Northern Ireland (Devine and Lloyd 2012), Israel (Olenik-Shemesh et al. 2012), Canada (Bonanno and Hymel 2013), Czech Republic (Macháčková et al. 2013), China (Wong et al. 2014), Sweden (Slonje et al. 2012), Switzerland (Perren et al. 2010), Taiwan (Chang et al. 2013), Turkey (Aricak et al. 2008), etc.

However, the effects suffered by cyberbullying victims are more or less severe depending on a series of situational factors, such as whether anonymity exists or not, or the number of bystanders (Dredge et al. 2014a). For example, if one effect of bullying is increased anxiety in victims (Garnefski and Kraaij 2014), this anxiety becomes even more acute in cyberbullying as victims do not know who actually bullies them and think that it can be anyone. It is also a very psychosocial matter in that one of the most painful aspects for victims is feeling exposed and that other people can see them, and there are potentially many more in cyberbullying than in traditional bullying.

Among the effects caused by cyberbullying, the following stand out:

(a) *Physical*: headache, stomachache, sleep disorders, tiredness, backache, loss of appetite, digestion problems, etc. (Gradinger et al. 2009; Sourander et al. 2010).
(b) *Psychological and emotional*: fear, and even feelings of terror, anxiety, anguish, sadness, stress, symptoms of depression (Ayas 2014; DeHue et al. 2008; Hinduja and Patchin 2010; Katzer et al. 2009; Kowalski and Limber 2013; Livingstone and Smith 2014; Machmutow et al. 2012; Nixon 2014; Perren et al. 2010; Price and Dalgleish 2010; Schultze-Krumbholz and Scheithauer 2009; Vazsonyi et al. 2012), more frequent ideas of suicide (Bauman et al. 2013; Hinduja and Patchin 2010; Kim and Leventhal 2008; Meltzer et al. 2011), and even committing suicide (Bonanno and Hymel 2013; Hinduja and Patchin 2010; Kirby 2008; Messias et al. 2014; Price and Dalgleish 2010). More specifically, in a recent meta-analysis done in Holland, Sonawane (2014) found that those who are electronically bullied are twice as likely to have suicidal thoughts, and 2.5 times more likely to actually commit suicide, than those who are not cyberbullying victims. Van Geel et al. (2014) found that having suicidal ideas was more likely among people who had experienced bullying and cyberbullying, followed by those who had suffered only cyberbullying, and finally by those who had been victims only of traditional bullying (see Pendergrass and Wright 2014 for some cases of suicide due to cyberbullying).
(c) *School-related*: one effect of cyberbullying is feeling less motivated about school, which entails academic performance problems (Bargh and Mckenna 2004; Beran and Li 2005; Hinduja and Patchin 2011; Price and Dalgleish 2010; Willard 2012; Ybarra and Mitchell 2004). So, although cyberbullying occurs outside school, schools should take this problem very seriously (Hinduja and Patchin 2011; Willard 2012).

(d) *Psychosocial*: more feelings of isolation and solitude, ostracism, and even social rejection (Wright and Li 2013). These effects are particularly harmful because they attack the individuals' social center, which involves psychosocial requirements, in particular belonging, positive identity, and self-esteem (Baumeister and Leary 1995; Williams 2007). Here, the harm caused to victims stands out (Brighi et al. 2012; Kowalski and Limber 2007; Kowalski and Limber 2007; Patchin and Hinduja 2010).

Moreover, the group of obese individuals is a particular target of bullying of both the traditional (DeSmet et al. 2014; Brixval et al. 2011; Eisenberg et al. 2006; Gray et al. 2009; Kukaswadia et al. 2011) and online (DeSmet et al. 2014; Mishna et al. 2012) kinds.

Yet as Özdemir (2014) points out, cybervictimization does not influence all victims in the same way (see Mckenna and Bargh 1998; Van der Aa et al. 2009): it depends on factors such as gender, the quantity and quality of social support that one has, the type of relationship victims have with their parents, their age, or the time they spend using electronic communication media. It is known that cyberbullied females experience more negative effects than males (Brown et al. 2014), and that the more time adolescents spend on the Internet and its various forms (cell phones, emails, text messages, chats, etc.), the more likely it is that they get involved in cases of cyberbullying (Levy et al. 2012; Staksrud et al. 2013). Even the number of friends on Facebook appears to be a predictor of cybervictimization (Dredge et al. 2014b; Staksrud et al. 2013). According to some studies (Burgess-Proctor et al. 2009; Dredge et al. 2014a; Patchin and Hinduja 2006; Ybarra et al. 2006), around half the victims state that the cyberbullying they experienced had no impact on their lives. This is perhaps because many victims reject bullies and consider them stupid, boring, and as having nothing better to do (Burgess-Proctor et al. 2009). So, then the question is, why is that some victims suffer so much and others are simply not affected by bullying? This question still needs clarifying and further research is necessary (Kiriakidis and Kavoura 2010).

1.6 The Social Psychology of Cyberbullying

We often believe that both traditional and online bullying are matters that occur between a bully (aggressor) and a bullied person (victim). Yet the situation is more complex, so we need an ecological model to be able to understand this phenomenon well (Espelage and Swearer 2004). First, it is more of a group phenomenon than an individual one; second, it always occurs in a sociocultural context, so analyzing the role played by the family, school, and community as a whole is essential. Social psychology has a great deal to say about the bullying and cyberbullying fields as both phenomena always take place in a highly specific psychosocial context, to the extent that to properly understand them, we need to analyze the cultural, social-community, family, school, and group contexts (see Ovejero 2013). Hence, many social and psychological themes are most interesting to help understand cyberbullying. These themes include those related with the group, family, aggressive conduct, gender, attitudes, communication processes, help-seeking behavior, values, moral disengagement, psychosocial needs, or power over the situation. Briefly:

1. *Psychology of groups*: We know that if a group of peers plays a key role in bullying (Salmivalli 2013), it also does in cyberbullying (boyd 2014). Indeed, adolescents never live on the fringe of the groups they form part of. Hence, at times a matter which adults consider is a case of bullying, adolescents may believe it to be merely a conflict of interpersonal relationships within the group (Marwick and boyd 2011).

2. *Aggressive and violent conduct*: Cyberbullying is related with other forms of violent and aggressive conduct (Calvete et al. 2010; Park et al. 2014; Sticca et al. 2013; Ybarra and Mitchell 2004). So, applying cyberbullying to existing models of violent conduct is most useful (see Ovejero 2010, Chap. 11), in particular, matters such as power over the situation (Zimbardo, 2007) or inhibitory effects caused by empathy (Castillo et al. 2013; Gini et al. 2007; Steffgen et al. 2011). The potential bully's concept of what is right and wrong will also have an influence (Fuchs et al. 2009) as it will facilitate or hinder moral disengagement (Bandura 1999).

3. *Feelings of empathy*: There is evidence of a clear association between antisocial behavior and low levels of empathy (Jolliffe and Farrington 2004). Nevertheless, it has been indicated that antisocial behavior in bullying is associated only with affective empathy (Caravita et al. 2009; Jolliffe and Farrington 2011) and not with cognitive empathy (Jolliffe and Farrington 2011), unlike in cyberbullying where it is associated with both empathy types (Ang and Goh 2010; Schultze-Krumbholz and Scheithauer 2009; see Baroncelli and Ciucci 2014).

4. *Moral disengagement*: It has been frequently discovered that moral disengagement correlates with antisocial behavior (Yadava et al. 2001) and bullying of both the traditional (Perren et al. 2011) and online (Bauman 2010; Pornari and Wood 2010) types. However, other studies have not found this relationship (Perren and Gutzwiller-Helfenfinger 2012). Yet evidently, the fact that cyberbullies neither see their victims nor witness the negative effects they cause them facilitates moral disengagement. As Milgram (1974) showed, his subjects administered more electric charges to their victims when they could not see them.

5. *Moral judgments and values*: Walrave and Heirman (2011) indicated that individuals who perform cyberbullying also tend to minimize the effects that their conduct has on victims. To date, very few studies into the moral aspects of cyberbullying are available (Bauman 2010; Gerbino et al. 2008; Menesini et al. 2011; Perren and Gutzwiller-Helfenfinger 2012; Pornari and Wood 2010; Steffgen et al. 2011; Talwar et al. 2014). We still know very little about the moral evaluations that adolescents make of cyberbullying situations. We are aware that bullies themselves often morally justify bullying (Burton et al. 2013; Williams and Guerra 2007), and when people's moral principles are not consistent with their own conduct, they use moral disengagement as a mediator between both aspects

(Bandura 2002), which thus legitimizes immoral conduct. Therefore, people who participate in cases of cyberbullying feel less guilty than those who take part in traditional bullying (Elledge et al. 2013; Wachs 2012), among other aspects, because of the ease with which they can disengage morally as they do not see the effect that their behavior has on victims (Perren and Gutzwiller-Helfenfinger 2012; Pettalia et al. 2013). Indeed, merely knowing that the teacher can intervene reduces cyberbullying conduct (Elledge et al. 2013).

6. *The family context*: Despite the changes to the traditional family in recent decades, the role that the family plays in the socialization processes of children and adolescents is still crucial. So, no one should be surprised that the family today plays a key role in cases of school bullying of both the traditional and online kinds. There are at least three reasons for this: (1) Children learn the models they later deploy at school from their family, which may be violent or altruistic, especially if these models are reinforced; (2) the family is still the main authority of social support and affection that people receive, especially when they are young. So, the family also plays an absolutely critical role in a child's socialization; therefore, the family will also be the main authority to prevent cyberbullying; and (3) similarly, the role played by the family in cyberbullying—and in preventing it— is essential, and is done by monitoring children's online behavior to a greater or lesser extent. As cyberbullying tends to take place outside school, the role played by parents here is much more relevant than that played by teachers. In many studies it has been observed that, compared with those who do not get involved in cyberbullying, those who do report weaker emotional links with parents, parents who punish them more, and parents who give them less advice about their online activities (Aoyama et al. 2012; Stadler et al. 2010; Taiariol 2010; Wade and Beran 2011; Ybarra and Mitchell 2004). Hinduja and Patchin (2013) stated that the mere perspective that parents could punish them dissuaded them from cyberbullying others. After conducting a meta-analysis on this subject, Lereya et al. (2013) stated that the three family factors that most protect children and adolescents from the negative effects of being a victim of school bullying are, and in his order: having good, affective relationships with parents; communicating well with parents; and parents suitably supervising them. Yet despite the benefit of telling parents their experiences on the Internet, particularly the social support that this gives (Özdemir 2014), adolescents do not usually do this.

7. *Gender*: If studies into traditional school bullying have clearly evidenced that boys bully more than girls (Dehue et al. 2008) and do so more directly, while females get more involved in indirect forms of aggression (Dilmac 2009), we would expect girls to use cyberbullying more than boys as it is an indirect form of aggression to a point. Unfortunately, things are much more complex. Some studies have concluded that more boys are cyberbullies than girls (Bartlett 2014; Erdur-Baker 2010; Låftman et al. 2013; Olweus and Limber 2010; Slonje and Smith 2008; Wong et al. 2014), while others have found no significant differences in either bullying rates or victimization rates. After reviewing the existing literature, Nixon (2014) concluded that for cybervictimization, there were no gender differences, which is something that many other studies have also

shown (Aricak et al. 2008; Beran and Li 2007; Didden et al. 2009; Li 2007; Hinduja and Patchin 2008; Juvonen and Gross 2008; Katzer et al. 2009; Patchin and Hinduja 2006; Slonje et al. 2012; Varjas et al. 2009; Williams and Guerra 2007). Nevertheless, others have indicated that females are more victimized than males (Ayas 2014; Dehue et al. 2008; Låftman et al. 2013; Wang et al. 2011), and even cyberbully more than males (Jones et al. 2012; Kowalski and Limber 2007). An example of the complexity of the situation is that some authors have indicated that females are more victimized than males by emails (Hinduja and Patchin 2008), while boys are more victimized by text messages (Slonje and Smith 2008).

Furthermore, research has not found a clear gender difference in terms of cyberbullying effects. As Nixon (2014) stated, while some authors have found that cyberbullying is more harmful for females than for males (Campbell et al. 2012; Ovejero et al. 2013; Machmutow et al. 2012), others have not found gender differences (Wigderson and Lynch 2013). A recent study by Kowalski and Limber (2013) revealed that when adolescents were both bullies and victims, males suffered more negative psychological effects (e.g., depression or anxiety) and more physical health problems (e.g., headaches, sleep disorders, skin problems) than females.

1.7 How to Prevent Cyberbullying and Face its Negative Effects

As cyberbullying harms its victims very much, evidently the main objective of research into this matter should be to prevent cyberbullying conduct to avoid as much harm as possible. Such prevention must come from the family, school, or community. We also know that psychology can be a great help when designing and setting up prevention programs in which encouraging good family relations is essential (Law et al. 2010). We are also well aware that having been previously involved in cases of bullying is the most important risk factor to get involved in cyberbullying (Sticca et al. 2013). So, it is obvious that antibullying programs can also prevent cyberbullying (Ovejero et al. 2013; Salmivalli et al. 2011; Smith 2014).

However, if we stated that in order to suitably understand cyberbullying it is necessary to embed it in an ecological model, which takes into account interpersonal and group relations, the atmosphere at school, the family context, and the community, we must underline that any prevention and/or intervention program that is to be effective in the cyberbullying field must also bear these variables in mind. So, we must include school, family, and psychosocial factors (see Davis and Nixon 2013 for a comparative analysis of the various strategies used in traditional and online bullying):

1. *School intervention*: Since cyberbullying occurs outside school (Snakenborg et al. 2011), both teachers and principals of schools could feel tempted to ignore this matter. But if they did, it would be a serious mistake because, as we previ-

ously mentioned, it is not only extremely harmful for schoolchildren's physical health, and especially their psychic health, but it also relates to school in different ways: first, it often continues from school bullying; second, it is more frequent in centers with a conflictive and unsatisfactory atmosphere; third, it has strong effects on schooling, for example, those bullied may leave school or display worse academic performance. Therefore, the role that schools play in cyberbullying is relevant (Mora-Merchán et al. 2010), which means having to train school personnel to face this phenomenon. For example, as a crucial factor in increasing cyberbullying is the anonymity that the new technologies facilitate, school prevention programs should show potential cyberbullies that cell phones and the Internet do not ensure anonymity and that it is possible to catch them at any time. In a recent study conducted with a sample of 308 principals of primary and secondary education schools in Flanders (Belgium), Vandebosch and Poels (2014) found that most schools considered that cyberbullying was a serious problem, and that it was their duty to tell students about this theme and to help seek solutions. Apart from requesting help from experts, they also stated that they would welcome scientific intervention and empirically backed programs.

Notwithstanding, Smith et al. (2012) indicated that many schools in the UK had policies against face-to-face bullying, but very few mentioned cyberbullying, and fewer still proposed measures to prevent it. Something similar occurred in Canada (Cassidy et al. 2012) or the USA (Orobko 2010). Furthermore, of the schools that had implemented cyberbullying prevention programs (Hunley-Jenkins 2013), very few had examined their effectiveness (see the guidelines about bullying and cyberbullying for educators by Bhat 2008 and by Willard 2005). A very efficient school method used to reduce bullying in schools, regardless of it being traditional or online, is to implement cooperative learning in the classroom (see Aronson 2000; Cowie et al. 1994; Ovejero 1990).

2. *Family intervention*: To prevent both bullying kinds, the work done at school must continue at students' homes. In this field, as in many others, cooperation between school and family is vital. It is essential that parents supervise how their children use the information and communication technologies. They must also watch for any changes in their children's moods after receiving a message or a phone call, or when they use the Internet because this could indicate cyberbullying problems. Specifically, all cyberbullying prevention programs should necessarily include family intervention to better address parents–children relationships, especially the communication type, and to show parents the importance of the role they play in this field to prevent cyberbullying and to mitigate its negative effects.

3. *Psychosocial intervention*: Although we are aware of the seriously negative effects that cyberbullying has on the health of children and adolescents, as we mentioned earlier, not all victims of cyberbullying suffer negative effects. For instance, it would be interesting to clarify the exact factors that make some adolescents immune to the negative effects of cyberbullying as this could help adolescents resist its effects. In this field, just as in others, it seems that resilience

depends above all on psychosocial factors, such as social support, feelings of self-efficacy, victims' social capital, their empathy and moral engagement, and self-esteem. To these, we need to add another more individual factor, that of being able to use problem-centered coping techniques.

4. *Increasing and improving social support*: One of the most important factors to prevent cyberbullying and to mitigate its effects is encouraging social support, especially when we know that cyberbullied adolescents tend to seek help from friends, but not from parents, and certainly not from teachers (Aricak et al. 2008; Smith et al. 2008; Ybarra and Mitchell 2007). Perhaps the reasons why cyberbullied adolescents do not tell adults about their situation are the following (Nixon 2014): (1) They feel they do not connect well with adults; finding the solution depends on adults (especially parents and teachers) making the effort to improve their relationships and connection with them; (2) adolescents tend to believe that cyberbullying is not a serious matter (Agatston et al. 2007), which suggests that parents and teachers should talk to their children or students about the serious consequences of cyberbullying; (3) cyberbullied adolescents do not often tell people about their experience because they feel ashamed (Wang et al. 2011), which we can overcome if there are trustful relationships between them and parents (and teachers). *ALSO FEAR LOSING DEVICE / ACCESS*

Despite being aware that various forms of support can mitigate the effects of bullying on psychological well-being (Davidson and Demaray 2007; Holt and Espelage 2007; Kochenderfer-Ladd and Skinner 2002), very few studies have analyzed this relation for the specific case of cyberbullying, and the few that have found that support provided to victims by peers or parents reduces the effects of cyberbullying (Machmutow et al. 2012; Fanti et al. 2012). In fact even though bullied youngsters complain that their peers "do nothing" to help them and even "ignore what is happening" (Davis and Nixon 2013), Bastiaensens et al. (2014) stated that in Belgium, bystanders were willing to help cybervictims when they noticed that cyberbullying was bad and its consequences could be serious. This indicates that a great deal can be done to prevent the terrible effects of electronic bullying.

5. *Increasing feelings of self-efficacy*: One of the effects of cyberbullying with more mid- and long-term negative consequences is learnt defenselessness, which makes them experience strong feelings of fatalism and symptoms of depression; both these feelings make victims suffer, and it is hard for them to make the effort to overcome the situation they face. It is important to encourage their feelings of self-efficacy, especially when we know about the positive effects that self-efficacy feelings have (Bandura 1986; Maddux and Gosselin 2003).

6. *Improving social capital or the social connection network*: A fundamental trait to prevent bullying and cyberbullying consists in helping adolescents obtain a good social connection (Davis and Nixon 2012); that is, a good network of social relations or "social capital" (Bourdieu 1983; Coleman 1988; Putnam 2000). It is necessary to bear in mind what type of social connection one has. Hinduja and Patchin (2013) discovered that adolescents who believed that their friends were involved in cases of cyberbullying were very likely to cyberbully others. Ado-

lescents who believed that the adults related to them (particularly their parents) disapproved their implication in cases of cyberbullying were less likely to participate in it. It is vital to bear this in mind when designing prevention programs.

7. *Encouraging empathy and moral engagement*: If moral disengagement is a risk factor in bullying and cyberbullying, then moral engagement in and empathy with others will be relevant prevention factors (Topcu and Erdur-Baker 2012). This is very important because the fact that bullies cannot see the verbal and non-verbal signs that cyberbullying victims display, because if they could, these signs could inhibit their violent behavior, it is less likely that they empathize with their victims. So, this aspect facilitates their moral disengagement and, consequently, cyberbullying is more likely.

8. *Improving self-esteem*: It is necessary to encourage this psychosocial trait given its importance in cyberbullying. A study by Modecki et al. (2013) showed that low self-esteem in adolescents predicted their future involvement in cyberbullying as either bullies or victims.

9. *Coping strategies*: Although very few research studies on the efficiency of various coping strategies in cases of cyberbullying have been conducted, more and more exist (Dooley et al. 2012; Machackova et al. 2013; Price and Dalgleish 2010; Vazsonyi et al. 2012). By coping strategies, we understand all those conducts, emotional or cognitive responses to stress made by individuals (Lazarus and Folkman 1984), which help them to eliminate or amend a problem by neutralizing its negative effects. Cyberbullying victims use different responses (Parris et al. 2012), which Perren et al. (2012) classify into these four categories: (1) responses that address the cyberbully, such as taking reprisals; (2) those that imply ignoring the aggressor; (3) the support-seeking kind (from peers, parents, or teachers); and (4) those that attempt to use technical cybernetic techniques to block the bully's account (see Aricak et al. 2008; Juvonen and Gross 2008; Kowalski et al. 2008; Livingstone et al. 2011; Smith et al. 2008; Stacey 2009). Although some of these strategies are efficient, others are not (Livingstone et al. 2011). Those that manage to block the aggressor's account or seek social support are efficient, whereas responses that entail direct confrontations with the aggressor are not and are used less frequently. Those that consist in doing nothing or ignoring the situation are not efficacious but are widely used (Dehue et al. 2008; Hoff and Mitchell 2009; Livingstone et al. 2011; Price and Dalgleish 2010; Smith et al. 2008; Šléglová and Černá 2011).

As Lazarus and Folkman pointed out (1987), coping has two main functions: changing the terms of the person-setting relation that existed when stress began (problem-centered coping) and controlling emotional troubles (emotional- or cognition-centered coping). Indeed a fact in itself is not harmful, threatening, or challenging, but the way we evaluate it confers it's one meaning or another. For instance, an adolescent can evaluate his/her photo that has been uploaded on the Internet as a joke, insult, or praise. This evaluation has one effect or another on the adolescent (feeling hurt or even proud to appear on the Internet). The coping strategies to be used will depend on the victims' interpretation. The longer the cyberbullying experience, the more likely emotion-centered coping strategies are used rather than problem-centered ones. However, the former are less efficient than the latter.

Indeed those who adopt problem-centered coping strategies (facing the situation) tend to better adapt to the stressful situation than those who deploy emotion-centered strategies (e.g., running away from the situation; Lazarus and Folkman 1987). The same can be said of cases of both traditional (Black et al. 2010; Burton et al. 2004; Cassidy and Taylor 2005; Hunter et al. 2004; Smith et al. 2001) and online (Cassidy and Taylor 2005; Lodge and Frydenberg 2007; Riebel et al. 2009; Schenk and Fremouw 2012; Völlink et al. 2013) bullying. In their cyberbullying study with females aged 11–17 years, Lodge and Frydenberg (2007) indicated that those who adopted emotion-centered coping strategies, such as worrying excessively, making self-accusations, or running away from the situation (e.g., hiding the problem from everyone or not seeking help), made their psychological well-being worse. Yet adolescents tend to use poorly efficient or even counterproductive coping strategies. Black et al. (2010) discovered that most victims (52%) responded aggressively or denied talking about the matter with their families (44%) or peers (42%). The results of Schenk and Fremouw (2012) ran along the same lines.

Briefly, existing data in this field lead us, along with Völlink et al. (2013), to stress the importance of teaching children to defend themselves and to employ efficient coping strategies to face cyberbullying. Self-confidence must be the basis of these strategies, which must be problem-centered rather than emotion-centered. Feeling of uselessness and learnt defenselessness are the worst that can happen to victims as they transmit a feeling of weakness to the bully, which only encourages the aggressor to continue attacking. This is the start of a dreadful vicious circle.

1.8 Need for Further Research

As Kowalski et al. (2014) pointed out, it is particularly necessary to further investigate some cyberbullying-related matters, among which the following stand out:

1. Longitudinal research is necessary to allow us to better know the way cyberbullying actually works as most former studies are cross-sectional and merely correlational. This will permit us to know the direction that the effects take.
2. We know that a relation between attitudes to violence and cyberbullying exists (Burton et al. 2013; Elledge et al. 2013), but very few studies have analyzed the existing relation between the degree of violence in society, attitudes to violence, and the more or less likely cyberbullying is. We need to improve our knowledge in this field.
3. It is necessary to further study the incidence of situational factors, such as exposure to media (e.g., TV or video games). Some studies have found a relation between getting involved in cases of bullying and watching violent video games (Dittrick et al. 2013; Lam et al. 2013). Nevertheless, we need more research, especially of the longitudinal type, to know if violence from media leads people

to get involved in bullying or cyberbullying, or vice versa. Other situational factors could be the adolescent's own group and its values, the time spent on the Internet, the most frequent type of online activities, etc.

4. We also need to conduct more research on cyberbullying through different electronic media (email, chat, text messages, etc.) and the different consequences they have on victims. As Smith (2013) reminds us, there is evidence to suggest that bullying performed on web sites, particularly in social networks, has become a usual form of aggression as adolescents employ these social networks more and more (Patchin and Hinduja 2010).

5. There should be more transcultural research to compare the cyberbullying that exists in more individualist cultures and that in more collectivistic cultures; or in more developed countries versus less developed ones (Shapka and Law 2013).

6. Very few studies on the relation between cyberbullying in adolescents and cyberbullying in adults have been carried out, especially in workplaces (cybermobbing). Indeed, in many countries, the Internet is now the main means of communication between workers (Lim and Teo 2009). According to Kowalski et al. (2014), it is important to determine whether the children and adolescents involved in cyberbullying as aggressors or victims are also involved in it when they start work. We hypothesize that a continuum exists in an individual's experiences in bullying from childhood, in the family, which later moves on through this person's experiences at school and, finally, at work. During this process, it is quite feasible that children learn to bully their siblings at home as they imitate models (older siblings or even parents). If their bullying behavior is reinforced in the family context, they can be involved as bullies at school and, years later, at work. Thus, the importance of preventive work that schools could undertake because it would stop not only school bullying but also workplace harassment, and the awful effects they have. Olweus (1993) indicated that it was quite likely that people who persistently bullied others at school would continue doing so in adulthood. Smith (1997) believed that we can learn a lot from schoolbullying for the workplace harassment problem and vice versa.

Hence, it would be most interesting to move in these still poorly explored directions. This would allow us to better know how bullying and cyberbullying processes really function and would, therefore, help to efficiently prevent them.

References

Agatston, P. W., Kowalski, R., & Limber, S. (2007). Students perspectives on cyber bullying. *Journal of Adolescent Health, 41*(6), S59–S60. doi:10.1016/j.jadohealth.2007.09.003.

Almeida, A., Correia, I., Marinho, S., & Garcia, D. (2012). Virtual but not less real: A study of cyberbullying and its relations to moral disengagement and empathy. In Q. Li, D. Cross, & P. K. Smith (Eds.), *Cyberbullying in the global playground: Research from international perspectives* (pp. 223–244). Malden: Blackwell.

Ang, R. P., & Goh, D. H. (2010). Cyberbullying among adolescents: The role of affective and cognitive empathy, and gender. *Child Psychiatry and Human Development, 41*, 387–397. doi:10.1007/s10578-010-0176-3.

Aoyama, I., Utsumi, S., & Hasegawa, M. (2012). Cyberbullying in Japan: Cases, government reports, adolescent relational aggression, and parental monitoring roles. In Q. Li, D. Cross, & P. K. Smith (Eds.), *Cyberbullying in the global playground: Research from international perspectives* (pp. 183–201). Malden: Blackwell.

Aricak, T., Siyahhan, S., Uzunhasanoglu, A., Saribeyoglu, S., Ciplak, S., Yilmaz, N., & Memmedov, C. (2008). Cyberbullying among Turkish adolescents. *CyberPsychology & Behavior, 11*, 253–261. doi:10.1089/cpb.2007.0016.

Arıcak, O. T. (2009). Psychiatric symptomatology as a predictor of cyberbullying among university students. *Eurasian Journal of Educational Research, 34*, 167–184.

Aronson, E. (2000). *Nobody left to hate: Teaching compassion after columbine*. New York: Freeman and Co.

Ayas, T. (2014). Prediction cyber bullying with respect to depression, anxiety and gender variables. Online Journal of Technology Addiction & Cyberbullying, (July, 2014).

Bandura, A. (1986). *Social foundations of thought and action*. Englewood Cliffs: Prentice-Hall.

Bandura, A. (1999). Moral disengagement in the perpetration of inhumanities. *Personality and Social Psychology Review, 3*, 193–209. doi:10.1207/s15327957pspr0303_3.

Bandura, A. (2002). Selective moral disengagement in the exercise of moral agency. *Journal of Moral Education, 31*(2), 101–119. http://dx.doi.org/10.1080/0305724022014322.

Bargh, J. A., & McKenna, K. Y. A. (2004). The Internet and social life. *Annual Review of Psychology, 55*, 573–590.

Baroncelli, A., & Ciucci, E. (2014). Unique effects of different components of trait emotional intelligence in traditional bullying and cyberbullying. *Journal of Adolescence, 37*, 807–815.

Bartlett, C. (2014). A meta-analysis of sex differences in cyber-bullying behavior: The moderating role of age. *Aggressive Behavior, 40*, 474–488.

Bastiaensens, S., Vandebosch, H., Poels, K., Van Cleemput, K., DeSmet, A., & De Bourdeaudhuij, I. (2014). Cyberbullying on social network sites. An experimental study into bystanders' behavioural intentions to help the victim or reinforce the bully. *Computers in Human Behavior, 31*, 259–271. doi:10.1016/j.chb.2013.10.036.

Bauman, S. (2009). Cyberbullying in a rural intermediate school: An exploratory study. *Journal of Early Adolescence, 30*(6), 803–833.

Bauman, S. (2010). Cyberbullying in a rural intermediate school: An exploratory study. *Journal of Early Adolescence, 30*, 803–833. doi:10.1177/0272431609350927.

Bauman, S., Toomey, R. B., & Walker, J. L. (2013). Associations among bullying, cyberbullying, and suicide in high school students. *Journal of Adolescence, 36*, 341–350.

Baumeister, R. F., & Leary, M. R. (1995). The need to belong: Desire for interpersonal attachment as a fundamental human motivation. *Psychological Bulletin, 117*, 497–529.

Baumeister, R. F., DeWall, C. N., Ciarocco, N. J., & Twenge, J. M. (2005). Social exclusion impairs self-regulation. *Journal of Personality and Social Psychology, 88*(4), 589–604.

Belsey, B. (2005). *Cyberbullying: An emerging threat to the "always on" generation*. http://www.cyberbullying.ca.

Beran, T., & Li, Q. (2005). Cyber-harassment: A study of a new method for an old behavior. *Journal of Educational Computing Research, 32*, 265–277. doi:10.2190/8YQM-B04H-PG4D-BLLH.

Beran, T., & Li, Q. (2007). The relationship between cyberbullying and school bullying. *Journal of Student Wellbeing, 1*, 15–33.

Bhat, C. S. (2008). Cyber bullying: Overview and strategies for school counselors, guidance officers, and all school personnel. *Australian Journal of Guidance and Counselling, 18*(1), 53–66.

Black, S., Weinles, D., & Washington, E. (2010). Victim strategies to stop bullying. *Youth Violence and Juvenile Justice, 8*(2), 138–147.

Bonanno, R. A., & Hymel, S. (2013). Cyber bullying and internalizing difficulties: Above and beyond the impact of traditional forms of bullying. *Journal of Youth and Adolescence, 42*(5), 685–697. http://dx.doi.org/10.1007/s10964-013-9937-1.

Bourdieu, P. (1983). Forms of capital. In J. G. Richardson (Ed.), *Handbook of theory and research for the sociology of education* (pp. 241–258). New York: Greenwood Press.

boyd, d. (2014). *It's complicated: The social lives of networked teens*. New Haven: Yale University Press.

Brighi, A., Melotti, G., Guarini, A., Genta, M. L., Ortetga, R., Mora-Merchán, J., Smith, P.K., & Thompson, F. (2012). Self-esteem and loneliness in relation to cyberbullying in three European countries. In Q. Li, D. Cross & P. K. Smith (Eds.), *Cyberbullying in the global playground: Research from international perspectives* (pp. 32–56). London: Wiley-Blackwell.

Brixval, C. S., Rayce, S. L. B., Rasmussen, M., Holstein, B. E., & Due, P. (2011). Overweight, body image and bullying—an epidemiological study of 11- to 15-year olds. *European Journal of Public Health, 22,* 126–130.

Brown, C. F., DeMaray, M., & Secord, S. M. (2014). Cyber victimization in middle school and relations to social emotional outcomes. *Computers in Human Behavior, 35,* 12–21. doi:10.1016/j.chb.2014.02.014.

Bureau, P. M. (2013). Canadians' usage of social media. http://www.pmb.ca/public/e/product_data/social_media.pdf.

Burgess-Proctor, A., Patchin, J., & Hinduja, S. (2006). Cyberbullying: The victimization of adolescent girls. http://www.cyberbullying.us/cyberbullying_girls_victimization.pdf.

Burgess-Proctor, A., Patchin, J., & Hinduja, S. (2009). Cyberbullying and online harassment: Reconceptualizing the victimization of adolescent girls. In V. Garcia & J. Clifford (Eds.), *Female crime victims: Reality reconsidered* (pp. 1–30). Upper Saddle River: Prentice Hall.

Burton, E., Stice, E., & Seeley, J. R. (2004). A prospective test of the stress-buffering model of depression in adolescent girls; no support once again. *Journal of Consulting and Clinical Psychology, 72,* 689–697.

Burton, K. A., Florell, D., & Wygant, D. B. (2013). The role of peer attachment and normative beliefs about aggression on traditional bullying and cyberbullying. *Psychology in the Schools, 50*(2), 103–115.

Calvete, E., Orue, I., Estévez, A., Villardón, L., & Padilla, P. (2010). Cyberbullying in adolescents: Modalities and aggressors' profile. *Computers in Human Behavior, 26,* 1128–1135. doi:10.1016/j.chb.2010.03.017.

Campbell, M. S. (2005). Cyberbullying: An old problem in a new guise? *Australian Journal of Guidance and Counselling, 15*(1), 68–76.

Campbell, M., Spears, B., Slee, P., Butler, D., & Kift, S. (2012). Victims' perceptions of traditional and cyberbullying and the psychosocial correlates of their victimization. *Emotional and Behavioral Difficulties, 17,* 389–401.

Campbell, M. A., Slee, P. T., Spears, B., Butler, D., & Kift, S. (2013). Do cyberbullies suffer too? Cyberbullies' perceptions of the harm they cause to others and to their own mental health. *School Psychology International, 34*(6), 613–629.

Cappadocia, M. C., Craig, W. M., & Pepler, D. (2013). Cyberbullying prevalence, stability, and risk factors during adolescence. *Canadian Journal of School Psychology, 28,* 171–192.

Caravita, S. C. S., Di Blasio, P., & Salmivalli, C. (2009). Unique and interactive effects of empathy and social status on involvement in bullying. *Social Development, 18*(1), 140–163.

Carr, N. (2010). *The shallows: What the Internet is doing to our our brains*. New York: W.W. Norton.

Carroll, D. C. (2008). Cyber bullying and victimization: Psychosocial characteristics of bullies, victims, and bully/victims. http://gradworks.umi.com/33/24/3324499.html.

Cassidy, T., & Taylor, L. (2005). Coping and psychological distress as a function of the bully victim dichotomy in older children. *Social Psychology of Education, 8,* 249–262.

Cassidy, W., Brown, K., & Jackson, M. (2012). "Under the radar": Educators and cyberbullying in schools. *School Psychology International, 33,* 520–532. doi:10.1177/0143034312445245.

Cassidy, W., Faucher, C., & Jackson, M. (2013). Cyberbullying among youth: A comprehensive review of current international research and its implications and application to policy and practice. *School Psychology International, 34,* 575–612.

Castells, M. (2001). *La Galaxia Internet: Reflexiones sobre Internet, empresa y sociedad*. Madrid. Areté.

Castillo, R., Salguero, J. M., Fernández-Berrocal, P., & Balluerka, N. (2013). Effects of an emotional intelligence intervention on aggression and empathy among adolescents. *Journal of Adolescence, 36*(5), 883–892. http://dx.doi.org/10.1016/j.adolescence. 2013.07.001.

Chang, F. C., Lee, C. M., Chiu, C. H., Hs, i, W. Y., Huang, T. F., & Pan, Y. C. (2013). Relationships among cyberbullying, school bullying, and mental health in Taiwanese adolescents. *Journal of School Health, 83*(6), 454–462.

Coleman, J. S. (1988). Social capital in the creation of human capital. *American Journal of Sociology, 94*, 95–120.

Collier, A. (2009). A better safety net. *School Library Journal, 55*(11), 36–38.

Cook, C. R., Williams, K. R., Guerra, N. G., & Kim, T. E. (2010). Variability in the prevalence of bullying and victimization: A cross-national and methodological analysis. In S. R. Jimerson, S. B. Swearer, & D. L. Espelage (Eds.), *Handbook of bullying in schools: An international perspective* (pp. 347–362). New York: Routledge.

Copeland, W. E., Wolke, D., Angold, A., & Costello, E. J. (2013). Adult psychiatric outcomes of bullying and being bullied by peers in childhood and adolescence. *JAMA Psychiatry*. http:// dx.doi.org/10.1001/jamapsychiatry.2013.504 1–8.

Cowie, H., Smith, P. K., Boulton, M. J., & Laver, R. (1994). *Co-operative group work in the multi-ethnic classroom*. London: David Fulton.

Davidson, L. M., & Demaray, M. K. (2007). Social support as a moderator between victimization and internalizing-externalizing distress from bullying. *School Psychology Review, 36*(3), 383.

Davis, S., & Nixon, C. (2012). Empowering bystanders. In J. V. Patchin, & S. Hinduja (Eds.), *Cyberbullying prevention and response: Expert perspectives.* (pp. 93–109). New York: Sage.

Davis, S., & Nixon, C. L. (2013). *Youth voice project: Student insights into bullying and peer mistreatment*. Champaign: Research Press Publishers.

Dehue, F., Bolman, C., & Völlink, T. (2008). Cyberbullying: Youngsters' experiences and parental perception. *CyberPsychology & Behavior, 11*, 217–223. doi:10.1089/cpb.2007.0008.

DeSmet, A., Deforche, B., Hublet, A., Tanghe, A., Stremersch, E., & De Bourdeaudhuij, I. (2014). Traditional and cyberbullying victimization as correlates of psychosocial distress and barriers to a healthy lifestyle among severely obese adolescents—a matched case-control study on prevalence and results from a cross-sectional Study. *BMC Public Health, 14*, 224. doi:10.1186/1471-2458-14-224.

Devine, P., & Lloyd, K. (2012). Internet use and psychological well-being among 10-year-old and 11-year-old children. *Child Care in Practice, 18*(1), 5–22.

Didden, R., Scholte, R. H. J., Korzilius, H., de Moor, J. M. H., Vermeulen, A., O'Reilly, M., & Lancioni, G. E. (2009). Cyberbullying among students with intellectual and developmental disability in special education settings. *Developmental Neurorehabilitation, 12*, 146–151. doi:10.1080/17518420902971356.

Dilmac, B. (2009). Psychological needs as a predictor of cyber bullying: A preliminary report on college students. Educational sciences. *Theory and Practice, 9*, 1307–1325.

Dittrick, C. J., Beran, T. N., Mishna, F., Hetherington, R., & Shariff, S. (2013). Do children who bully their peers also play violent video games? A Canadian national study. *Journal of School Violence, 12*, 297–318. doi:10.1080/15388220.2013.803244.

Dooley, J. J., Shaw, T., & Cross, D. (2012). The association between the mental health and behavioural problems of students and their reactions to cyber-victimization. *European Journal of Developmental Psychology, 9*, 275–289. doi:10.1080/17405629.2011.648425.

Dredge, R., Gleeson, J., & de la Piedad Garcia, X. (2014a). Cyberbullying in social networking sites: An adolescent victim's perspective. *Computers in Human Behavior, 36*, 13–20.

Dredge, R., Gleeson, J., & de la Piedad Garcia, X. (2014b). Risk factors associated with impact severity of cyberbullying victimization: A qualitative study of adolescent online social networking. *Cyberpsychology, Behavior and Social Networking, 17*(5), 287–291. doi:10.1089/ cyber.2013.0541.

Duggan, M., & Smith, A. (2014). Pew research center—Social media update 2013. http://pewinternet.org/Reports/2013/Social-Media-Update/Main-Findings.aspx.

Eisenberg, M. E., Neumark-Sztainer, D., Haines, J., & Wall, M. (2006). Weight-teasing and emotional well-being in adolescents: Longitudinal findings from project EAT. *Journal of Adolescence Health, 38*, 675–683.

Elledge, L.C., Williford, A., Boulton, A., DePaolis, K., Little, T., & Salmivalli, C. (2013). Individual and contextual predictors of cyberbullying: The influence of children's provictim attitudes and teachers' ability to intervene. *Journal of Youth and Adolescence, 42*(5), 698–710. http://dx.doi.org/10.1007/s10964-013-9920-x.

Erdur-Baker, Ö. (2010). Cyberbullying and its correlation to traditional bullying, gender and frequent and risky usage of Internet-mediated communication tools. *New Media & Society, 12*, 109–125. doi:10.1177/1461444809341260.

Espelage, D. L., & Swearer, S. M. (2004). *Bullying in American schools: A social-econological perspective on prevention and intervention*. Mahwah: Lawrence Erlbaum.

Estévez, A., Villardón, L., Calvete, E., Padilla, P., & Orue, I. (2010). Adolescentes víctimas de cyberbullying: Prevalencia y características [Adolescent victims of cyberbullying. *Prevalence and characteristics*]. *Behavioral Psychology/Psicología Conductual, 18*, 73–89.

Fanti, K. A., Demetriou, A. G., & Hawa, V. V. (2012). A longitudinal study of cyberbullying: Examining riskand protective factors. *European Journal of Developmental Psychology, 9*(2), 168–181. doi:10.1080/17405629.2011.643169.

Festl, R., & Quandt, T. (2013). Social relations and cyberbullying: The influence of individual and structural attributes on victimization and perpetration via the internet. *Human Communication Research, 39*(1), 101–126. http://dx.doi.org/10.1111/j.1468–2958.2012.01442.x.

Finkelhor, K., Mitchell, K., & Wolak, J. (2000). *Online victimization: A report on the nation's youth*. Alexandria: National Center for Missing and Exploited Children.

Floros, G. D., Siomos, K. E., Fisoun, V., Dafouli, E., & Geroukalis, D. (2013). Adolescent online cyberbullying in Greece: The impact of parental online security practices, bonding, and online impulsiveness. *Journal of School Health, 83*(6), 445–453.

Fredstrom, B. K., Adams, R. E., & Gilman, R. (2011). Electronic and school-based victimization: Unique contexts for adjustment difficulties during adolescence. *Journal of Youth and Adolescence, 40*, 405–415. doi:10.1007/s10964-010-9569-7.

Fuchs, C., Bichler, R. M., & Raffl, C. (2009). Cyberethics and co-operation in the information society. *Science and Engineering Ethics, 15*(4), 447–466.

Garbarino, J. (1999). *Lost boys: Why our sons turn violent and how we can save them*. New York: Free Press.

Garbarino, J., & deLara, E. (2003a). *And words can hurt forever: How to protect adolescents from bullying, harassment, and emotional violence*. New York: Free Press.

Garbarino, J., & deLara, E. (2003b). Lost boys: Why our sons turn violent and how we can save them. *Paediatrics and Child Health, 10*(8), 447–450.

Garnefski, N., & Kraaij, V. (2014). Bully victimization and emotional problems in adolescents: Moderation by specific cognitive coping strategies? *Journal of Adolescence, 37*(7), 1153–1160. doi:10.1016/j.adolescence.2014.07.005.

Genta, M. L., Brighi, A., & Guarini, A. (2013). *Cyberbullismo: Ricerche e strategie di intervento*. Milano. Franco Angeli.

Gerbino, M., Alessandri, G., & Caprara, G. V. (2008). Valori, disimpegno morale e violenza nei giovani adulti. [*Values, moral disengagement and violence in young adults*]. *Età Evolutiva, 90*, 88–96.

Gini, G., Albiero, P., Benelli, B., & Altoè, G. (2007). Does empathy predict adolescents' bullying and defending behavior? *Aggressive Behavior, 33*(5), 467–476. http://dx.doi.org/10.1002/ab.20204.

Gladden, R. M., Vivolo-Kantor, A. M., Hamburger, M. E., & Lumpkin, C. (2014). Bullying surveillance: Uniform definitions and recommended data elements, Version 1.0. Atlanta.

Gradinger, P., Strohmeier, D., & Spiel, C. (2009). Traditional bullying and cyberbullying: Identification of risk groups for adjustment problems. *Zeitschrift für Psychologie/Journal of Psychology, 217*, 205–213. doi:10.1027/0044-3409.217.4.205.

Gradinger, P., Strohmeier, D., & Spiel, C. (2010). Definition and measurement of cyberbullying. *Cyberpsychology: Journal of Pyschosocial research on cyberspace, 4*(2). http://www.cyber-psychology.eu/view.php?cisloclanku=2010112301&article=1.

Gray, W. N., Kahhan, N. A., & Janicke, D. M. (2009). Peer victimization and pediatric obesity: A review of the literature. *Psychology in the Schools, 46,* 720–726.

Hemphill, S. A., Kotevski, A., Tollit, M., Smith, R., Herrenkohl, T. I., Toumbourou, J. W., & Cata-lano, R. F. (2012). Longitudinal predictors of cyber and traditional bullying perpetration in Australian secondary school students. *Journal of Adolescent Health, 51,* 59–65. doi:10.1016/j.jadohealth.2011.11.019.

Hinduja, S., & Patchin, J. W. (2008). Cyberbullying: An exploratory analysis of factors related to of-fending and victimization. *Deviant Behavior, 29,* 129–156. doi:10.1080/01639620701457816.

Hinduja, S., & Patchin, J. W. (2010). Bullying, cyberbullying, and suicide. *Archives of Suicide Research, 14,* 206–221. doi:10.1080/13811118.2010.494133.

Hinduja, S., & Patchin, J. W. (2011). Cyberbullying: A review of the legal issues facing educators. *Preventing School Failure: Alternative Education for Children and Youth, 55*(2), 71–78. http://dx.doi.org/10.1080/1045988X.2011.539433.

Hinduja, S., & Patchin, J. (2013). Social influences on cyberbullying behaviors among middle and high school students. *Journal of Youth and Adolescence, 42,* 711–722. doi:10.1007/s10964-012-9902-4.

Hoff, D. L., & Mitchell, S. N. (2009). Cyberbullying: Causes, effects, and remedies. *Journal of Educational Administration, 47,* 652–665.

Holfeld, B., & Grabe, M. (2012). An examination of the history, prevalence, characteristics, and reporting of cyberbullying in the United States. In Q. Li, D. Cross, & P. K. Smith (Eds.), *Cy-berbullying in the global playground: Research from international perspectives* (pp. 117–142). Malden: Blackwell.

Holt, M. K., & Espelage, D. L. (2007). Perceived social support among bullies, victims, and bully-victims. *Journal of Youth and Adolescence, 36*(8), 984–994. doi:10.1007/s10964-006-9153-3.

Hunley-Jenkins, K. (2013). *Principal perspectives about policy components and practices for reducing cyberbullying in urban schools* (Doctoral dissertation). Available from Dissertation Abstracts International.

Hunter, S. C., Mora-Merchan, J., & Ortega, R. (2004). The long-term effects of coping strategy use in victims of bullying. *The Spanish Journal of Psychology, 7,* 3–12.

INE. (2008). *Encuesta sobre equipamientos y uso de tecnologías de la información y comuni-cación en los hogares, 2008.* http://www.ine.es/jaxi/menu.do?type=pcaxisypath=%2Ft25/p450yfile=inebaseyL=0.

Jolliffe, D., & Farrington, D. P. (2004). Empathy and offending: A systematic review and meta-analysis. *Aggressive and Violent Behavior, 9,* 441–476.

Jolliffe, D., & Farrington, D. P. (2011). Is low empathy related to bullying after controlling for individual and social background variables? *Journal of Adolescence, 34,* 59–71.

Jones, L. M., Mitchell, K., & Finkelhor, D. (2012). Trends in youth internet victimization: Find-ings from three youth internet safety surveys 2000–2010. *Journal of Adolescent Health, 50*(2), 179–186.

Juvonen, J., & Gross, E. F. (2008). Extending the school grounds? Bullying experiences in cyber-space. *Journal of School Health, 78,* 496–505. doi:10.1111/j.1746-1561.2008.00335.x.

Kann, L., Kinchen, S., Shanklin, S. L., Flint, K. H., Hawkins, J., et al. (2014). Youth risk behavior surveillance—United States, 2013. *MMWR Surveillance Summaries, 63*(SS-04), 1–168.

Kapatzia, A., & Syngollitou, E. (2007). *Cyberbullying in middle and high schools: Prevalence, gender and age differences (Manuscript unpublished).* Thessaloniki: University of Thessa-loniki.

Katzer, C., Fetchenhauer, D., & Belschak, F. (2009). Cyberbullying: Who are the victims? A com-parison of victimization in Internet chatrooms and victimization in school. *Journal of Media Psychology, 21,* 25–36. doi:10.1027/1864-1105.21.1.25.

Katzer, C., Fetchenhauer, D., & Belschak, F. (2009). Cyberbullying: Who are the victims? A com-parison of victimization in Internet chatrooms and victimization in school. *Journal of Media Psychology, 21*(1), 25–36. http://dx.doi.org/10.1027/1864-1105.21.1.25.

Kessel Schneider, S., O'Donnell, L., Stueve, A., & Coulter, R. W. S. (2012). Cyberbullying, school bullying, and psychological distress: A regional census of high school students. *American Journal of Public Health, 102*, 171–177. doi:10.2105/AJPH.2011.300308.

Kim, Y. S., & Leventhal, B. (2008). Bullying and suicide. A review. *International Journal of Adolescence Medical Health, 20*, 133–154.

Kirby, E. (2008). Eliminate bullying—A legal imperative. *A Legal Memorandum, 8*(2), 1–6.

Kiriakidis, S. P., & Kavoura, A. (2010). Cyberbullying: A review of the literature on harassment through the internet and other electronicmeans. *Family & Community Health, 33*, 82–93. http://dx.doi.org/10.1097/FCH.0b013e3181d593e4.

Kochenderfer-Ladd, B., & Skinner, K. (2002). Children's coping strategies: moderators of the effects of peer victimization?. *Developmental psychology, 38*(2), 267–278. doi:10.1037/0012-1649.38.2.267.

Kowalski, R. M., & Limber, S. P. (2007). Electronic bullying among middle school students. *Journal of Adolescent Health, 41*(Suppl. 6), S22–S30. doi:10.1016/j.jadohealth.2007.08.017.

Kowalski, R. M., & Limber, S. P. (2013). Psychological, physical, and academic correlates of cyberbullying and traditional bullying. *Journal of Adolescent Health, 53*, S13–S20. doi:10.1016/j.jadohealth.2012.09.018.

Kowalski, R. M., Limber, S. E., & Agatston, P. W. (2012). *Cyberbullying: Bullying in the digital age* (2nd edn.). Malden: Wiley-Blackwell.

Kowalski, R. M., Morgan, C. A., & Limber, S. E. (2012). Traditional bullying as a potential warning sign of cyberbullying. *School Psychology International, 33*, 505–519. doi:10.1177/0143034312445244.

Kowalski, R. M., Giumetti, G. W., Schroeder, A. N., & Lattanner, M. R. (2014). Bullying in the digital age: A critical review and meta-analysis of cyberbullying research among youth. *Psychological Bulletin, 140*(4), 1073–1137. doi:10.1037/a0035618.

Kraft, E. M., & Wang, J. (2009). Effectiveness of cyber bullying prevention strategies: A study on students' perspectives. *International Journal of Cyber Criminology, 3*(2), 513–535.

Kukaswadia, A., Craig, W., Janssen, I., & Pickett, W. (2011). Obesity as a determinant of two forms of bullying in Ontario youth: A short report. *Obesity Facts, 4*, 469–472.

Kumazaki, A., Suzuki, K., Katsura, R., Sakamoto, A., & Kashibuchi, M. (2011). The effects of netiquette and ICT skills on school-bullying and cyber-bullying: The two-wave panel study of Japanese elementary, secondary, and high school students. Procedia. *Social and Behavioral Sciences, 29*, 735–741.

Kwan, G. C. E., & Skoric, M. M. (2013). Facebook bullying: An extension of battles in school. *Computers in Human Behavior, 29*(1), 16–25. http://dx.doi.org/10.1016/j.chb. 2012.07.014.

Låftman, S. B., Modin, B., & Östberg, V. (2013). Cyberbullying and subjective health: A large-scale study of students in Stockholm, Sweden. *Children and Youth Services Review, 35*(1), 112–119. http://dx.doi.org/10.1016/j.childyouth.2012. 10.020.

Lam, L. T., Cheng, Z., & Liu, X. (2013). Violent online games exposure and cyberbullying/victimization among adolescents. *Cyberpsychology, Behavior, and Social Networking, 16*, 159–165. doi:10.1089/cyber.2012.0087.

Landstedt, E., & Persson, S. (2014). Bullying, cyberbullying, and mental health in young people. *Scandinavian Journal of Public Health, 42*(4), 393–399. doi:10.1177/1403494814525004.

Laval, P., & Dardot, C. (2010). *La nouvelle raison du monde. Essai sur la société néolibérale.* Paris: La Découberte.

Law, D. M., Shapka, J. D., & Olson, B. F. (2010). To control or not to control? Parenting behaviours and adolescent online aggression. *Computers in Human Behavior, 26*, 1651–1656.

Lazarus, R. S., & Folkmann, S. (1984). *Stress, appraisal and coping.* New York: Springer.

Lazarus, R. S., & Folkman, S. (1987). Transactional theory and research on emotions and coping. *European Journal of Personality, 1*, 141–169.

Lazzarato, M. (2011). *La fabrique de l'homme endetté: Essai sur la condition néoliberale.* Paris: Amterdam.

Lereya, S. T., Samara, M., & Wolke, D. (2013). Parenting behavior and the risk of becoming a victim and a bully/victim: A meta-analysis study. *Child Abuse & Neglect, 37*, 1091–1108.

Leung, L., & Lee, P. (2012). The influences of information literacy, internet addiction and parenting styles on internet risks. *New Media & Society, 14*(1), 117–136.

Levy, N., Cortesi, S., Gasser, U., Crowley, E., Beaton, M., Casey, J., & Nolan, C. (2012). *Bullying in a networked era: A literature review 2012*. Cambridge: Berkman Center for Internet & Society.

Li, Q. (2006). Cyberbullying in schools: A research of gender differences. *School Psychology International, 27*, 157–170. doi:10.1177/0143034306064547.

Li, Q. (2007). Bullying in the new playground: Research into cyberbullying and cyber victimization. *Australasian Journal of Educational Technology, 23*, 435–454.

Lim, V. K. G., & Teo, T. S. H. (2009). Mind your E-manners: Impact of cyber incivility on employees' work attitude and behavior. *Information & Management, 46*, 419–425. doi:10.1016/j.im.2009.06.006.

Livingstone, S., & Smith, P. K. (2014). Annual research review: Harms experienced by child users of online and mobile technologies: The nature, prevalence and management of sexual and aggressive risks in the digital age. *Journal of Child Psychology and Psychiatry, 55*, 635–654.

Livingstone, S., Haddon, L., Görzig, A., & Ólafsson, K. (2011) Risks and safety on the internet: The perspective of European children: Full findings. http://eprints.lse.ac.uk/33731/.

Lodge, J., & Frydenberg, E. (2007). Cyber-bullying in Australian schools: Profiles of adolescent coping and insights. *Australian Educational and Developmental Psychologist, 24*, 45–58.

Machackova, H., Cerna, A., Sevcikova, A., Dedkova, L., & Daneback, K. (2013). Effectiveness of coping strategies for victims of cyberbullying. *Cyberpsychology: Journal of Psychosocial Research on Cyberspace, 7*(3), article 5. doi:10.5817/CP2013-3-5.

Machmutow, K., Perren, S., Sticca, F., & Alsaker, F. D. (2012). Peer victimisation and depressive symptoms: Can specific coping strategies buffer the negative impact of cybervictimisation? *Emotional and Behavioural Difficulties, 17*, 403–420. doi:10.1080/13632752.2012.704310.

Maddux, J. E., & Gosselin, J. T. (2003). Self-efficacy. In M. R. Leary & J. P. Tangney (Eds.), *Handbook Of Self and Identity* (pp. 218–238). New York: Guilford Press.

Marwick, A., & boyd, d. (2011). The drama! Teen conflict, gossip, and bullying in networked publics. A decade in internet time: Symposium on the dynamics of the Internet and society, September 2011. http://papers.ssrn.com/sol3/papers.cfm?abstract_id=1926349.

McKenna, K. Y. A., & Bargh, J. A. (1998). Coming out in the age of the Internet: Identity 'demarginalization' through virtual group participation. *Journal of Personality and Social Psychology, 75*(3), 681–694.

Mehari, K. R., Farrell, A. D., & Le, A. H. (2014). Cyberbullying among adolescents: Measures in search of a construct. *Psychology of Violence*. doi:10.1037/a0037521.

Meltzer, H., Vostanis, P., Ford, T., Bebbington, P., & Dennis, M. S. (2011). Victims of bullying in childhood and suicide attempts in adulthood. *European Psychiatry, 26*, 498–503.

Menesini, E., & Nocentini, A. (2009). Cyberbullying definition and measurement: Some critical considerations. *Zeitschrift für Psychologie/Journal of Psychology, 217*, 230–232. doi:10.1027/0044-3409.217.4.230.

Menesini, E., Nocentini, A., & Calussi, P. (2011). The measurement of cyberbullying: Dimensional structure and relative item severity and discrimination. *Cyberpsychology, Behavior, and Social Networking, 14*, 267–274. doi:10.1089/cyber.2010.0002.

Menesini, E., Calussi, P., & Nocentini, A. (2012). Cyberbullying and traditional bullying: Unique, additive, and synergistic effects on psychological health symptoms. In Q. Li, D. Cross, & P. K. Smith (Eds.), *Cyberbullying in the global playground: Research on international perspectives* (pp. 245–262). Malden: Blackwell.

Menesini, E., Nocentini, A., & Camodeca, M. (2013). Morality, values, traditional bullying, and cyberbullying in adolescence. *British Journal of Developmental Psychology, 31*, 1–14. Advance online publication. doi:10.1111/j.2044-835X.2011.02066.x.

Messias, E., Kindrick, K., & Castro, J. (2014). School bullying, cyberbullying, or both: Correlates of teen suicidality in the 2011 CDC youth risk behavior survey. *Comprehensive Psychiatry, 55*(5), 1063–1068. doi:10.1016/j.comppsych.2014.02.005.

Milgram, S. (1974). *Obedience to authority: An experimental view*. New York: Harpercollins.

Mishna, F., Cook, C., Gadalla, T., Daciuk, J., & Solomon, S. (2010). Cyber bullying behaviors among middle and high school students. *American Journal of Orthopsychiatry, 80*, 362–374. doi:10.1111/j.1939-0025.2010.01040.x.

Mishna, F., Khoury-Kassabri, M., Gadalla, T., & Daciuk, J. (2012). Risk factors for involvement in cyber bullying: Victims, bullies and bully– victims. *Children and Youth Services Review, 34*, 63–70. doi:10.1016/j.childyouth.2011.08.032.

Mitchell, K. J., Finkelhor, D., Wolak, J., Ybarra, M. L., & Turner, H. (2011). Youth Internet victimization in a broader victimization context. *Journal of Adolescent Health, 48*, 128–134. doi:10.1016/j.jadohealth.2010.06.009.

Mnet. (2001). Young Canadians in a wired world. http:/www.media-awareness.ca/English/special_initiatives/surveys/index.cfm.

Modecki, K. L., Barber, B. L., & Vernon, L. (2013). Mapping developmental precursors of cyber-aggression: Trajectories of risk predict perpetration and victimization. *Journal of Youth and Adolescence, 42*(5), 651–661. doi:10.1007/s10964-012-9887-z.

Modecki, K. L., Minchin, J., Harbaugh, A. G., Guerra, N. G., & Runions, K. C. (2014). Bullying prevalence across contexts: A meta-analysis measuring cyber and traditional bullying. *Journal of Adolescent Health*. doi:10.1016/j.jadohealth.2014.06.007.

Monks, C. P., Robinson, S., & Worlidge, P. (2012). The emergence of cyberbullying: A survey of primary school pupils' perceptions and experiences. *School Psychology International, 33*, 477–491. doi:10.1177/0143034312445242.

Mora-Merchán, J., Ortega, R., Calmaestra, J., & Smith, P. K. (2010). El uso violento de la tecnología: el cyberbullying. In E. R. Ortega (Ed.), *Agresividad injustificada, byllying, y violencia escolar (189–209)*. Madrid: Alianza.

Navarro, R., Yubero, S., Larrañaga, E., & Martínez, V. (2012). Children's cyberbullying victimization: Associations with social anxiety and social competence in a Spanish sample. *Child Indicators Research, 5*, 281–295. doi:10.1007/s12187-011-9132-4.

Navarro, R., Serna, C., Martínez, V., & Ruiz-Oliva, R. (2013). The role of Internet use and parental mediation on cyberbullying victimization among Spanish children from rural public schools. *European Journal of Psychology of Education, 28*, 725–745. doi:10.1007/s10212-012-0137-2.

Nixon, C. (2014). Current perspectives: The impact of cyberbullying on adolescent health. *Adolescent Health, Medicine and Therapeutics, 5*, 143–158. doi:10.2147/AHMT.S36456.

Noret, N., & Rivers, I. (2006). The prevalence of bullying by text message or email: Results of a four year study. Póster presented at the British Psychological Society Annual Conference, Cardiff.

Olenik-Shemesh, D., Heiman, T., & Eden, S. (2012). Cyberbullying victimisation in adolescence: Relationships with loneliness and depressive mood. *Emotional and Behavioural Difficulties, 17*(3–4), 361–374.

Olin, F. (2003). Digital bullying: Harassments amongst youths through Internet and SMS. Karlsrad University. http://www.digitalkultur.se/pdf/Digial1%20mobbing.pdf.

Olweus, D. (1993). Victimisation by peers: Antecedents and long-term outcomes. In K. H. Rubin & J. B. Asendorpf (Eds.), *Social withdrawal, inhibition and shyness in childhood*. Hillsdale: Erlbaum.

Olweus, D. (2012). Cyberbullying: An overrated phenomenon? *European Journal of Developmental Psychology, 9*, 520–538. doi:10.1080/17405629.2012.682358.

Olweus, D. (2013). School bullying: Development and some important challenges. *Annual Review of Clinical Psychology, 9*, 751–780. doi:10.1146/annurev-clinpsy-050212-185516.

Olweus, D., & Limber, S. P. (2010, November). What do we know about bullying: Information from the Olweus Bullying Questionnaire. Seattle, WA: Paper presented at the meeting of the International Bullying Prevention Association.

Orobko, A. (2010). *An examination of policies, programs, and strategies that address bullying in Virginia public school systems* (Doctoral dissertation). Available from Dissertation Abstracts International.

Ortega, R., Elipe, P., Mora-Merchán, J. A., Calmaestra, J., & Vega, E. (2009). The emotional impact on victims of traditional bullying and cyberbullying: A study of Spanish adolescents. *Zeitschrift für Psychologie/Journal of Psychology, 217*, 197–204. doi:10.1027/0044-3409.217.4.197.

Ovejero, A. (1990). *El aprendizaje cooperativo: Una alternativa eficaz a la enseñanza tradicional. Barcelona*. P.P.U.

Ovejero, A. (2010). *Psicología Social: Algunas claves para entender la conducta humana*. Madrid: Biblioteca Nueva.

Ovejero, A. (2013). El acoso escolar: Cuatro décadas de investigación internacional. En A. Ovejero. In P. K. Smith & S. Yubero (Eds.), *El acoso escolar y su prevención: Perspectivas internacionales* (pp. 11–56). Madrid: Biblioteca Nueva.

Ovejero, A. (2014). *Perdedores del nuevo capitalismo. Devastación del mundo del trabajo*. Madrid: Biblioteca Nueva.

Ovejero, A., Yubero, S., Larrañaga, E., & Navarro, R. (2013). Sexismo y comportamiento de acoso escolar en adolescentes. *Behavioral Psychology/Psicología Conductual, 2*(1), 157–171.

Ovejero, A., Smith, P. K., & Yubero, S. (2013). (Eds.). *El acoso escolar y su prevención: Perspectivas internacionales*. Madrid: Biblioteca Nueva.

Özdemir, Y. (2014). Cyber victimization and adolescent self-esteem: The role of communication with parents. *Asian Journal of Social Psychology*. doi:10.1111/ajsp.12070.

Park, S., Na, E.-Y., & Kim, E.-m (2014). The relationship between online activities, netiquette and cyberbullying. *Children and Youth Services Review, 42*, 74–81.

Parris, L., Varjas, K., Meyers, J., & Cutts, H. (2012). High school students' perceptions of coping with cyberbullying. *Youth & Society, 44*, 284–306. doi:10.1177/0044118×11398881.

Patchin, J. W., & Hinduja, S. (2006). Bullies move beyond the schoolyard: A preliminary look at cyberbullying. *Youth Violence and Juvenile Justice, 4*, 148–169. doi:10.1177/1541204006286288.

Patchin, J. W., & Hinduja, S. (2010). Cyberbullying and self-esteem. *Journal of School Health, 80*, 614–621. doi:10.1111/j.1746-1561.2010.00548.x.

Patchin, J. W., & Hinduja, S. (2012). Cyberbullying: An update and synthesis of the research. In J. W. Patchin & S. Hinduja (Eds.), *Cyberbullying prevention and response: Expert perspectives* (pp. 13–36). New York: Routledge.

Pendergrass, W. S., & Wright, M. (2014). Cyberbullied to death: An analysis of victims taken from recent events. *Issues in Information Systems, 15*, 32–140.

Perren, S., & Gutzwiller-Helfenfinger, E. (2012). Cyberbullying and traditional bullying in adolescence: Differential roles of moral disengagement, moral emotions, and moral values. *European Journal of Developmental Psychology, 9*, 195–209. doi:10.1080/17405629.2011.643168.

Perren, S., Dooley, J., Shaw, T., & Cross, D. (2010). Bullying in school and cyberspace: Associations with depressive symptoms in Swiss and Australian adolescents. *Child and Adolescent Psychiatry and Mental Health, 4*, Article 28. doi:10.1186/1753-2000-4-28.

Perren, S., Gutzwiller-Helfenfinger, E., Malti, T., & Hymel, S. (2011). Moral reasoning and emotion attributions of adolescent bullies, victims, and bully-victims. *British Journal of Developmental Psychology*. doi:10.1111/j.2044-835X.2011.02059.x. Published online first.

Perren, S., Corcoran, L., Cowie, H., Dehue, F., Garcia, D. J., Mc Guckin, C., et al. (2012). Tackling cyberbullying: Review of empirical evidence regarding successful responses by students, parents, and schools. *International Journal of Conflict and Violence, 6*, 283–292.

Pettalia, J. L., Levin, E., & Dickinson, J. (2013). Cyberbullying: Eliciting harm without consequence. *Computers in Human Behavior, 29*(6), 2758–2765.

Pew. (2009). Home broadband adoption. Paper presented at Pew Internet & American Life project. Washington, DC. http://pewinternet.org/Reports/2009/10-Home-Broadband-Adoption-2009.aspx.

Pornari, C. D., & Wood, J. (2010). Peer and cyber aggression in secondary school students: The role of moral disengagement, hostile attribution bias, and outcome expectancies. *Aggressive Behavior, 36*, 81–94. doi:10.1002/ab.20336.

Price, M., & Dalgleish, J. (2010). Cyberbullying: Experiences, impacts and coping strategies as described by Australian young people. *Youth Studies Australia, 29*, 51–59.

Privitera, C., & Campbell, M. A. (2009). Cyberbullying: The new face of workplace bullying? *CyberPsychology & Behavior, 12*, 395–400. doi:10.1089/cpb.2009.0025.

Putnam, R. (2000). *Bowling alone. The collapse and revival of American community.* New York: Simon & Schuster.

Raskauskas, J., & Stoltz, A. D. (2007). Involvement in traditional and electronic bullying among adolescents. *Developmental Psychology, 43,* 564–575. doi:10.1037/0012-1649.43.3.564.

Riebel, J., Jäger, R. S., & Fischer, U. C. (2009). Cyberbullying in Germany—An exploration of prevalence, overlapping with real life bullying and coping strategies. *Psychology Science Quarterly, 51,* 298–314.

Rivers, I. (2013). What to measure? In S. Bauman, D. Cross, & J. Walker (Eds.), *Principles of cyberbullying research: Definitions, measures, and methods* (pp. 222–237). New York: Routledge.

Robers, S., Kemp, J., Rathbun, A., & Morgan, R. E. (2014). *Indicators of School Crime and Safety: 2013 (NCES 2014-042/NCJ 243299). National Center for Education Statistics, U.S. Department of Education, and Bureau of Justice Statistics.* Washington, DC: Office of Justice Programs, U.S. Department of Justice.

Sabella, R. A., Patchin, J. W., & Hinduja, S. (2013). Cyberbullying myths and realities. *Computers in Human Behavior, 29*(6), 2703–2711. http://dx.doi.org/10.1016/. j.chb.2013.06.040.

Sakellariou, T., Carroll, A., & Houghton, S. (2012). Rates of cyber victimization and bullying among male Australian primary and high school students. *School Psychology International, 33,* 533–549. doi:10.1177/0143034311430374.

Salmivalli, C. (2013). El acoso y el grupo de iguales. En A. Ovejero. In P. K. Smith & S. Yubero (Eds.), *El acoso escolar y su prevención: Perspectivas internacionales* (pp. 111–130). Madrid: Biblioteca Nueva.

Salmivalli, C., Kärnä, A., & Poskiparta, E. (2011). Counteracting Bullying in Finland: The KiVa Program and Its Effects on Different Forms of Being Bullied. *International Journal of Behavioral Development, 35,* 405–411.

Schenk, A. M., & Fremouw, W. J. (2012). Prevalence, psychological impact, and coping of cyberbully victims among college students. *Journal of School Violence, 11,* 21–37. doi:10.1080/15 388220.2011.630310.

Schneider, S. K., O'Donnell, L., Stueve, A., & Coulter, R. W. S. (2012). Cyberbullying, school bullying, and psychological distress: A regional census of high school students. *American Journal of Public Health, 102*(1), 171–177. http://dx.doi.org/ 0.2105/AJPH.2011.300308.

Schultze-Krumbholz, A., & Scheithauer, H. (2009). Social-behavioral correlates of cyberbullying in a German student sample. *Zeitschrift für psychologie/Journal of Psychology, 217,* 224–226. doi:10.1027/0044-3409.217.4.224.

Ševčíková, A., Šmahel, D., & Otavová, M. (2012). The perception of cyberbullying in adolescent victims. *Emotional and Behavioural Difficulties, 17,* 319–328. doi:10.1080/13632752.2012.7 04309.

Shapka, J. D., & Law, D. M. (2013). Does one size fit all? Ethnic differences in parenting behaviors and motivations for adolescent engagement in cyberbullying. *Journal of Youth and Adolescence, 42,* 723–738. doi:10.1007/s10964-013-9928-2.

Šléglová, V., & Černá, A. (2011). Cyberbullying in adolescent victims: Perception and coping. *Cyberpsychology: Journal of Psychosocial Research on Cyberspace, 5*(2), article 4. http://www.cyberpsychology.eu/view.php?cisloclanku=2011121901&article=4.

Slonje, R., & Smith, P. K. (2008). Cyberbullying: Another main type of bullying? *Scandinavian Journal of Psychology, 49,* 147–154. doi:10.1111/j.1467-9450.2007.00611.x.

Slonje, R., Smith, P. K., & Frisén, A. (2012). Processes of cyberbullying, and feelings of remorse by bullies: A pilot study. *European Journal of Developmental Psychology, 9,* 244–259. doi:10 .1080/17405629.2011.643670.

Smith, P. K. (1997). Commentary III. Bullying in life-span perspective: What can studies of school bullying and workplace bullying learn from each other? *Journal of Community & Applied Social Psychology, 7,* 249–255.

Smith, P. K. (2013). Cyberbullying y ciberagresión. A. Ovejero, P. K. Smith, & S. Yubero (Eds.), *El acoso escolar y su prevención: Perspectivas internacionales* (pp. 173–190). Madrid: Biblioteca Nueva.

Smith, P. K. (2014). *Understanding school bullyhing: Its nature & prevention strategies*. London: Sage.

Smith, P. K., & Slonje, R. (2010). Cyberbullying: The nature and extent of a new kind of bullying, in and out of school. In S. Jimerson, S. Swearer, & D. Espelage (Eds.), *Handbook of bullying in schools* (pp. 249–262). New York: Routledge.

Smith, P. K., Shu, S., & Madsen, K. (2001). Characteristics of victims of schoolbullying: Developmental changes in coping strategies and skills. In J. Juoven & S. Graham (Eds.), *Peer Harassment at School: The Plight of the Vulnerable and Victimised* (pp. 332–352). New York: Guilford.

Smith, P., Mahdavi, J., Carvalho, M., & Tippett, N. (2006). An investigation into cyberbullying, its forms, awareness and impact, and the relationship between age and gender in cyberbullying. A Report to the Anti-Bullying Alliance. http://www.dcsf.gov.uk/research/data/uploadfiles/RBX03-06.pdf.

Smith, P. K., Mahdavi, J., Carvalho, M., Fisher, S., Russell, S., & Tippett, N. (2008). Cyberbullying: Its nature and impact in secondary school pupils. *Journal of Child Psychology and Psychiatry, 49*, 376–385. doi:10.1111/j.1469-7610.2007.01846.x.

Smith, P. K., Smith, C., Osborn, R., & Samara, M. (2008). A content analysis of school antibullying policies: Progress and limitations. *Educational Psychology in Practice, 24*, 1–12. http://dx.doi.org/10.1080/02667360701661165.

Smith, P. K., del Barrio, C., & Tokunaga, R. (2012). Definitions of bullying and cyberbullying: How useful are the terms? In S. Bauman, D. Cross, & J. Walker (Eds.), *Principles of cyberbullying research: Definition, measures, and methods* (pp. 29–40). Philadelphia: Routledge.

Smith, P. K., Kupferberg, A., Mora-Merchan, J. A., Samara, M., Bosley, S., & Osborn, R. (2012). A content analysis of school anti-bullying policies: A follow-up after six years. *Educational Psychology in Practice, 28*, 61–84.

Snakenborg, J., Van Acker, R., & Gable, R. A. (2011). Cyberbullying: Prevention and Intervention to Protect Our Children and Youth. *Preventing School Failure, 55*(2), 88–95 doi:10.1080/1045988X.2011.539454.

Sonawane, V. (2014, March 11). Cyber bullying increases suicidal thoughts and attempts: Study. HNGN. http://www.hngn.com/articles/26245/20140311/cyber-bullying-increases-suicidal-thoughtsattempts-study.htm.

Sourander, A., Brunstein Komek, A., Ikonen, M., et al. (2010). Psychosocial risk factors associated with cyberbullying among adolescents: A population-based study. *Archives of General Psychiatry, 67*(7), 720–728.

Stacey, E. (2009). Research into cyberbullying: Student perspectives on cybersafe learning environments. *Informatics in Education-An International Journal, 8*, 115–130.

Stadler, C., Feifel, J., Rohrmann, S., Vermeiren, R., & Poustka, F. (2010). Peer-victimization and mental health problems in adolescents: Are parental and school support protective? *Child Psychiatry & Human Development, 41*(4), 371–386. doi:10.1007/s10578-010-0174-5.

Staksrud, E., Olafsson, K., & Livingstone (2013). Does the use of social networking sites increase children's risk of harm? *Computers in Human Behavior, 29*(1), 40–50.

Steffgen, G., König, A., Pfetsch, J., & Melzer, A. (2011). Are cyberbullies less empathic? Adolescents' cyberbullying behavior and empathic responsiveness. *Cyberpsychology, Behavior, and Social Networking, 14*, 643–648. doi:10.1089/cyber.2010.0445.

Stewart, D. M., & Fritsch, E. J. (2011). School and law enforcement efforts to combat. *Cyberbullying, Preventing School Failure, 55*(2), 79–87.

Sticca, F., Ruggieri, S., Alsaker, F., & Perren, S. (2013). Longitudinal risk factors for cyberbullying in adolescence. *Journal of Community & Applied Social Psychology, 23*, 52–67. doi:10.1002/casp.2136.

Taiariol, J. (2010). *Cyberbullying: The role of family and school* (Doctoral dissertation). Available from Dissertation Abstracts International.

Talwar, V., Gomez-Garibello, C., & Shariff, S. (2014). Adolescents' moral evaluations and ratings of cyberbullying: The effect of veracity and intentionality behind the event. *Computers in Human Behavior, 36*, 122–128.

Tokunaga, R. S. (2010). Following you home from school: A critical review and synthesis of research on cyber bullying victimization. *Computers in Human Behavior, 26,* 277–287. doi:10.1016/j.chb.2009.11.014.

Topcu, Ç., & Erdur-Baker, Ö. (2012). Affective and cognitive empathy as mediators of gender differences in cyber and traditional bullying. *School Psychology International, 33*(5), 550–561. doi:10.1177/0143034312446882.

Twenge, J. M., Catanese, K. R., & Baumeister, R. F. (2002). Social exclusion causes self-defeating behavior. *Journal of Personality and Social Psychology, 83*(3), 606–615.

Twenge, J. M., Catanese, K. R., & Baumeister, R. F. (2003). Social exclusion and the deconstructed state: Time perception, meaninglessness, lethargy, lack of emotion, and self-awareness. *Journal of Personality and Social Psychology, 85*(3), 409–442.

Twenge, J. M., Baumeister, R. F., DeWall, C. N., Ciarocco, N.J., & Bartels, J. M. (2007). Social exclusion decreases prosocial behavior. *Journal of Personality and Social Psychology, 92*(1), 56–66.

van Geel, M., Vedder, P., & Tanilon, J. (2014). Relationship between peer victimization, cyberbullying, and suicide in children and adolescents: A meta-analysis. *JAMA Pediatrics, 168*(5), 435–442. doi:10.1001/jamapediatrics.2013.4143.

Van de bosch, H., & Poels, K. (2014). Schools and cyberbullying: Problem perception, current actions and future needs. International. *Journal of Cyber Society and Education, 7,* 29–48.

Van den Eijnden, R. J. J. M., Vermulst, A., Van Rooij, T., & Meerkerk, G. J. (2006). *Monitor Internet en jongeren: Pestem op Internet en het psychosociales welbevinden van jogeren.* Rotterdam: IVO Facrsheer.

Van der Aa, N., Overbeek, G., Engels, R. C., Scholte, R. H., Meerkerk, G. J., & van den Eijnden, R. (2009). Daily and compulsive Internet use and well-being in adolescence: A diathesis-stress model based on big five personality traits. *Journal of Youth and Adolescence, 38,* 765–776.

Vandebosch, H., & Van Cleemput, K. (2009). Cyberbullying among youngsters: Profiles of bullies and victims. *New Media & Society, 11,* 1349–1371. doi:10.1177/1461444809341263.

Varjas, K., Henrich, C. C., & Meyers, J. (2009). Urban middle school students' perceptions of bullying, cyberbullying, and school safety. *Journal of School Violence, 8,* 159–176. doi:10.1080/15388220802074165.

Vazsonyi, A. T., Machackova, H., Sevcikova, A., Smahel, D., & Cerna, A. (2012). Cyberbullying in context: Direct and indirect effects by low self-control across 25 European countries. *European Journal of Developmental Psychology, 9,* 210–227. doi:10.1080/17405629.2011.644919.

Vivolo-Kantor, A. M., Martell, B. N., Holland, K. M., & Westby, R. (2014). A systematic review and content analysis of bullying and cyber-bullying measurement strategies. *Aggression and Violent Behavior, 19,* 423–434.

Völlink, T., Bolman, C. A. W., Dehue, F., & Jacobs, N. C. L. (2013). Coping with cyberbullying: Differences between victims, bully-victims and children not involved in bullying. *Journal of Community & Applied Social Psychology Journal of Community Applied Social Psychology, 23,* 7–24. doi:10.1002/casp.2142.

Wachs, S. (2012). Moral disengagement and emotional and social difficulties in bullying and cyberbullying: Differences by participant role. *Emotional and Behavioral Difficulties, 17,* 347–360. doi:10.1080/13632752.2012.704318.

Wade, A., & Beran, T. (2011). Cyberbullying: The new era of bullying. Canadian. *Journal of School Psychology, 26,* 44–61. doi:10.1177/0829573510396318.

Walrave, M., & Heirman, W. (2011). Cyberbullying: Predicting victimisation and perpetration. *Children & Society, 25,* 59–72. doi:10.1111/j.1099-0860.2009.00260.x.

Wang, J., Nansel, T. R., & Iannotti, R. J. (2011). Cyber and traditional bullying: Differential association with depression. *Journal of Adolescent Health, 48,* 415–417. doi:10.1016/j.jadohealth.2010.07.012.

Wegge, D., Vandebosch, H., & Eggermont, S. (2013). Offline netwerken, online pesten: Een sociale netwerkanalyse van cyberpesten in de schoolcontext [Offline networking. *online bullying: A social network analysis of cyberbullying in the school context*]. *Tijdschrift voor Communicatiewetenschap, 41*(1), 15.

Wigderson, S., & Lynch, M. (2013). Cyber- and traditional peer victimization: Unique relationships with adolescent well-being. *Psychology of Violence, 3*(4), 297–309.

Willard, N. (2005). *An educators guide to cyberbullying.* Center for safe and responsible Internet use. http://www.cyberbully.org/docs/cpct.educators.pdf. Accessed: 15. Sept 2005

Willard, N. (2012). Cyberbullying and the law. In J. W. Patchin & S. Hinduja (Eds.), *Cyberbullying. Prevention and response. Expert perspectives* (pp. 36–56). New York: Routledge.

Willemse, I., Waller, G., & Süss, D. (2010). *JAMES—Jugend. Aktivitäten, Medien—Erhebung Schweiz.* Zürich: Zürcher Hochschule für Angewandte Wissenschaften.

Williams, K. D. (2007). Ostracism. *Annual Review of Psychology, 58,* 525–552.

Williams, K. R., & Guerra, N. G. (2007). Prevalence and predictors of Internet bullying. *Journal of Adolescent Health, 41*(Suppl. 6), S14–S21. doi:10.1016/j.jadohealth.2007.08.018.

Wong, D. S. W., Chan, H. C., & Cheng, C. H. K. (2014). Cyberbullying perpetration and victimization among adolescents in Hong Kong. *Children and Youth Services Review, 36,* 133–140. http://dx.doi.org/10.1016/j.childyouth.2013.11.006.

Wright, M. F., & Li, Y. (2013). The association between cyber victimization and cyber aggression: The moderating effect of peer rejection. *Journal of Youth & Adolescence, 42*(5), 662–674.

Wright, V. H., Burnham, J. J., Inman, C. T., & Ogorchock, H. N. (2009). Cyberbullying: Using virtual scenarios to educate and raise awareness. *Journal of Computing in Teacher Education, 26,* 35–42.

Yadava, A., Sharma, N. R., & Gandhi, A. (2001). Aggression and moral disengagement. *Journal of Personality and Clinical Studies, 17,* 95–99.

Ybarra, M. L., & Mitchell, K. J. (2004). Online aggressor/targets, aggressors, and targets: A comparison of associated youth characteristics. *Journal of Child Psychology and Psychiatry, 45,* 1308–1316. doi:10.1111/j.1469-7610.2004.00328.x.

Ybarra, M. L., & Mitchell, K. J. (2007). Prevalence and frequency of Internet harassment instigation: Implications for adolescent health. *Journal of Adolescent Health, 41*(2), 189–195. doi:10.1016/j.jadohealth.2007.03.005.

Ybarra, M. L., & Mitchell, K. J. (2008). How risky are social networking sites? A comparison of places online where youth sexual solicitation and harassment occurs. *Pediatrics, 121*(2), e350–e357. http://dx.doi.org/10.1542/peds.2007–0693.

Ybarra, M. L., Mitchell, K. J., Wolak, J., & Finkelhor, D. (2006). Examining characteristics and associated distress related to Internet harassment: Findings from the Second Youth Internet Safety Survey. *Pediatrics, 118,* e1169–e1177. doi:10.1542/peds.2006–0815.

Ybarra, M. L., Boyd, D., Korchmaros, J. D., & Oppenheim, J. (2012). Defining and measuring cyberbullying within the larger context of bullying victimization. *Journal of Adolescent Health, 51,* 53–58. doi:10.1016/j.jadohealth.2011.12.031.

Zimbardo, P. (2007). *The Lucifer effect.* New York: Random House.

Part I
Gender, Family, and Psychosocial Issues

Chapter 2
Gender Issues and Cyberbullying in Children and Adolescents: From Gender Differences to Gender Identity Measures

Raúl Navarro

2.1 Introduction

Slightly more than a decade ago, when the first psychological research with child and adolescent samples into cyberbullying was done, gender played a key role in analyzing cyberbullying prevalence. The term "gender," in addition to recognizing the influence of biological factors, includes cultural and experiential factors to explain aggressive behavior. Thus, gender not only implies the categorization of people into male or female groups but also refers to the gender-typing process in which they acquire those motives, values, and behaviors viewed as appropriate for males and females within a given culture (Diamond 2002). Regarding cyberbullying research, the principal aim was to know if this form of aggression is a gender-specific behavior or if, on the contrary, both genders are involved and whether they develop different behavior patterns in their involvement (Connell et al. 2014). To meet this objective, research has analyzed differences in boys' and girls' implication in it by considering that if such differences existed, they would be linked to learning that derives from gender socialization. Nevertheless, most studies have limited their analysis of gender to classifying participants in accordance with sexual dimorphism, and have not analyzed how acquired gender-related beliefs can be linked to cyberbullying. Therefore, from our point of view, it is necessary to review the way in which gender has been included in research and to consider the need to examine how the gender norms that operate in peer groups can contribute to cyberbullying being manifested. An examination of these trends may serve as a reference for gender research in cyberbullying and might help enhance our understanding of the way in which gender-typing processes are related to these negative cyberinteractions.

Based on this notion, this chapter reviews gender research on cyberbullying and presents data never published before in order to present new ways to advance in

R. Navarro (✉)
Department of Psychology, Faculty of Education and Humanities,
University of Castilla-La Mancha, Avda. De los Alfares, 42, 16071 Cuenca, Spain
e-mail: Raul.Navarro@uclm.es

© Springer International Publishing Switzerland 2016
R. Navarro et al. (eds.), *Cyberbullying Across the Globe*,
DOI 10.1007/978-3-319-25552-1_2

gender studies into this aggressive phenomenon. The objectives are none other than generating debate on the state of the art of research in this area and helping researchers to also identify new directions in international research. First, we present studies that examine gender differences in roles and forms within cyberbullying. To this end, we offer an up-to-date literature review. Second, we review the gender identity concept, understood as private experience of the gender roles and traits learned during the socialization process, and present a preliminary study on the influence of gender identity on cyberbullying. We have examined the way in which the gender standards adopted or violated in peer groups can protect from or trigger cyberbullying. Finally, as the youths who move away from the social expectations for their gender are more exposed to various forms of aggression, studies that examine the victimization suffered by sexual and gender minorities are reviewed and new qualitative data on their exposure to cyberbullying are offered. Throughout this chapter, we accompany theoretical presentations with not only a description of the studies done in different countries but also with new data that allow us to extend the gender perspective to study cyberbullying.

2.2   Gender Differences in Cyberbullying

Analyses into gender differences in cyberbullying took the results found in traditional bullying as a starting point. In general, research has reported that boys tend to get involved in direct forms of physical or verbal aggression to a greater extent than girls (Griezel et al. 2012; Pereira et al. 2004). Conversely, however, girls have been reported to use indirect aggression to a greater extent, where the victim is excluded from the peer group or his/her personal and social reputation is attacked (Björkqvist et al. 1994; Crick et al. 2002; Owens et al. 2004). These results have supported the idea that direct aggression is more prototypical of the male gender, while indirect aggression is more prototypical of the female gender. Several factors have been used to explain this division between more masculine or feminine forms of aggression, including biological reasons (e.g., physically, girls have less strength) and interpersonal reasons (e.g., the social structure of groups of girls as these groups are smaller and more intimate if compared with groups of boys, which would make indirect aggression a more effective strategy). Finally, there are gender socialization factors, for example, adults being less tolerant about girls getting involved in physical aggression, which would mean them having to adopt subtler and less visible forms (Kistner et al. 2010).

These explanations, along with results from many studies, have generated a considerable generalized consensus about girls using more indirect forms of aggression within traditional bullying (Kowalski et al. 2014), which makes them the center of attention when it comes to analyzing the prevalence of cyberbullying. This starting point is not at all surprising if we consider that cyberbullying has been described as a type of psychological and emotional abuse, carried out through gossip or diffusing information on the Internet where the aggressor attacks victims' privacy and intimacy but remains anonymous (Beran and Li 2008). Similar characteristics to traditional indirect bullying led preliminary research on cyberbullying to assume that girls were implied to the same extent, or even to a greater extent, than boys were. However, empirical evidence has not always been available to back this premise. In fact, far from finding a clear gender pattern in being involved as aggressors or victims, research has provided quite contradictory information.

Generally speaking, some researchers have encountered that boys act more as aggressors than girls, but girls are more victimized than boys (Walrave and Heirman 2011). Other studies have reported that boys act more as aggressors, but found no significant differences in victimization (Smith et al. 2012). Some other studies have indicated that girls act more as both aggressors and victims than boys (Mark and Ratliffe 2011), or that boys act more as aggressors and victims (Fanti et al. 2012). Numerous studies have found no gender differences in victims and aggressors (Griezel et al. 2012; Hinduja and Patchin 2008), while some research has suggested that gender differences depend on the analyzed forms of cyberbullying (Monks et al. 2012).

These mixed results could be put down to differences in the theories and methodologies used to characterize the studies conducted on cyberbullying. For instance, definitions of cyberbullying have varied from one study to another; different cyberbullying types have been examined, for example, by means of mobile phones (e.g., phone calls and text messages) or through social networks (e.g., Facebook and Twitter); different measurement instruments have been used, and distinct procedures have also been followed, when categorizing victims and aggressors. However, yet even in the studies that we conducted only a few years ago in Spain, which followed an identical measuring instrument, and the same cyberbullying definition and the same procedure to categorize subjects, mixed results were also obtained as one study showed that gender differences did not exist (Navarro et al. 2012), while another study indicated that girls were more victimized than boys (Navarro et al. 2013). Lack of consistency among studies has led some authors to conclude that research on gender differences in cyberbullying is a fruitless research area (Tokunaga 2010), and has downplayed the importance of the analysis of gender in cyberbullying.

2.2.1 Is Cyberbullying a Gender-Specific Behavior?

In order to check whether more recent studies on cyberbullying still provide mixed results for gender differences, we did a systematic literature review, using PsycINFO, PsycARTICLES, and Google Scholar, of the studies published while this chapter was being written. The criteria adopted to include studies in the review were as follows: (a) the search was not limited to specific countries or cultures, but had to include international representation, although only those articles published in English were reviewed; (b) year of publication: The table below indicates that the search was limited to the years 2013 and 2015 (including in-press articles) in order to include only the most recent studies; (c) articles had to contain empirical studies, and no reviews on the subject were included; (d) for a study to be selected, it had to analyze gender differences in both aggressors and victims, and no articles that centered on only one of these roles were included; and (e) articles had to be published in peer reviewed journals. As the scope of our review is broad, we do not claim having been able to include a complete review of all existing topic-related publications.

Table 2.1 shows the studies we reviewed, along with the main results found for gender differences in cyberbullying. These studies were arranged by considering the similarity of the results obtained. As a whole, six different results categories appeared. There were more articles with similar results in the first category, after which the number of coincidences progressively lowered. The studies that found no gender differences in victimization and perpetration within cyberbullying are first presented. Those showing that boys acted more as aggressors and girls as victims are presented in the second place. Those studies indicating that boys are more involved as both victims and aggressors come third. Studies which revealed that boys act more as aggressors than girls are the fourth category, but they found no gender differences in victimization. In the fifth place appears the research which indicated that no gender differences appeared in perpetration, but stated that more girls were cyberbullying victims. Finally, there is a group of studies which reported that more girls acted as both aggressors and victims than boys.

As the systematic review indicates, the results are still mixed. However, far from not contributing to research on cyberbullying, these results may indicate that we have analyzed gender difference from an unsuitable viewpoint as we have looked to seek that certain gender trends found in research on traditional bullying are fulfilled. Trends may have become stereotyped. According to these stereotyped gender trends, cyberbullying has been seen as a more concealed psychological and emotional strategy, which entails greater planning and more premeditation, and it has been more stereotypically related with girls. On the contrary, boys would continue using direct forms of aggression, which are clearer, simpler, and more visible than those employed by girls. This stereotyped view has continued, even when some years ago international research denied that indirect aggression is a more prototypical conduct of girls and pointed out that such strategies are used by both genders and to the same extent (Archer 2004; Artz et al. 2008; Card et al. 2008). Indeed, some studies have even demonstrated that boys employ more indirect aggression than girls. Specifically, the transcultural study by Artz et al. (2013), conducted with 5789 adolescents from six countries including Canada and Spain, found that more boys (46.8%) than girls (31.7%) employed indirect aggression with peers. As the authors concluded, this result goes against generalized beliefs as indirect aggression was more of an issue among girls than it was for boys, and the same may be said of cyberbullying.

Yet, available data do not let us to state that cyberbullying is merely a girls' issue. Indeed, many studies have shown that boys stand out as aggressors. Likewise, a recent meta-analysis on the aggressor role by Barlett and Coyne (2014) concluded that males were more likely to be cyberbullies than females. However, this difference was moderated by age; indeed, females were more likely to report

Table 2.1 Cyberbullying and gender: Overview of studies (2013/2015) that analyzed gender differences in cyberbullying perpetration and victimization

Country	Study	Sample	Main results
Greece	Lazuras et al. (2013)	355 students aged 13–17 years	There were no gender differences in either experiencing or reporting cyberbullying
South Korea	Park et al. (2014)	1200 students aged 12–15 years	No gender differences were found in perpetration and victimization
Colombia	Mura and Diamantini (2014)	360 students aged 14–19 years	No gender differences were found in cyberbullying perpetration and victimization
Canada	Bonanno and Hymel (2013)	399 students in grades 8–10	No significant gender differences were found in cyberbullying victimization and perpetration
Switzerland	Sticca et al. (2013)	First assessment: 835 students in 6th grade. Second assessment: 820 students	No significant associations were found between gender and cyberbullying perpetration or victimization
USA	Kowalski and Limber (2013)	931 students in grades 6–12	No significant main gender effects were observed in perpetration and victimization
Spain	Navarro et al. (2015)	1058 students aged 10–12 years	No statistically significant differences were found between boys and girls in cyberbullying victimization and perpetration
South Korea	Shin and Ahn (2015)	1036 students aged 12–18 years	There was no gender effect on the classification of victims and bullies
Israel	Heiman and Olenik-Shemesh (2015)	507 students in grades 7–10. (242 typically achieving students, 149 LD students in general education classes, 116 LD comorbid in special education classes)	Girls were more likely to be cyberbullying victims than boys. Boys were more likely to be cyberbullying perpetrators. Girls in special education classes were at higher risk of being cyberbullying victims
USA	Navarro and Jasinski (2013)	1500 students aged 10–17 years	Girls were at higher risk of cyberbullying victimization than boys. Boys engaged significantly more in cyberbullying perpetration
Sweden	Låftman et al. (2013)	22,544 students aged 15–18 years	Girls tended to be cyberbullying victims more often than boys, while boys were more often perpetrators

Table 2.1 (continued)

Country	Study	Sample	Main results
Germany	Festl and Quandt (2013)	408 students aged 12–19 years	Boys were more frequently perpetrators, whereas girls were more frequently victims
Israel	Tarablus et al. (in press)	458 junior high students aged 11–13 years	Girls were more likely to be cybervictims than boys and that boys were more likely to be cyberbullies than girls
Israel	Heiman et al. (2015)	480 students aged 12–16 years. (342 typical achieving students and 140 students with ADHD)	Significantly more girls were cybervictims than boys
			Boys reported more involvement as cyberperpetrators than girls
			No significant interactions were obtained among gender, groups (ADHD/Non ADHD) and the two cyberbullying involvement types
Multiregion: six European countries	Schultze-Krumbholz et al. (2015)	6260 students aged 11–23 years	More often girls were victims and more often boys were perpetrators
Germany	Wachs et al. (2015)	1928 students aged 11–18 years	Boys were more likely than girls to be cyberbullies and girls were more likely than boys to be cybervictims
USA	Pelfrey and Weber (2013)	3403 students in grades 6–12	Male students were more likely to be perpetrators and victims of cyberbullying than females
China	Wong et al. (2014)	1917 students aged 12–15 years	Boy participants reported having significantly more frequent cyberbullying perpetration and victimization than their female counterparts
South Korea	Yang et al. (2013)	1344 students in grade 4	Male students reported being more involved as perpetrators and victims than female students
China	Zhou et al. (2013)	1483 students in grades 10–12	Boys were more likely to report being involved in cyberbullying as perpetrators than girls
			Boys were also more likely to be cybervictims than girls
Taiwan	Chin Yang et al. (2014)	837 students in grades 5–12	Boys were more likely to be perpetrators and victims than girls
Israel	Lapidot-Lefter and Dolev-Cohen (2015)	465 students in grades 7–12	No gender differences were found for victimization
			Boys reported being perpetrators more than girls did

Table 2.1 (continued)

Country	Study	Sample	Main results
Mexico	Gámez-Guadix et al. (2014)	1491 students aged 12–18 years	Perpetration was significantly higher for males than for females, whereas no differences were found for victimization
Italy	Baroncelli and Ciucci (2014)	529 students in grades 6–8	Males obtained higher scores for cyberbullying perpetration
			No differences were found in cyberbullying victimization
Greece	Kokkinos et al. (2013)	300 students aged 10–12 years	Boys reported more frequent involvement in cyberbullying perpetration, while no significant gender differences were found in cybervictimization terms
Canada	Cappadocia et al. (2013)	1972 students in grades 9–12	Boys and girls reported similar rates of cyberperpetration
			Girls reported more involvement in cybervictimization than boys
Sweden	Beckman et al. (2013)	2989 students aged 13–15 years	No significant gender differences were found for cyberbullies.
			Girls were significantly more likely to be cybervictims than boys
USA	Connell et al. (2014)	3867 students in grades 5–8	Girls were more likely to report having engaged in cyberbullying perpetration than boys
			Girls reported higher levels of cybervictimization than boys

ADHD Attention deficit hyperactivity disorder, *LD* is Learning Disabilities

cyberbullying in early adolescence, while males were more likely to be cyberbullies in later adolescence. Similarly, other studies have found that in middle childhood, cyberbullying is more of a girls' issue in both aggressor and victim roles (Connell et al. (2014). Thus, age could be a key factor when it comes to analyzing gender differences.

However, the previous systematic review presented in this chapter shows that recent studies conducted with different aged samples have found no gender differences. The examined results as a whole led us conclude that far from cyberbullying corresponding to the female dominion, it is an issue that concerns both genders and that both gender can sometimes be involved as aggressors or victims.

The results obtained by international researchers and the data provided herein do not allow us to conclude that a clear gender difference exists in cyberbullying behaviors. However, they allow us to draw some conclusions. First, contrary to the results found in traditional bullying, there are no clear differences between males and females in cyberbullying. The absence of differences may indicate that more females are actually victims of cyberbullying than traditional bullying (Kowalski et al. 2012). Second, past research has reported that more males apparently tend to exercise and suffer the form of cyberbullying that employs humiliating images or contains physical aggression than females. Males also tend to send more sexual or pornographic images, which is a form of cyberbullying to which females are more exposed (Cassidy et al. 2012). These new forms of sexual and gender harassment require more research efforts, which could be essential to understand the role that gender plays in cyberbullying. Third, researchers need to explore the role of gender in moderating the effects of different factors that may be related with cyberbullying victimization and perpetration (Wong et al. 2015). Finally, future research should also analyze differences in what behaviors are considered to be cyberbullying by each gender, as well as in the level of awareness about behaviors related to cyberbullying. These differences might influence their responses to cyberbullying measures (Akbaba et al. 2015).

2.2.2   What Do We Do Now with Gender?

The conclusion that cyberbullying is not a clearly gender-specific behavior must not lead us to believe that gender analyses are not useful and necessary. In fact, quite the opposite is true as these analyses are still a key dimension for understanding the cyberbullying phenomenon and, in particular, for comprehending which aspects linked to social pressures on gender learning can make boys and girls more vulnerable to cyberbullying, irrespective of the greater or lesser extent of their implication. In order to know more about the role that gender plays in cyberbullying, it is important that research goes beyond merely analyzing mean scores and measure how the internalization of gender-related beliefs and peer pressures toward gender norms are risk factors for involvement in cyberbullying.

From this perspective, research must be reinforced in methodological terms by including new measuring instruments of gender typification. Research also needs to be reinforced theoretically by adopting different gender development approaches that allow us to hypothesize about its relation with cyberbullying, and help to interpret the results obtained. Along these lines, some studies have already included gender theories in the analyses of their results. One example is the work of Navarro and Jasinski (2013), which adopted the cyberdystopian feminist perspective as a standpoint that girls are inherently more at cyberbullying risk because of their already disadvantaged position in society. However, as far as we are aware, no studies have examined the way in which beliefs, gender roles, or identities are risk or protection factors against cyberbullying. Studies that have adopted a qualitative methodology by questioning youths about these matters are also scarce. For this reason, the following sections present new data as an attempt to illustrate the predictive value of gender in cyberbullying beyond analyzing gender differences.

2.3 Cyberbullying and Gender Identity

Gender identity has been analyzed as an indicator of children's and adolescents' psychosocial adjustment and well-being in peer groups (Carver et al. 2003), and cyberbullying may be associated with gender identity in different ways. Traditionally speaking, gender identity is defined as an individual feeling of belonging to one gender and not to the other (Kohlberg 1966). Subsequently, gender identity has been defined as the extent to which people see themselves as being masculine or feminine when compared to the cultural stereotypes for their own gender (Bem 1981; Spence 1993). In line with this definition, gender identity will vary from one person to another according to the degree of adherence to culturally marked standards that offer different personality traits and conduct repertoires in accordance with gender. This "private or personal" identification with patterns and systems of beliefs that are considered appropriate for one sex or another also has a public expression, gender roles, which communicate the degree of adhesion that someone has or some people have to social prescriptions (Bem 1981).

Self-identification with socially prescribed stereotypes and gender roles has been more recently considered to be only one of the factors involved in constructing gender identity (Egan and Perry 2001). These authors argued that gender identity must be conceptualized as a multidimensional variable for whose knowledge we must contemplate five components: (1) membership knowledge in a gender category (the traditional view of gender identity), (2) gender typicality, self-perceived similarity with other members of the same gender category, (3) gender contentedness, an individual's satisfaction with his/her own gender, (4) felt pressure for gender conformity, and (5) intergroup bias, the belief that one gender is superior to the other gender. After developing a self-report measure to evaluate the last four of the above components, the authors found that gender typicality and gender contentment were related with a favorable psychosocial adjustment in boys and girls (in terms of greater self-esteem and peer acceptance), while felt pressure and intergroup bias were sometimes found to be negatively related with good psychosocial adjustment. Despite a few differences, these findings have been replicated in other samples (Carver et al. 2003) and in distinct cultures (Yu and Xie 2010) to show that identity development includes various components that go beyond self-identification as male or female. These studies also underline the importance of gender identity components on different personal and social adjustment indices in peer groups.

We will now review the studies that link bullying, understood as an indicator of a negative psychosocial adjustment, with both types of gender identity approaches. First, some studies that analyze gender identity as self-perceived similarity to gender stereotypes are presented. Second, there are studies that use the multidimensional gender identity model of Egan and Perry (2001). In our view, Egan and Perry's proposal more accurately and completely captures the elements that constitute gender identity. However, since studies into bullying have examined its relationship with the internalization of what we call from now gender-typed personality traits, we believe that it is relevant to continue considering them as part of gender studies in bullying behaviors. This review allows us to offer a comparison between both perspectives in the analysis of gender identity and its relationship with bullying. After reviewing these studies, the study conducted about the influence of components of gender identity, on the one hand, and the internalization of gender-typed personality traits, on the other hand, on cyberbullying victimization and perpetration is presented.

2.3.1 Gender-Typed Personality Traits and Bullying Behaviors

Past research has proposed that differences in aggressive conduct can derive, to some extent, from learning instrumental (masculine) traits or expressive (feminine) traits. Such traits determine that men must be assertive, aggressive, brave, and independent, while women must be sensitive, emotional, friendly, and concerned about looking after relationships. Although everyone differs insofar as the personal integration they make of these masculine and feminine traits, it has been hypothesized that those people who construct their identity on masculine traits, like dominance, intransigence, or self-expansion, can behave aggressively more easily in order to exert control over others or to affirm these masculine traits (Phillips 2007). Conversely, constructing identity on female traits that emphasize self-sacrifice, concern for others, and even passiveness might be related with a less hostile interaction style, inhibited aggression, or using indirect forms of aggression (Underwood et al. 2001). Following this argument, aggression could be a way of demonstrating adaptation to gender schemes to comply with social expectations (Eagly et al. 2004).

Young and Sweeting (2004) were the first to analyze the relationship between internalization of gender traits and school bullying among secondary school students. They found that masculine traits and the perpetrator role were positively related. Nonetheless, they did not find any relationship between feminine traits and bullying in both the perpetrator and victim roles. Later, Gini and Pozzoli (2006) encountered the same relationship between masculine traits and the role of aggressor in a sample of primary school students. Crothers et al. (2005) analyzed the relationship between feminine traits and bullying led by girls, based on the premise that feminine traits could also be related stereotypically with the relational aggression associated with females. And so it was that they found that adolescents who described themselves as having more feminine traits were more aggressive relationally. Unlike previous studies, they did not find any type of relationship with masculine traits. However, it should be stated that their study sample was integrated only by females and, perhaps, the masculine traits internalization results would have differed if the sample had included males.

Some years ago in Spain, we analyzed the relationship between gender traits and implication as aggressors or victims in direct (physical and verbal aggression) and indirect (conducts of social exclusion) forms of bullying. The results revealed that irrespective of participants' genders, those students who reported feeling very well identified with masculine traits exercise more physical harassment, verbal abuse, and social exclusion-type conduct than students who stated they feel less identified with these traits. Conversely, those students who identified themselves more clearly with feminine traits reported no, or very little, involvement in all the forms of bullying analyzed (Navarro et al. 2011). More recent studies in our country have also found a positive relationship between instrumental traits and attitudes that favor bullying at school, and also between feminine traits and unfavorable attitudes toward this conduct (Carrera-Fernández et al. 2013).

Some of the reviewed studies have also analyzed the relationship between victimization and behaviors or interests not traditionally associated with one's own gender, as well as internalization of non-prototypical traits for own gender. Young and Sweeting (2004), for instance, specifically investigated the link between atypical gender behaviors and bullying. Their results indicated that a high score of atypical behaviors for their gender, plus a low score in masculine traits, was closely related with the victimization that boys suffered. Navarro et al. (2011) found that boys displaying high internalization of feminine traits were more likely to be victims of bullying in the three aggressive forms examined. Additionally, those girls who reported feeling more identified with masculine traits were more victims of verbal aggression. Victimization appeared to be the way in which peers punished identification with non-prototypical traits for their own gender.

These studies have been criticized because they adopted measures analyzing gender typification in specific domains and did not consider gender identity as the diverse and abstract information about how one feels about their attachment to one gender category or another. It has also been pointed out that researchers attribute a motivational meaning to the masculinity and femininity patterns which are scored within these measures. For instance, just as Egan and Perry (2001, p. 452) explained, "Bem (1981) suggested that gender schematic people are motivated to adopt behaviors consistent with one sex role and to shun behaviors associated with the other. However, it seems gratuitous to assume that sex-typed self-perceptions necessarily reflect felt pressure for sex role conformity rather than derive from some other source (e.g.) temperamental proclivities." For these reasons, internalization of gender-typed personality traits must be considered as a gender typification measure and would only display one specific gender identity aspect.

2.3.2   The Multidimensional Gender Identity Model and Bullying Behaviors

The multidimensional gender identity model (Egan and Perry 2001) understands that we must not only pay attention to specific domains such as gender-typed personality traits, but more integrative measures that cover personal judgments must also be generated, which we can all form about our gender (e.g., do I fit well with my gender category? Is my gender superior to the other?). The model's different dimensions are related with children's psychological adaptation and can also be linked to victimization processes. The first dimension is gender typicality (the extent to which people feel they are a typical member of their own gender category). According to this model, youths with low gender typicality tend to be more prone to anxiety, sadness, and can even be rejected by peers. For this reason, they can be perceived as being easy victims for aggressive peers and being more easily victimized by others. This hypothesis has been corroborated by several studies which found that those who display greater gender typicity, or those who express more gender conformity, are less victimized by colleagues (Carver et al. 2003; Drury et al. 2013; Roberts et al. 2013) and feel less loneliness than those who exhibit less gender typicity (Yu and Xie 2010).

It has also been hypothesized that the other gender identity components can be related with aggression and victimization conducts among peers (Carver et al. 2003). Gender contentedness can be related with victimization if we consider that the youths who state that they are not satisfied with their own gender (the feeling of not being at home in one's body) might be exposed to negative social reactions and may feel more pressure to adapt to gender norms from peers. Along this line of thought, felt pressure to gender conformity might also be related with adopting stereotypical conducts for one gender or another (antisocial trends for boys and subordination conducts for girls). Intergroup bias can imply that children find it difficult to interact with peers because biased perception and negative attitudes toward the other sex can mean fewer respectful and cooperative interactions with other peers. Very little research has been conducted into these relationships; so it is still difficult to conclude whether the relationships hypothesized between gender identity and bullying actually take place. Previous studies have found that peers describe gender-dysphoric girls as being more aggressive and disruptive than other girls. Yet, it is still not clear whether aggression is a reaction to discontentment with own gender or whether gender discontentment is a rationalization by aggressive girls: "if only I were a boy, it would be okay for me to act like this" (Carver et al. 2003, p. 106). The work by Drury et al. (2013) found an indirect relationship between felt pressure and victimization when determining that the negative relationship between gender typicality and victimization was more pronounced in contexts with more pressure to conforming to gender norms. More recently, Navarro et al. (2015a) tested how gender identity measures were related to victims, bullies, and bully-victims of school bullying. The results showed that perceiving self as being a typical member of the same-sex group is a protective factor for victimization, whereas felt pressure to conform to the cultural stereotypes about gender and lack of satisfaction with one's gender are risk factors for perpetration.

Although not all studies have reported the same results because of, among other aspects, differences in the methodologies used and cultural differences between the countries they were conducted in, their results have revealed the usefulness of analyzing different gender constructs despite gender differences when analyzing the different ways boys and girls get involved in bullying. The relationship between the dimensions in the gender identity model of Egan and Perry (2001) and gender-typing process measures and cyberbullying is an issue which, as far as we are aware, has not yet been explored. For this reason, we now go on to present the preliminary results of a study that analyzed the association of cyberbullying with both constructs in an attempt to better understand the cyberbullying phenomenon as an indicator of psychosocial adaptation in its relationship with the gender variable.

2.3.3   The Role of Gender Identity Dimensions and Gender-Typed Personality Traits in Cyberbullying Victimization and Perpetration Among Spanish Children

Children's involvement in bullying behaviors is assumed to be associated with gender identity components, such as gender typicality, and also with sex-typing constructs, such as gender-typed personality traits. For example, high gender typicality is associated with less victimization and high levels of masculine traits are related to perpetration. Considering previous findings, it seems logical to explore whether these variables may function as protective or risk factors to engage in bullying behavior as victims or bullies, which would extend the analysis to cyberbullying, where studies for these relationships are still scarce. Therefore, this study aims to explore the relative contribution of gender identity components and gender-typed traits in predicting victimization and perpetration status in cyberbullying behaviors.

For this purpose, 445 schoolchildren in grades 5 and 6 at five primary education schools were asked to complete the Multidimensional Gender Identity Inventory (Egan and Perry 2001) and the Children's Personal Attributes Questionnaire (CAPQ; Hall and Halberstadt 1980). The Egan and Perry Inventory assesses multiple gender identity components, namely gender typicality, gender contentedness, felt pressure, and intergroup bias. CAPQ consists of separate masculine and feminine scales, and a third bipolar masculine–feminine traits scale. Schools were located in a city of central Spain with an approximate population of 60,000. Participants included 208 girls (M (age): 10.78, standard deviation (SD)=0.74) and 237 boys (M (age)=10.78, SD=0.68).

Relying on previous traditional bullying findings and considering that cyberbullying is not a completely different phenomenon from school bullying, it is assumed that results for this kind of bullying will be similar to those found in traditional forms. It was hypothesized that cybervictimization would be negatively related to gender typicality and masculinity traits, whereas perpetration would be positively related to masculine traits and negatively related to feminine traits. No predictions were made for the remaining gender identity components since it was considered that they are less explored in the review literature.

In order to examine the associations between independent variables (gender identity dimensions and gender-typed personality traits) and the dependent variable

Table 2.2 Logistic regression model predicting the associations among reports of cybervictimization, gender identity dimensions, and gender-typed personality traits

	B	SE	Wald	OR	95% CI	
					Lower	Upper
Gender	–	–	–	–		
Grade	–	–	–	–		
Gender identity						
Gender typicality	−0.61	−0.28	4.65	0.54*	0.31	0.94
Gender contentedness	−0.94	0.28	10.91	0.39**	0.22	0.68
Felt pressure	–	–	–	–		
Intergroup bias	−0.44	0.21	4.40	0.63*	0.42	0.97
Gender-typed traits						
Masculine traits	−0.54	0.27	3.80	0.58*	0.33	1.00
Feminine traits	–	–	–	–		
Masculine/feminine traits	–	–	–	–		
Constant	5.35	1.15	21.38	211.96		
−2 LL	273.36					
Nagelkerke R^2	0.197					

Model $\chi^2 = 47.58$, df=4, $p < 0.001$, $n = 445$
– not in the final model, *B* coefficient, *SE* standard error, *OR* odds ratio, *CI* confidence interval, *LL* log likelihood
*$p < 0.05$; **$p < 0.01$

(cyberbullying victimization and perpetration), logistic regression analyses were applied to the data. Table 2.2 presents the regression statistics for cybervictimization. Cyberbullying victimization was associated with gender typicality (OR = 0.54), gender contentedness (OR = 0.39), intergroup bias (OR = 0.63), and masculine traits (OR = 0.58). The overall data indicate that self-perceived similarity to other members of the same gender category, one's satisfaction with own gender, the belief that one's own gender is superior to the other, and self-description with masculine traits lowered the likelihood of cyberbullying victimization.

The data reveal that those children who feel more psychologically compatible with their own gender in terms of self-perceived gender typicality and gender contentedness suffer less cybervictimization. This result corroborates previous research that has indicated that good gender compatibility is beneficial for children's psychosocial adaptation (Carver et al. 2003; Egan and Perry 2001; Navarro et al. 2015a; Yu and Xie 2010), which, in our case, was measured in terms of less victimization among peers. The present study also backs studies which have indicated that children who report more typicality also report less victimization (Drury et al. 2013), which could also occur in online contexts. Thus, it can be stated that children who display an atypical gender conduct, that is, cross-sex-typed children, are more likely to feel rejected by their peers as a form of cyberaggression.

Similarly, the analyses have indicated that self-description regarding masculine traits is related to less victimization. Hence, masculine traits act as a protection factor against victimization, which might be related with greater gender typification, just as the results on the effect of the gender typicality dimension have shown. The regression analysis did not indicate if participants' gender had any effect on victimization. So, we do not know if the effect of masculine traits as a protector factor is clearer among boys or girls. Future research must investigate this aspect more thoroughly as these traits are more prototypical of boys than of girls, and when girls adhere to them, they could display cross-gender behavior, which can be penalized by peers as victimization, as previous studies have indicated (Navarro et al. 2011). Nevertheless, this does not seem the case in this study. We could examine whether adhesion to prototypically masculine traits, such as "feels superior," "feelings not easily hurt," and "not easily influenced," can lead peers to not choose these children as targets of aggression. It would also be interesting to analyze if, irrespective of gender, these children may even be victimized, and whether they do not perceive online attacks as attempts of aggression due to their feelings of superiority of being tougher. In any case, we cannot talk in terms of casualty in one direction or another, and knowing the reason for these results must lead us to conduct longitudinal studies, as well as qualitative research, to learn the opinions of those who participate in cyberbullying about such matters.

Intergroup bias has also been found to be a protection factor in the face of victimization. This is a surprising finding if we consider that it is a gender identity dimension associated with unfavorable adaptation with difficulties in interactions with peers (Egan and Perry 2001). Although this dimension needs examining more thoroughly, one possible explanation for these results is the fact that showing same-sex favoritism can be seen as a sign of adapting to own gender. In this way, peers may view boys and girls with more intergroup prejudices as being better adapted to their gender groups as they respond to gender stereotypes, and can be less exposed to online victimization. Conversely, showing cross-sex favoritism can be seen as less suitable behavior within the gender typification process and may be penalized through victimization. Nonetheless, these explanations can help understand the lack of aggression by own gender but, as a part of intergroup prejudice, cross-sex discrimination can cause aggression by peers of the opposite sex. Nonetheless, the very nature of cyberbullying in which most forms of aggression are anonymous makes this issue a difficult one to explore.

Table 2.3 presents perpetration statistics. Cyberbullying perpetration was associated negatively with gender (OR = 0.49), gender contentedness (OR = 0.30), and feminine traits (OR = 0.28), but positively with masculine traits (OR = 9.96). The results indicate that the odds of cyberbullying perpetration were higher for males than for females. Moreover, one's satisfaction with own gender and self-description with feminine traits lowered the likelihood of cyberbullying perpetration, whereas children who were self-described with masculine traits were at higher risk of participating as perpetrators in cyberbullying.

These results indicate that more boys tend to play the aggressor role and, once again, show a link between adhesion to prototypically masculine traits and perpetration of online bullying conducts. This result coincides with that found for traditional bullying conducts (Gini and Pozzoli 2006; Younger and Sweeting 2004), and this could be important to understand why boys are sometimes more implicated in

Table 2.3 Logistic regression model predicting the associations among reports of cyberperpetration, gender identity dimensions, and gender-typed personality traits

	B	SE	Wald	OR	95% CI	
					Lower	Upper
Gender	−0.69	0.35	3.80	0.49*	0.24	1.00
Grade	−	−	−	−		
Gender identity						
Gender typicality	−	−	−	−		
Gender contentedness	−1.17	0.47	6.00	0.30**	0.12	0.79
Felt pressure	−	−	−	−		
Intergroup bias	−	−	−	−		
Gender-typed traits						
Masculine traits	2.29	0.63	13.18	9.96***	2.88	34.45
Feminine traits	−1.26	0.44	8.18	0.28**	0.11	0.67
Masculine/feminine traits	−	−	−	−		
Constant	−2.98	2.44	1.49	0.05		
−2 LL	91.35					
Nagelkerke R²	0.294					

Model $\chi^2=33.05$, df=4, $p<0.001$, $n=445$
− not in the final model, *B* coefficient, *SE* standard error, *OR* odds ratio, *CI* confidence interval, *LL* log likelihood
*$p<0.05$; **$p<0.01$; ***$p<0.001$

cyberbullying perpetration than girls, given that the internalization of masculinity traits is more prototypical in males. Conversely, those who describe themselves in relation to feminine traits that are more linked to cooperative conducts and caring for interpersonal relations are seen as being less involved as aggressors in cyberbullying. This result also agrees with that found for school bullying (Navarro et al. 2011). A second protection factor emerged from the multidimensional gender identity model, which indicated that children with more gender contentedness display lesser aggression tendency within cyberbullying. Carver et al. (2003) found that those girls who are not content with their own gender are described by their peers as being more aggressive and troublesome than girls who do not display this dissatisfaction. Those children who are not content with their gender may possibly react aggressively, given their feeling of discontent since they have not adapted to what is socially expected of them, and possibly also due to the social rejection they may be suffering. However, from the data obtained, we cannot conclude that this relation is taking place, and future research needs to deal with this issue. At any rate, and as Carver et al. (2003) pointed out, these data reveal that at least in social interactions, those children who show greater compatibility with their gender better adapt since they are neither aggressors nor victims with cyberbullying.

Despite all these results being preliminary, they provide interesting information about the gender relation and cyberbullying and also suggest that gender variables operate similarly in real and virtual settings.

2.4   Cyberbullying and Sex and Gender Minorities

In recent decades, several studies on bullying have analyzed the victimization that youths belonging to sexual minorities and gender minorities have suffered (Collier et al. 2013). In line with these authors, the term "sexual minority" has been used in this chapter to denote those youths who may be attracted to people of the same sex; have had sexual relationships with people of their own sex; or who define themselves as lesbians, gays, bisexuals, or questioning. The term "gender minority" has been employed to refer to transgender individuals and gender nonconforming individuals who do not self-identify as transgenders but whose gender identity or expression does not conform to cultural norms for their birth sex.

Generally speaking, research has informed that lesbian, gay, bisexual, and transgender (LGBT) youths suffer more victimization than their heterosexual peers (Berlan et al. 2010; Mitchell et al. 2014; Russell et al. 2012). Among its consequences, it has been consistently found that this type of victimization is related with less sense of belonging to their schools, higher levels of depression, and higher suicidal proclivity (Collier et al. 2013). Most studies describe such bullying as being homophobic. However, exactly as we can see in the review by Rivers (2013), it is important to consider that not all victims identify themselves with homosexuals or transgenders, but some people are simply bullied because they are perceived as being different in some way. This fact is normally attributed to their sexual orientation when this difference may be due only to them showing atypical gender behavior that does not conform to gender roles.

The distinction between sexual orientation and gender identity is important if we consider that research has found differences in the risk of suffering victimization for each minority type, and that transgender youths and gender nonconforming youths tend to be more victimized if compared with lesbian, gay, and bisexual youths. For example, transgender students and gender atypical students are more physically harassed and received degrading insults like "faggot," given its perceived expression of gender or sexual orientation (Greytak et al. 2009). It has been recently found that these youths also suffer more sexual harassment in both real and virtual situations (Mitchell et al. 2014).

Several studies have also documented differences according to age and sex in the victimization of these minorities by demonstrating that boys are victimized more than girls, and victimization indices are higher in the first years of adolescence, which seems to be related with a drop in homophobic and discriminatory attitudes among students in grades 7–12 (Poteat et al. 2009). Yet, the study carried out by Russell et al. (2014) demonstrated that even though physical aggression shown against these minorities diminishes with age, indirect aggressions (e.g., stealing or damaging their belongings) remain more persistent among sexual and gender minorities, even when such aggressions diminish for the general population. These results make us think that the offline bullying suffered by these minorities could be transferred to online contexts where they would become more indirect and would, therefore, become more persistent harassment due to the anonymity that the Internet offers and due to the difficulties of this means to control it. This argument is also supported in the study by Rivers and Noret (2010), who found a relation between online bullying and offline bullying suffered by these minorities. Their results indicate that boys received more insulting text messages and e-mails if they had been previously harassed for their physical appearance, perceived sexually orientation, or the clothes they wore, while girls suffer more online victimization if they had been harassed for getting good results at school or performing well in sports beforehand.

Although few studies that systematically study such online interactions have been done to date, what comes over clearly, as Rivers explained (2014, p. 28–29), is that "sexuality, sexual orientation, gender typicality and atypicality are aspects of young people's lives that constantly appear in developmental literature. The Internet provides an environment in which it is possible for young people to explore these most personal aspects of lives often anonymously. However, the Internet also provides forums where others can express their likes and dislikes, their prejudices and their suspicions [sic] about others without having the social cues and restrictions that regulate face-to-face interactions."

2.4.1 Student's Perceptions of Cyberbullying Directed to Sexual and Gender Minorities

There were two reasons for including this section in this chapter. First, because results in Sect. 2.2. indicate that those boys and girls who are gender typified (i.e., who show more interests, attitudes, or conducts that are stereotypically associated with own gender) suffer less online victimization. Second, but no less important, while forming the focal groups for another chapter of this book, some participants talked about the aggressions that those people considered different, either due to their sexual orientation or due to their conducts, which peers do not consider gender-adequate, suffer on the Internet. Although the participants did not use the terms employed in this chapter in their discussions, they actually referred to sexual and gender minorities. One of the male participants in the secondary education groups identified himself as being homosexual and talked about the harassment he had suffered for years, first in real contexts like school and later in virtual contexts like social networks. His testimony was taken as a highly valuable contribution to the discourse generated on cyberbullying, and it led us to include a series of questions on the cyberbullying that sex and gender minorities face in the other groups formed. The intention of these questions was to know what perception the participants have of cyberbullying prevalence among LGBT youths, the forms it takes, the motivations of those who undertake such aggression, and the confrontation strategies that can be adopted.

Table 2.4 includes all the different categories into which the participants' responses were grouped, along with fragments that exemplify them, as well as grade from which similar ideas were collected and the gender of the participants who

Table 2.4 Students' perceptions of cyberbullying in sexual and gender minorities

Categories	Subcategories	Examples	Grade	Gender
Forms of cyberbullying	Private messages sent to the victim (over the phone or on social networks)	"Just like they laugh at them at school and call them queers, weirdos, etc., they do the same on the Internet. They send them messages to insult them or blackmail them by threatening with what they'd tell their families if they don't do what they want. I've also seen comments on photos on Instagram."—a 14-year-old girl	Primary Secondary	Boys Girls
	Public messages in third-party accounts, posts in forums where others can include comments, taped conversations that are then uploaded on the Internet, fixed photos, etc	"I've seen in Twitter that they said someone was gay, and they've even included the email of this person so people can write."—a 12-year-old boy "People who also act as though they were gay speak with a boy who is gay, they record their conversations or copy messages to then send them to others and mess things up." —a 13-year-old boy	Primary Secondary	Boys Girls
Factors linked to cyberbullying	Directionality: offline harassment that becomes an online kind	"Sometimes someone starts insulting you on Facebook or on any other forum because someone you know has told them something because they don't know you directly. So it almost always starts with something at school, then they start sending you messages or post things on social networks. At least that's my case." —a 15-year-old boy	Primary Secondary	Boys Girls
	Mediation technology: facilitated through anonymity and greater tolerance on the Internet	"The Internet is great for picking on someone because you don't have to say who you are or you can use profiles. It's great for laughing at someone, especially if you want to laugh at a gay because it's much easier." —a 14-year-old boy	Secondary	Boys Girls
	Real or perceived sexual orientation	"It doesn't matter if someone is gay or not. If people think someone is, they say it so that others believe it. They can also do this to convince their friends that that person is weird so they don't mix with him or her." —a 14-year-old girl	Secondary	Boys Girls

Table 2.4 (continued)

Categories	Subcategories	Examples	Grade	Gender
Cyberbullies' motives	Discrimination: stereotypes and homophobic attitudes	"Those who pick on them think they are different from everyone else. Obviously they are homophobes, they don't like them because they think they are abnormal and they pick on them." —a 12-year-old girl	Primary Secondary	Boys Girls
	Aggressors have problems with their own sexual orientation	"Often when they pick on others they do it to hide something. People who are frightened of coming out of the closet or have doubts keep picking on those who have accepted it." —a 14-year-old girl	Secondary	Girls
	For fun	"People love gossip and the gay theme gives plenty of gossip. People have fun with it on social networks." —a 13-year-old boy	Primary	Boys
	Harming social reputation	"People use this subject to be nasty with people. It's a very delicate subject. It doesn't matter if you're gay or not because if they say it about you, they make your life at school very difficult because everyone else will always smell a rat. Sometimes they won't want to get on with you." —a 14-year-old girl "If think it's just as harmful whether you're gay or not. Perhaps it affects you more if you're not because you think: God, why do they have to say these things about me if they aren't true. But it's harmful anyway. It's just as harmful because the person who's insulting you doesn't really know if you're gay or not and he or she will carry on saying these things." —a 15-year-old girl	Secondary	Girls

shared these views. In general, many similarities were found in the discourse with participants, regardless of the grade they were in and their gender. In general, girls contributed more ideas and it was more a matter of concern for those who were in the first year of secondary education.

First, it is important to point out that the participants did not clearly differentiate between sexual minorities and gender minorities. They normally spoke about the people who aggressors believed were gays or lesbians. The term "transgender" or "transsexual" was not employed, but in most cases, there was talk about attacks or aggressions made on the Internet against those who were seen differently because of their real or perceived sexual orientation. Nonetheless, they expressed the idea that it did not matter if the victim was really homosexual as cyberbullying addresses anyone whose conduct is gender atypical (e.g., boys who only have girl friends, people whose body language suggests affectations, or those who do not participate in sports like soccer).

2.4.1.1   The Factors Linked to This Type of Cyberbullying

According to the discourse that took place, the participants seemed to coincide in that it was quite a normal issue, although more boys were victims of such aggression because, in their opinion, the behaviors classified as atypical are more noticeable among boys. They did not believe that aggressions began online, but that insults and aggressions had occurred in places like school. If this were the case, cyberbullying would, thus, be the continuation of school bullying. So, it is most interesting to observe that such discourses show no clear distinction between cyberbullying and school bullying as both forms of bullying are treated like a continuum. Nevertheless, the participants believed that the Internet facilitates such aggression because greater tolerance to such display is found on it, and also because it is much more difficult to identify harassers and to take measures against them.

2.4.1.2   Forms That This Type of Cyberbullying Takes

The participants explained that the Internet offers many ways to harm minorities, for example, through private messages to victims or public messages in third-party accounts or forums from where they are submitted to these aggressions. In such cases, cyberbullying includes insults about sexual orientation, like "faggot" or "dyke"; strongly sexually related nicknames like "pillow biter" and "neck blower"; threats to make them come out of the closet at home if they refuse to do what the aggressor wants; fixed photos showing them fondling or kissing other people; and videos showing how they are insulted and even physically harassed. In other words, harassment can even take a more direct nuance on the Internet when the aggressor(s) direct(s) aggressive interactions exclusively to the victim, or indirectly when messages are made public and other Internet users can participate in some way.

2.4.1.3 Cyberbullies' Motives

The participants believe that sexual orientation is a subject that provides plenty of gossip and that it might be used on social networks simply as a bit of fun, something that gives people a lot to talk about on Facebook, Twitter, etc., even though the people who participate do not consider what the person who is the center of all the comments may feel. Other students think that the Internet can be a very fruitful place to attack the reputation of other students, and sexual orientation is a very sensitive subject for many youths' identity. Envy and jealousy of another person's success in areas like studies or sports can be a reason for cyberbullies to damage the image of those with a better social reputation and one way to damage it is questioning their sexual orientation. Nevertheless, according to the participants, the main reason for these aggressions is the stereotypes and prejudices of harassed people being different. This result coincides with former research, which has indicated that "bothering someone who is different" is among the most widely argued reasons for getting involved in cyberbullying (Willton and Campbell 2011). Some youths' lack of tolerance of sexual diversity and gender is the reason for most aggressions and, in this case, cyberbullying is a way to punish or penalize not adapting to traditional sexual and gender roles. In some cases, girls who participate in groups of secondary education students point out that this kind of cyberbullying could also be the result of those with sexual orientation problems feeling frustration, so they attack those who live or behave in the way they would also like to live or behave.

In general, cyberbullying these minorities is considered something that habitually occurs, is the continuation of harassment that previously occurred face-to-face, and can result from some form of prejudice and discrimination of those who do not conform to traditional gender norms, do not feel that their gender corresponds to their biological sex, or show sexual interest in people of their own sex. This type of bullying has, according to previous research, more serious consequences for those who suffer it than other forms of bullying not based on discrimination (Russell et al. 2012).

2.5 Conclusion

Both the literature review and the new data presented in this chapter allow us to state that the inclusion of gender variables in research on cyberbullying offers a more complete picture of the many factors that intervene in such aggressive dynamics. The findings reported in this chapter highlight the importance of moving beyond the analysis of gender differences to analyze how gender variables (e.g., gender identity) are associated with the youths involved in cyberbullying. The above findings suggest that being a typical member of the same-sex peer group is important for psychosocial adjustment in both boys and girls, at least in terms of suffering less victimization. In parallel, our findings indicate that, especially for boys, felt pressure for gender conformity may make them confront social expectations through ways that damage their self-concepts (e.g., adopting an aggressive role). Regarding self-attribution of gender-typed personality traits, the results reveal that internalization of gender cues is associated with risk behaviors, such as cyberbullying perpetration. This implies that it is important for parents, educators, and other professionals to show them ways to establish a sense of compatibility with one's gender category, and to provide children with other forms to confront peer pressure, while offering spaces that are free of social expectations to explore cross-sex behaviors.

References

Akbaba, S., Peker, A., Eroğlu, Y., & Yaman, E. (2015). Cross-gender equivalence of cyber bullying and victimization. *Participatory Educational Research, 2*(2), 59–69. doi:http://dx.doi.org/10.17275/per.15.15.2.2

Archer, J. (2004). Sex differences in aggression in real-world settings: A meta-analytic review. *Review of General Psychology, 8*, 291–322. doi:10.1037/1089-2680.8.4.291.

Artz, S., Nicholson, D., & Magnuson, D. (2008). Examining sex differences in the use of direct and indirect aggression. *Gender Issues, 25*(4), 267–288. doi:10.1007/s12147-008-9065-5.

Artz, S., Kassis, W., & Moldenhauer, S. (2013). Rethinking indirect aggression: The end of the mean girl myth. *Victims & Offenders, 8*(3), 308–328. doi:10.1080/15564886.2012.756842.

Barlett, C., & Coyne, S. M. (2014). A meta-analysis of sex differences in cyber-bullying behavior: The moderating role of age. *Aggressive Behavior, 40*(5), 474–488. doi:10.1002/ab.21555.

Baroncelli, A., & Ciucci, E. (2014). Unique effects of different components of trait emotional intelligence in traditional bullying and cyberbullying. *Journal of Adolescence, 37*(6), 807–815. doi:10.1016/j.adolescence.2014.05.009.

Beckman, L., Hagquist, C., & Hellström, L. (2013). Discrepant gender patterns for cyberbullying and traditional bullying–An analysis of Swedish adolescent data. *Computers in Human Behavior, 29*(5), 1896–1903. doi:10.1016/j.chb.2013.03.010.

Bem, S. L. (1981). Gender schema theory: A cognitive account of sex typing. *Psychological Review, 88*(4), 354–364. doi:10.1037/0033-295X.88.4.354.

Beran, T., & Li, Q. (2008). The relationship between cyberbullying and school bullying. *The Journal of Student Wellbeing, 1*(2), 16–33.

Berlan, E. D., Corliss, H. L., Field, A. E., Goodman, E., & Bryn Austin, S. (2010). Sexual orientation and bullying among adolescents in the growing up today study. *Journal of Adolescent Health, 46*(4), 366–371. doi:10.1016/j.jadohealth.2009.10.015.

Björkqvist, K., Osterman, K., & Lagerspetz, K. M. (1994). Sex differences in covert aggression among adults. *Aggressive Behavior, 20*(1), 27–33. doi:10.1002/1098-2337(1994)20:1%3C27::AID-AB2480200105%3E3.0.CO;2-Q.

Bonanno, R. A., & Hymel, S. (2013). Cyber bullying and internalizing difficulties: Above and beyond the impact of traditional forms of bullying. *Journal of Youth and Adolescence, 42*(5), 685–697. doi:10.1007/s10964-013-9937-1.

Cappadocia, M. C., Craig, W. M., & Pepler, D. (2013). Cyberbullying prevalence, stability, and risk factors during adolescence. *Canadian Journal of School Psychology, 28*(2), 171–192. doi:10.1177/0829573513491212.

Card, N. A., Stucky, B. D., Sawalani, G. M., & Little, T. D. (2008). Direct and indirect aggression during childhood and adolescence: A meta-analytic review of gender differences, intercorrelations, and relations to maladjustment. *Child Development, 79*(5), 1185–1229. doi:10.1111/j.1467-8624.2008.01184.x.

Carrera-Fernández, M. V., Lameiras-Fernández, M., Rodríguez-Castro, Y., & Vallejo-Medina, P. (2013). Bullying among spanish secondary education students the role of gender traits, sexism, and homophobia. *Journal of Interpersonal Violence, 28*(14), 2915–2940. doi:10.1177/0886260513488695.

Carver, P. R., Yunger, J. L., & Perry, D. G. (2003). Gender identity and adjustment in middle childhood. *Sex Roles, 49*(3–4), 95–109. doi:10.1023/A:1024423012063.

Cassidy, W., Brown, K., & Jackson, M. (2012). 'Under the radar': Educators and cyberbullying in schools. *School Psychology International, 33*(5), 520–532. doi:10.1177/0143034312445245.

Collier, K. L., van Beusekom, G., Bos, H. M., & Sandfort, T. G. (2013). Sexual orientation and gender identity/expression related peer victimization in adolescence: a systematic review of associated psychosocial and health outcomes. *Journal of Sex Research, 50*(3–4), 299–317. doi :10.1080/00224499.2012.750639.

Connell, N. M., Schell-Busey, N. M., Pearce, A. N., & Negro, P. (2014). Badgrlz? Exploring sex differences in cyberbullying behaviors. *Youth Violence and Juvenile Justice, 12*(3), 209–228. doi:10.1177/1541204013503889

Crick, N. R., Casas, J. F., & Nelson, D. A. (2002). Toward a more comprehensive understanding of peer maltreatment: Studies of relational victimization. *Current Directions in Psychological Science, 11*(3), 98–101. doi:10.1111/1467-8721.00177.

Crothers, L. M., Field, J. E., & Kolbert, J. B. (2005). Navigating power, control, and being nice: Aggression in adolescent girls' friendships. *Journal of Counseling & Development, 83*(3), 349–354. doi:10.1002/j.1556-6678.2005.tb00354.x.

Diamond, M. (2002). Sex and gender are different: Sexual identity and gender identity are different. *Clinical Child Psychology and Psychiatry, 7*(3), 320–334. doi:10.1177/1359104502007003031.

Drury, K., Bukowski, W. M., Velásquez, A. M., & Stella-Lopez, L. (2013). Victimization and gender identity in single-sex and mixed-sex schools: Examining contextual variations in pressure to conform to gender norms. *Sex Roles, 69*(7–8), 442–454. doi:10.1007/s11199-012-0118-6.

Eagly, A. H., Wood, W., & Johannesen-Schmidt, M. C. (2004). Social role theory of sex differences and similarities. A. H. Eagly, A. E. Beall, & R. J. Sternberg (Eds), *The psychology of gender* (pp. 269–295) New York: Guilford Press.

Egan, S. K., & Perry, D. G. (2001). Gender identity: A multidimensional analysis with implications for psychosocial adjustment. *Developmental Psychology, 37*(4), 451–463. doi:10.1037//0012-1649.37.4.451.

Fanti, K. A., Demetrious, A. G., & Hawa, V. V. (2012). A longitudinal study of cyberbullying: Examining risk and protective factors. *European Journal of Developmental Psychology, 9*, 168–181. doi:10.1080/17405629.2011.643169.

Festl, R., & Quandt, T. (2013). Social relations and cyberbullying: The influence of individual and structural attributes on victimization and perpetration via the internet. *Human Communication Research, 39*(1), 101–126. doi:10.1111/j.1468-2958.2012.01442.x.

Gámez-Guadix, M., Villa-George, F., & Calvete, E. (2014). Psychometric properties of the Cyberbullying Questionnaire (CBQ) among Mexican adolescents. *Violence and Victims, 29*(2), 232–247. doi:10.1891/0886-6708.VV-D-12-00163R1.

Gini, G., & Pozzoli, T. (2006). The role of masculinity in children's bullying. *Sex Roles, 54*(7–8), 585–588. doi:10.1007/s11199-006-9015-1.

Greytak, E. A., Kosciw, J. G., & Diaz, E. M. (2009). *Harsh realities: The experiences of transgender youth in our nation's schools.* New York: Gay, Lesbian and Straight Education Network.

Griezel, L., Finger, L. R., Bodkin-Andrews, G. H., Craven, R. G., & Yeung, A. S. (2012). Uncovering the structure of gender and developmental differences in cyber bullying. *The Journal of Educational Research, 105*(6), 442–455. doi:10.1080/00220671.2011.629692.

Guerra, N. G., Williams, K. R., & Sadek, S. (2011). Understanding bullying and victimization during childhood and adolescence: A mixed methods study. *Child Development, 82*(1), 295–310. doi:10.1111/j.1467-8624.2010.01556.x.

Hall, J. A., & Halberstadt, A. G. (1980). Masculinity and femininity in children: Development of the children's personal attributes questionnaire. *Developmental Psychology, 16*(4), 270–280. doi:10.1037/0012-1649.16.4.270.

Heiman, T., & Olenik-Shemesh, D. (2015). Cyberbullying experience and gender differences among adolescents in different educational settings. *Journal of Learning Disabilities, 48*(2), 146–155. doi:10.1177/0022219413492855.

Heiman, T., Olenik-Shemesh, D., & Eden, S. (2015). Cyberbullying involvement among students with ADHD: Relation to loneliness, self-efficacy and social support. *European Journal of Special Needs Education, 30*(1), 15–29. doi:10.1080/08856257.2014.943562.

Hinduja, S., & Patchin, J. W. (2008). Cyberbullying: An exploratory analysis of factors related to offending and victimization. *Deviant Behavior, 29*(2), 129–156. doi:10.1080/01639620701457816.

Kapatzia, A., & Syngollitou, E. (2007). Cyberbullying in middle and high schools: Prevalence, gender and age differences. Unpublished manuscript based on MSc Thesis of A. Kaptazia, University of Thessaloniki.

Kistner, J., Counts-Allan, C., Dunkel, S., Drew, C. H., David-Ferdon, C., & Lopez, C. (2010). Sex differences in relational and overt aggression in the late elementary school years. *Aggressive Behavior, 36*, 282–291. doi:10.1002/ab.20350.

Kohlberg, L. (1966). A cognitive-developmental analysis of children's sex-role concepts and attitudes. In E. E. Maccoby (Ed.), *The developmental of sex differences* (pp. 82–173). Stanford: Stanford University Press.

Kokkinos, C. M., Antoniadou, N., Dalara, E., Koufogazou, A., & Papatziki, A. (2013). Cyber-bullying, personality and coping among pre-adolescents. *International Journal of Cyber Behavior, Psychology and Learning (IJCBPL), 3*(4), 55–69. doi:10.4018/ijcbpl.2013100104.

Kowalski, R. M., & Limber, S. P. (2013). Psychological, physical, and academic correlates of cyberbullying and traditional bullying. *Journal of Adolescent Health, 53*(1), 13–S20. doi:10.1016/j.jadohealth.2012.09.018.

Kowalski, R. M., Morgan, C. A., & Limber, S. P. (2012). Traditional bullying as a potential warning sign of cyberbullying. *School Psychology International, 33*(5), 505–519. doi:10.1177/0143034312445244.

Kowalski, R. M., Giumetti, G. W., Schroeder, A. N., & Lattanner, M. R. (2014). Bullying in the digital age: A critical review and meta-analysis of cyberbullying research among youth. *Psychological Bulletin, 140*(4), 1073–1137. doi:10.1037/a0035618.

Låftman, S. B., Modin, B., & Östberg, V. (2013). Cyberbullying and subjective health: A large-scale study of students in Stockholm, Sweden. *Children and Youth Services Review, 35*(1), 112–119. doi:10.1016/j.childyouth.2012.10.020.

Lapidot-Lefler, N., & Dolev-Cohen, M. (2015). Comparing cyberbullying and school bullying among school students: Prevalence, gender, and grade level differences. *Social Psychology of Education, 18*(1), 1–16. doi:10.1007/s11218-014-9280-8.

Law, D. M., Shapka, J. D., Hymel, S., Olson, B. F., & Waterhouse, T. (2012). The changing face of bullying: An empirical comparison between traditional and internet bullying and victimization. *Computers in Human Behavior, 28*(1), 226–232. doi:10.1016/j.chb.2011.09.004.

Lazuras, L., Barkoukis, V., Ourda, D., & Tsorbatzoudis, H. (2013). A process model of cyberbullying in adolescence. *Computers in Human Behavior, 29*(3), 881–887. doi:10.1016/j.chb.2012.12.015.

Mark, L., & Ratliffe, K. T. (2011). Cyber worlds: New playgrounds for bullying. *Computers in Schools, 28*, 92–116. doi:10.1080/07380569.2011.575753.

Mitchell, K. J., Ybarra, M. L., & Korchmaros, J. D. (2014). Sexual harassment among adolescents of different sexual orientations and gender identities. *Child Abuse & Neglect, 38*(2), 280–295. doi:10.1016/j.chiabu.2013.09.008.

Monks, C. P., Robinson, S., & Worlidge. P. (2012). The emergence of cyberbullying: A survey of primary school pupil's perceptions and experiences. *School Psychology International, 33*(5), 477–491. doi:10.1177/0143034312445242.

Mura, G., & Diamantini, D. (2014). Cyberbullying among Colombian students: An exploratory investigation. *European Journal of Investigation in Health, Psychology and Education, 3*(3), 249–256.

Navarro, J. N., & Jasinski, J. L. (2013). Why girls? Using routine activities theory to predict cyberbullying experiences between girls and boys. *Women & Criminal Justice, 23*(4), 286–303. doi:10.1080/08974454.2013.784225.

Navarro, R., Larrañaga, E., & Yubero, S. (2011). Bullying-victimization problems and aggressive tendencies in Spanish secondary schools students: The role of gender stereotypical traits. *Social Psychology of Education, 14*(4), 457–473. doi:10.1007/s11218-011-9163-1.

Navarro, R., Yubero, S., Larrañaga, E., & Martínez, V. (2012). Children's cyberbullying victimization: Associations with social anxiety and social competence in a Spanish sample. *Child Indicators Research, 5*(2), 281–295. doi:10.1007/s12187-011-9132-4.

Navarro, R., Serna, C., Martínez, V., & Ruiz-Oliva, R. (2013). The role of internet use and parental mediation on cyberbullying victimization among Spanish children from rural public schools. *European Journal of Psychology Education, 28*, 725–745. doi:10.1007/s10212-012-0137-2.

Navarro, R., Larrañaga, E., & Yubero, S. (2015a). Gender identity, gender-typed personality traits and school bullying: Victims, bullies and bully-victims. *Child Indicators Research.* Advance online publication. doi:10.1007/s12187-015-9300-z.

Navarro, R., Ruiz-Oliva, R., Larrañaga, E., & Yubero, S. (2015b). The impact of cyberbullying and social bullying on optimism, global and school-related happiness and life satisfaction among 10–12-year-old schoolchildren. *Applied Research in Quality of Life, 10*(1), 15–36. doi:10.1007/s11482-013-9292-0.

Owens, L., Shute, R., & Slee, P. (2004). Girls' aggressive behavior. *Prevention Researcher, 11*(3), 9–10.

Park, S., Na, E. Y., & Kim, E. M. (2014). The relationship between online activities, netiquette and cyberbullying. *Children and Youth Services Review, 42*, 74–81. doi:10.1016/j.childyouth.2014.04.002.

Pelfrey, W. V. Jr., & Weber, N. L. (2013). Keyboard gangsters: Analysis of incidence and correlates of cyberbullying in a large urban student population. *Deviant Behavior, 34*(1), 68–84. doi:10.1080/01639625.2012.707541.

Pereira, B., Mendonca, D., Neto, C., Valente, L., & Smith, P. K. (2004). Bullying in Portuguese schools. *School Psychology International, 25*(2), 241–254. doi:10.1177/0143034304043690.

Phillips, D. A. (2007). Punking and bullying strategies in middle school, high school, and beyond. *Journal of Interpersonal Violence, 22*(2), 158–178. doi:10.1177/0886260506295341.

Poteat, V. P., Espelage, D. L., & Koenig, B. W. (2009). Willingness to remain friends and attend school with lesbian and gay peers: Relational expressions of prejudice among heterosexual youth. *Journal of Youth and Adolescence, 38*(7), 952–962. doi:10.1007/s10964-009-9416-x.

Rivers, I. (2013). El bullying homofóbico. In A. Ovejero, P. K. Smith, & S. Yubero (Eds.), *El acoso escolar y su prevención. Perspetivas Internacionales* (pp. 131–143). Madrid: Biblioteca Nueva.

Rivers, I. (2014). Cyberbullying and cyberagression. Sexualised and gendered experiences explore. In I. Rivers & N. Duncan (Eds.), *Bullying. Experiences and discourses of sexuality and gender* (pp. 17–30). London: Routledge.

Rivers, I., & Noret, N. (2010). 'I h8 u': Findings from a five-year study of text and email bullying. *British Educational Research Journal, 36*(4), 643–671. doi:10.1080/01411920903071918.

Roberts, A. L., Rosario, M., Slopen, N., Calzo, J. P., & Austin, S. B. (2013). Childhood gender nonconformity, bullying victimization, and depressive symptoms across adolescence and early adulthood: An 11-year longitudinal study. *Journal of the American Academy of Child & Adolescent Psychiatry, 52*(2), 143–152. doi:10.1016/j.jaac.2012.11.006.

Russell, S. T., Sinclair, K. O., Poteat, V. P., & Koenig, B. W. (2012). Adolescent health and harassment based on discriminatory bias. *American Journal of Public Health, 102*(3), 493–495. doi:10.2105/AJPH.2011.300430.

Russell, S. T., Everett, B. G., Rosario, M., & Birkett, M. (2014). Indicators of victimization and sexual orientation among adolescents: Analyses from youth risk behavior surveys. *American Journal of Public Health, 104*(2), 255–261. doi:10.2105/AJPH.2013.301493.

Schultze-Krumbholz, A., Göbel, K., Scheithauer, H., Brighi, A., Guarini, A., Tsorbatzoudis, H., Barkoukis, V., Pyzalski, J., Plichta, P., Del Rey, R., Casas, J. A., Thompson, F, & Smith, P. K.

(2015). A comparison of classification approaches for cyberbullying and traditional bullying using data from six European countries. *Journal of School Violence, 14*(1), 47–65. doi:10.108 0/15388220.2014.961067.

Shin, N., & Ahn, H. (2015). Factors affecting adolescents' involvement in cyberbullying: What divides the 20% from the 80%? *Cyberpsychology, Behavior, and Social Networking, 18*(7), 393–399. doi:10.1089/cyber.2014.0362.

Smith, P. K., Thompson, F., & Bhatti, S. (2012). Ethnicity, gender, bullying and cyberbullying in English secondary school pupils. *Studia Edukacyjne, 23*, 7–18.

Spence, J. T. (1993). Gender-related traits and gender ideology: Evidence for a multifactorial theory. *Journal of Personality and Social Psychology, 64*(4), 624–635. doi:10.1037//0022-3514.64.4.624.

Sticca, F., Ruggieri, S., Alsaker, F., & Perren, S. (2013). Longitudinal risk factors for cyberbullying in adolescence. *Journal of Community & Applied Social Psychology, 23*(1), 52–67. doi:10.1002/casp.2136.

Tarablus, T., Heiman, T., & Olenik-Shemesh, D. (in press). Cyber bullying among teenagers in Israel: An examination of cyber bullying, traditional bullying, and socioemotional functioning. *Journal of Aggression, Maltreatment & Trauma* (online first) doi:10.1080/10926771.2015.10 49763.

Tokunaga, R. S. (2010). Following you home from school: A critical review and synthesis of research on cyberbullying. *Computers in Human Behavior, 26*, 277–287. doi:10.1016/j. chb.2009.11.014.

Underwood, M. K., Galenand, B. R., & Paquette, J. A. (2001). Top ten challenges for understanding gender and aggression in children: Why can't we all just get along? *Social Development, 10*(2), 248–266. doi:10.1111/1467-9507.00162.

Vanden Abeele, M., & De Cock, R. (2013). Cyberbullying by mobile phone among adolescents: The role of gender and peer group status. *Communications, 38*(1), 107–118. doi:10.1515/commun-2013-0006.

Wachs, S., Junger, M., & Sittichai, R. (2015). Traditional, cyber and combined bullying roles: Differences in risky online and offline activities. *Societies, 5*(1), 109–135. doi:10.3390/soc5010109.

Walrave, M., & Heirman, W. (2011). Cyberbullying: Predicting victimization and perpetration. *Children & Society, 25(1)*, 59–72. doi:10.1111/j.1099-0860.2009.00260.x.

Wilton, C., & Campbell, M. A. (2011). An exploration of the reasons why adolescents engage in traditional and cyber bullying. *Journal of Educational Sciences & Psychology, 1*(2), 101–109.

Wong, D. S., Chan, H. C. O., & Cheng, C. H. (2014). Cyberbullying perpetration and victimization among adolescents in Hong Kong. *Children and Youth Services Review, 36*, 133–140. doi:10.1016/j.childyouth.2013.11.006.

Wong, R. Y., Cheung, C. M., Xiao, S. B., & Chan, T. K. (2015). The instigating, impelling, and inhibiting forces in cyberbullying perpetration across gender. *PACIS 2015 Proceedings*. Paper 109. http://aisel.aisnet.org/pacis2015/109.

Yang, S. J., Stewart, R., Kim, J. M., Kim, S. W., Shin, I. S., Dewey, M. E., & Yoon, J. S. (2013). Differences in predictors of traditional and cyber-bullying: A 2-year longitudinal study in Korean school children. *European Child & Adolescent Psychiatry, 22*(5), 309–318. doi:10.1007/s00787-012-0374-6.

Yang, S. C., Lin, C. Y., & Chen, A. S. (2014). A study of Taiwanese teens' traditional and cyberbullying behaviors. *Journal of Educational Computing Research, 50*(4), 525–552. doi:10.2190/EC.50.4.e.

Young, R., & Sweeting, H. (2004). Adolescent bullying, relationships, psychological well-being, and gender-atypical behavior: A gender diagnosticity approach. *Sex Roles, 50*(7–8), 525–537. doi:10.1023/B:SERS.0000023072.53886.86.

Yu, L., & Xie, D. (2010). Multidimensional gender identity and psychological adjustment in middle childhood: A study in China. *Sex Roles, 62*(1–2), 100–113. doi:10.1007/s11199-009-9709-2.

Zhou, Z., Tang, H., Tian, Y., Wei, H., Zhang, F., & Morrison, C. M. (2013). Cyberbullying and its risk factors among Chinese high school students. *School Psychology International, 34*(6), 630–647. doi:10.1177/0143034313479692.

Chapter 3
Gender Variables and Cyberbullying in College Students

Elisa Larrañaga, Santiago Yubero and Anastasio Ovejero

3.1 Introduction

The increased use of information and communications technologies (ICTs) is a phenomenon that is taking place globally and that has brought a new kind of bullying, even more harmful than face-to-face aggression: cyberbullying. Cyberbullying is behavior generated by electronic and/or digital means by one or more individuals that address aggressive messages or hostile communications repeatedly aiming at harming and bothering other/s (Smith et al. 2008; Tokunaga 2010).

According to the review of Kiriakidis and Kavoura (2010), cyberbullying increases with age. Walrave and Heirman (2011) explain that this fact is due to less supervision by parents regarding how their children use the Internet. Likewise, senior school and college students are the groups that use the Internet and social media more often, namely e-mail, instant messaging, and chats (Palfrey and Gasser 2008). As stated by Baldasare et al. (2012), college students are nowadays digital natives (Prensky 2001) since they have integrated digital technologies in all aspects of their lives. Almost all of them have smartphones; therefore, they have continuous access to the Internet at hand. College students have just completed secondary education, where they may be familiar with cyberbullying, use Internet resources very often, and are becoming increasingly independent from their parents. These circumstances make analyzing cyberbullying in the college environment more important. On the other hand, some authors (Chapell et al. 2006; Kraft and Wang 2010; Paullet and

E. Larrañaga (✉)
Department of Psychology, Faculty of Social Work, University of Castilla-La Mancha,
Camino del Pozuelo s/n., 16071 Cuenca, Spain
e-mail: elisa.larranaga@uclm.es

S. Yubero
Department of Psychology, Faculty of Education and Humanities,
University of Castilla-La Mancha, 16071 Cuenca, Spain

A. Ovejero
Department of Psychology, University of Valladolid, Valladolid, Spain

© Springer International Publishing Switzerland 2016
R. Navarro et al. (eds.), *Cyberbullying Across the Globe,*
DOI 10.1007/978-3-319-25552-1_3

Pinchot 2014; Zacchilli and Valerio 2011; Zalaquett and Chatters 2014) have found that there is continuity between bullying and cyberbullying at high school and college. Nevertheless, as stated by Zalaquett and Chatters (2014), there are few studies on cyberbullying among college students; therefore, little is known of the features of this phenomenon in the college context (Smith and Yoon 2013).

3.2 Prevalence of Cyberbullying Among College Students

In this section, we will be reviewing the main quantitative studies that inform on the prevalence of cyberbullying at college. Studies generally find the need to further analyze this phenomenon since it can be noted that cyberbullying is also an important issue in the college context.

Although the first study on cyberbullying was made by Finn in 2004, research on this issue was not very common in the USA until the tragic events that occurred in 2010, when two students killed themselves as a result of the aggression suffered by them via the Internet. This first study showed that between 10 and 15 % of the 339 New Hampshire college students that participated in this study had suffered harassment by e-mail and instant messaging (Finn 2004). Nevertheless, the outcome of the research does not show any uniform data allowing for comparisons among different studies to date. This fact is mainly due to three factors:

1. Different criteria have been used when considering participation in acts of cyber-bullying (for example, Akbulut and Eristi 2011; Faucher et al. 2014; Hoff and Mitchell 2009) and/or when considering and identifying the feeling of participation in acts of cyberbullying (for example, Mateus et al. 2015; Molluzzo and Lawler 2012; Schenk et al. 2013).
2. Different scales of measurement have been used because some of them include more cyberbullying behaviors than others. In fact, Vandebosch and Van Cleemput (2009) proved that on asking about different behaviors, there are more affirmative answers than on including a direct question on participation in acts of cyber-bullying. Cyberbullying victims also do not sometimes notice attacks (Sevcikova et al. 2012), therefore Nocentini et al. (2010) consider that victims perception of the acts suffered can also be relevant to measure and define cyberbullying.
3. The time period assessed throughout research, which ranges through lifetime (for example, Akbulut and Eristi 2011; Dilmac 2009; Mateus et al. 2015), over the last year (for example, Aricak 2009; Faucher et al. 2014; Tomsa et al. 2013), over the last 6 months (for example, Zacchilli and Valerio 2011), or at present (for example, Paullet and Pinchot 2014).

In Table 3.1, we intended to represent a short review of the studies on cyberbullying performed in the college context, in increasing chronological order. Most of them focused on the incidence of victimization, with less data on perpetration and the aggressor/victim role (mixed).

As we can see, Hoff and Mitchell (2009) collected data from 351 college students and informed that 56 % of them participated in cyberbullying dynamics. In

Table 3.1 Main studies on the incidence cyberbullying

Author/s	Year	Country	N	Incidence (%)		
				Perpetrators	Victims	Mixed
Hoff and Mitchell	2009	USA	351		56	
Dilmac	2009	Turkey	666		53	
Aricak	2009	Turkey	695		36.7	17.7
Englander et al.	2009	USA	283	3	8	
Kraft and Wang	2010	USA	471		10	
MacDonald and Roberts-Pittman	2010	USA	439	9	21.5	
Walker et al.	2011	USA	120		11	
Molluzzo and Lawler	2012	USA	110	3.6	9	
Turan et al.	2011	Turkey	579		60	
Akbulut and Eristi	2011	Turkey	254		81	
Schenk and Fremouw	2012	USA	799		8.6	
Schenk et al.	2013	USA	799	7.5		2.4
Smith and Yoon	2013	USA	276		10	
Tomsa et al.	2013	Bulgaria	92	2.2	8.7	
Washington	2014	USA	140		12	
Zalaquett and Chatters	2014	USA	613		19	
Paullet and Pinchot	2014	USA	168		9	
Faucher et al.	2014	Canada	1733		55	
Selkie et al.	2015	USA	265	3	17	7.2
Mateus et al.	2015	Portugal	519	8	27.4	

2009, Dilmac asked 666 college students from the Faculty of Education of Selçuk University (Turkey) if they had experienced cyberbullying in their lives; the prevalence was very high because 55.3% had suffered acts of cyberbullying and 22.5% suffered these acts over their senior year at college. Also in Turkey, Aricak (2009) performed a study with 695 college students from Selçuk University; in this case, 17.7% participated as perpetrators and victims, while 36.7% were victims. That same year, Englander et al. (2009) did some research on the frequency of bullying and cyberbullying in 283 college students from Massachusetts, 8% of them saw themselves as victims of aggression and 3% informed that they were conducting online aggression.

As mentioned above, a greater number of studies on cyberbullying have been performed since 2010, especially in certain colleges in the USA. Kraft and Wang (2010), with a sample of 471 college students from New Jersey (USA), found a 10% prevalence of victims of cyberbullying. MacDonald and Roberts-Pittman (2010), with a sample of 439 students from western USA, found that 38% knew someone who had been a victim of cyberbullying, 21.9% reported being victimized (21.9% of men, 22% of women), and almost 9% of the students who participated in this study reported to be bullies. Most of the students were victimized through social media (25%), as well as through text messages (21.2%), e-mail (16.1%), instant messaging (13.2%), in chats (9.9%), and through websites (6.8%). Based on the information provided by 131 college students, Walker et al. (2011) reported that 11% of students were victims of cyberbullying at college, and more than 30% declared to have suffered incidents online. Half of them stated that they were bullied by classmates, 57% by people outside college, 43% did not know the bully's identity, and, besides, 54% knew someone that had been a victim of cyberbullying. Molluzzo and Lawler (2012), with a sample of 121 students from the Pace University (New York), found that 9% of students reported to be cyberbullies, 7% reported to be cybervictims, and 29% reported arguments online with teachers. Zacchilli and Valerio (2011) found that 9% of students felt being a victim of cyberbullying, while 3.6% reported to be cyberbullies. Turan et al. (2011), who performed a study with 579 students from Istanbul Bilgi University (Turkey), found that almost 60% had been victimized by electronic means, while 20.7% had acted as aggressors over the Internet, 27.7% via cell phone, and 51% using both means. Schenk and Fremouw (2012), with 799 students from the University of Virginia (USA) interviewed over the Internet, made a joint consideration of information on cyberbullying behaviors and the perception of participation and found that 8.6% of students had been victims. In a subsequent study, Schenk et al. (2013) reported that 7.5% of students see themselves as cyberbullies and 2.4% see themselves as both bullies and victims. Smith and Yoon (2013) found that 10% of students reported to feel they were victims of cyberbullying at college, while 25% reported cyberbullying behaviors. In Bulgaria, Tomsa et al. (2013), with 92 students from the University of Bucharest, found that 8.7% of students had suffered cyberbullying, while 2.2% saw themselves as cyberbullies over the past year.

One of the most recent research performed with students from different colleges was conducted by Gilroy (2013) in Indiana University (USA). This study reported that 22% of students had suffered cyberbullying. Zalaquett and Chatters (2014), with a sample of 613 students from the University of Pennsylvania (USA), reported that 19% of students felt they were victims of cyberbullying, while 28% declared to know a classmate who was suffering cyberbullying behaviors at that time. Regarding their perpetrator, 44% were harassed by a classmate, 42% by a friend, 22.6% by his/her boyfriend/girlfriend, and 22.6% did not know his/her identity. Paullet and Pinchot (2014) reported that 21% of the 168 students of Robert Morris University who participated in their study declared they had been victims of cyberbullying, 9% were victims at that time, while 37% reported to be victimized by a friend and 31% were victimized by his/her boyfriend/girlfriend. In Canada, Faucher et al. (2014) performed their study with 1733 students. The results showed that 24.1% of college students had suffered some cyberbullying behavior over the past 12 months, mainly through social media (55%), e-mail (47%), and text messages (43%) and, to a lesser extent, through forums, blogs, and chats (25%). A total of 5.1% reported having had cyberbullying behaviors against classmates and 2% reported having had cyberbullying behaviors against teachers and tutors.

By using a sample of women only, Selkie et al. (2015) analyzed cyberbullying among 265 college students from Washington. The results showed that 27.2% reported that they were involved in cyberbullying, that 3% were perpetrators, 17% were victims, and 7.2% turned to play a mixed role of victimization and aggression. Mateus et al. (2015) informed about the prevalence of cyberbullying in the

University of Lisbon. Of the 519 students who completed the study, 8% were cyberbullies, while 27.94% were victims of some kind of cyberbullying behavior. The behaviors reported more frequently were insults (73.7%), spreading rumors (59.3%), and mockery (55.8%). More than 50% of aggressors were classmates, while 33.3% did not know the identity of their aggressor.

As far as the gender of college students involved in cyberbullying behaviors is concerned, we cannot assure the results obtained are very consistent. While in some cases, there are significant differences that show a greater victimization of women (for example, Faucher et al. 2014; Paullet and Pinchot 2014; Zalaquett and Chatters 2014), in other cases, there are no differences between men and women (for example, MacDonald and Roberts-Pittman 2010; Schenk and Fremouw 2012). Paullet and Pinchot (2014) assure that women are more linked to victimization, 57% in comparison to 43% of men. Faucher et al. (2014) obtain similar values: 57% in comparison to 41%; while Zalaquett and Chatters (2014) found an incidence in women that is five times that found in men because 15.5% of women reported to be victims of cyberbullying in comparison to 3.6% of men. Nevertheless, in their study, Schenk and Fremouw (2012) report a similar percentage of victims of cyberbullying, between men (8.4%) and women (8.7%). Other studies, such as that of Schenk et al. (2013) regarding the bully role, found a greater participation of women (56.7%) in comparison to men (43.3%).

As can be seen, studies do not show clear differences by gender in cases of cyberbullying behaviors, nor in the case of bullies or victims. Additionally, only few studies analyze gender differences according to the different behavior that cyberbullying may adopt. Among these studies, Aricak (2009), with a sample of 695 undergraduate students in Turkey, found that males were more likely than females to pretend to be someone else on the Internet. Faucher et al. (2014), with 1925 college students in Canada, showed that females were much more likely than males to report having experienced cyberbullying over social networkings and vita text messages, whereas males were more likely than females to report cyberbullying on non-course-related blogs, forums, or chat rooms. Turan et al. (2011), in a sample of 579 students in the range of 18–30 years old from Turkey, showed that females were more disturbed on the Internet about their sexuality. Again, the literature on gender differences in specific types of cyberbullying indicates that more research needs to be conducted before conclusions can be drawn.

3.3 Same-Sex and Cross-Sex Cyberbullying Among College Students

Although research has demonstrated that cross-sex cyberbullying is less prevalent among college students than same-sex cyberbullying, cross-sex cyberbullying it is usual. Cyberbullies among higher education students are more often people that victims know, even someone victims thought was supposed to be a friend (Faucher et al. 2014). Indeed, previous studies have shown that an important percentage of youth victims report that they have been cyberbullied by their romantic partners (Spitzberg 2002). Romantic partners are also identified as the targets of many of the cyberbullying behaviors (Alexy et al. 2005). Therefore, research analyzing cyberbullying in college students has begun to study to what extent cyberbullying is part of romantic relationships. For example, Crosslin and Crosslin (2014) in an open-ended questions inquiry found that some participants reported that cyberbullying sometimes occurs after a romantic relationship ended. Several of these breakups were described with a violent nature (e.g., "angry ex-boyfriend made late night calls and sent MySpace messages that were hateful and vulgar"). Others described that friends of the ex-boyfriend/girlfriend carried out threats to the participants in the study (e.g., "a female friend of my ex was upset with me for ending the relationship, which hurt her friend, threatened to kill me"). Additionally, Crosslin and Golman (2014) showed that according to 30% of participants, cyberbullying may be used to create disagreement or harm romantic relationships by friends, acquaintances, and ex-significant others. For example, an ex-boyfriend of a student attempted to become Facebook friends with all of their friends to share the truth about their relationship.

In Spain, Durán and Martínez-Pecino (2015) analyzed cybervictimization and cyberperpetration in dating relationships among 336 college students in the range of 18–30 years old. They found that 57.2% of the participants were victimized through the cell phone, whereas 27.4% were victimized through the Internet by their romantic partners. A total of 47.6% of the participants reported to harass their romantic partners through the cell phone and 14% through the Internet. Regarding gender differences, males reported higher levels of victimization than females did, through both the cell phone and Internet. Males also informed of higher levels of harassment directed to their romantic partners during the last year through the cell phone and Internet. These results show that males report higher levels of cyberbullying in dating relationships both as victims and as perpetrators (Burke et al. 2011; Durán and Martínez-Pecino 2015). However, it is not clear if females are less exposed to this type of cyberbullying or they are unreporting these behaviors. Future research should analyze in detail gender differences in cyberbullying in dating relationships considering that cyberbullying may be becoming a new way for abuse in couples.

3.4 Consequences of Cyberbullying in College Students

Zalaquett and Chatters (2014) state that cyberbullying can be of a more emotional nature for college students than for high school students. The psychological effects, therefore, are greater in the first case. Several research (for example, Dilmac 2009; Hartwell-Walter 2010; Lindsay and Krysik 2012; Zacchilli and Valerio 2011) show that cyberbullying in the college stage can result in mental health problems and even in suicide.

The college students who participated in the study of Smith and Yoon (2013) reported the following effects of cybervictimization: 21% had diminished self-esteem; 18.5% had negative impact on their academic performance, even abandon-

Table 3.2 Effects of cyberbullying by gender (%)

	Male	Female	Total
Emotional security or physical safety threatened	21	44	39
Affected ability to do assignments (productivity, loss of confidence, concentration problems, etc.)	28	45	41
Grades suffered as a result	17	26	24
Felt like dropping out of the university	8	17	14
Missed classes as a result	9	20	17
Affected friendships at the university	17	30	27
Affected personal relationships outside of the university	25	47	41
Mental health issues (anxiety, depression, emotional outbursts, etc.)	25	47	42
Physical health issues (headaches, stomach problems, nausea, heart palpitations or chest pain, sweating, etc.)	10	30	26
Felt suicidal or thought about harming self	7	17	14

ment of studies; 15.5% had diminished social contacts; and 13.2% had depression. Schenk and Fremouw (2012) also report that those college students who suffer cyberbullying also suffer depression and anxiety; they also state that 10.1% of victims had suicidal ideations, while no differences were found in terms of gender. In their study, they included a question to assess how students perceive the impact of being victim of cyberbullying. The students admitted they would feel frustrated (46.2%), stressed (40.9%), aggressive (33.8%), and have trouble concentrating (23.4%). In 2013, Schenk et al. analyzed the consequences of college cyberbullies and cyberbullies/victims. The results showed that cyberbullies and cyberbullies/victims scored significantly higher than control participants did on the clinical scales of interpersonal sensitivity, depression, hostility, phobic anxiety, and psychoticism. In suicidal behaviors, the results were indicative of these individuals experiencing more tendencies than control participants did. Cyberbully/victims group was involved in more violent and drug-related crimes than participants who only cyberbullied others. The group also scored higher on proactive and total aggression than pure cyberbullies.

Faucher et al. (2014) include impacts on social relationships both at college and outside it among the consequences identified above. The effects of cyberbullying on college students, 75% of the sample being women, are shown in Table 3.2.

3.5   Predictive Factors of Cyberbullying in College Students

Research shows that there is a certain consistency between "online and offline" lives in terms of behavior (Subrahmanyam et al. 2006). Those studies that have jointly analyzed bullying and cyberbullying found a correlation in the participation between both types of aggression (Baroncelli and Ciucci 2014; Jang et al.

2014). MacDonald and Roberts-Pittman (2010) also found a correlation between cyberbullying and bullying behaviors of college students, ranging between 0.22 and 0.65. Tomsa et al. (2013) reported that 31.5% of cybervictims suffered bullying to; as far as aggression is concerned, 10.9% of cyberbullies also got involved in traditional bullying behaviors.

On the other hand, other studies performed with teenagers and youngsters have found that being a victim of cyberbullying was the best predictive factor of aggression online and vice versa (Bauman 2010; Dilmac 2009; Zacchilli and Valerio 2011).

It would, therefore, be interesting to know the features of those college students suffering victimization in order to obtain a better understanding of cyberbullying in adulthood and to establish prevention and action programs at college. Faucher et al. (2014) believe that the college context may give continuity to cyberbullying behaviors from preadolescence to youth. Several studies show that involvement in bullying processes at high school has continuity at college. Some authors such as Zalaquett and Chatters (2014) report that 50% of cyberbullying victims at college had already suffered cyberbullying at high school. Paullet and Pinchot (2014) also reported the existence of a significant statistical relation between being a victim of cyberbullying at high school and having some kind of incident at high school. Zacchilli and Valerio (2011) also reported the relation between cyberbullying at college and involvement in bullying processes in the early years of primary education.

Nevertheless, some youngsters at college lose the momentum of bullying they were involved in at high school because their context has changed. This is a very interesting fact when intending to isolate the predictive factors of cyberbullying at college. The objective thereof is understanding why some students are still victimized once their context has changed and they are interacting with different people. We need to know what makes victims vulnerable to establish proper prevention and providing them with strategies to face cyberbullying (Schenk and Fremouw 2012). In this sense, several studies have analyzed the predictive value of certain personal variables. Aricak (2009) analyzed the psychiatric symptomatology to predict cyberbullying in college students through the *Symptom Check List-90-Revised Form*. The results showed that students who do not participate in cyberbullying dynamics had significantly less symptoms; hostility and psychoticism were predictive factors of cyberbullying. Dilmac (2009) analyzed psychological needs as predictive factors of cyberbullying through the *Adjective Check List*. The results showed that aggressors have greater dominance. Those students who did not participate in cyberbullying processes had a greater network of social support. Problems in relationships are one of the key cybervictimization factors (Hoff and Mitchell 2009). Pellegrini and Bartini (2002) had already pointed out that social support inhibits victimization. Several researches also confirmed that having friends protects against victimization (Dilmac 2009). Nevertheless, as stated by Salmivalli (2010), there is little research on the importance of social support in cyberbullying processes. Social support has shown itself as the best protective factor against bullying in college students, especially support from their friends (Eisenberg et al. 2007; Holt et al. 2014; Meriläinen et al. 2015; Myers and Cowie 2013; Rivituso 2014). Tokunaga (2010) assures that college students believe that turning to their parents is childish, and they thus seek support from their friends. As far as the advantages of having their friends' support as a protective factor against cyberbullying is concerned, Rivituso (2014) reported that, in the opinion of college students, being a victim of cyberbullying notably results in a decrease in self-esteem in an indirect way. Jacobs et al. (2014) reported that high self-esteem is a relevant protective factor against cyberbullying.

3.6   Cyberbullying Among College Students from a Qualitative Perspective

Given that research on cyberbullying among college students is very recent, the use of qualitative methods has been essential to explore this emerging phenomenon within the college community and to understand the existing differences when it manifests during this period, in comparison to other development moments that have been analyzed more often, such as preadolescence and adolescence. There are few qualitative studies to date. Nevertheless, available research allows knowing how college students perceive and define this phenomenon, to what extent they consider it is a problem present in their academic and social environment, their view on the features and reasons of people involved in those dynamics, and the differences with cyberbullying in primary and secondary schools. In this section, we are presenting a short review on the main results of each field of study analyzed in studies of a qualitative nature.

3.6.1   The Use of the Term "Cyberbullying"

College students generally believe that "cyberbullying" is a very broad term that covers mockery, threats, attempts to undermine social reputation or exclusion patterns through social media, texts messages, blogs, videos, and digital learning platforms. The wide range of reasons and the different forms under which it may appear make them think that the term "cyberbullying" does not accurately cover bullying behaviors that are actual forms of aggression via the Internet or cell phones (Baldasare et al. 2012; Crosslin and Golman 2014). This difficulty to define the term is governed by the features inherent to communications via the Internet (for example, the absence of visual keys), making that messages sent may be perceived ambiguously as threats or forms of aggression, despite the sender not intending to do so. From this point of view, cyberbullying may be something very common because anyone can send messages or post some information on social media that can be understood by others as harmful. On the other hand, they discuss the need for a specific term for aggression via the Internet because they find it difficult to separate the events that take place in online contexts from those that take place in offline contexts. Both contexts form part of a continuum whereby they develop social relationships and build their identity; for this reason, it might be more appropriate to use a term that does not emphasize the means by which aggression takes place (Crosslin and Golman 2014). Furthermore, many students believe that the term "cyberbullying" is more appropriate when applied to the secondary education stage because the term "bullying" is linked to behaviors that they see as childish whereby some students have fun at the expense of others. Nevertheless, college students point out that this kind of behavior, which they see as childish, also takes place at college (Baldasare et al. 2012; Crosslin and Golman 2014).

3.6.2   Features of the Definition of Cyberbullying

College students agree that cyberbullying is a subjective term that is interpreted depending on the sender and the receiver of the messages, and also on those who can gain access to them as observers (Baldasare et al. 2012). Cyberbullying would be defined by the possibility to remain anonymous and its repetition over time. However, the most important factor to define it would be the aggressor's intention. If the sender's intention is not to attack or threaten, many students do not see that behavior as bullying (Baldasare et al. 2012; Kota et al. 2014). Students point out that cyberbullying is sometimes part of jokes that go too far and, in consequence, they understand that the target, therefore, can feel bad. For this reason, some students believe that the victim perspective must be also taken into account to define what is cyberbullying (Baldasare et al. 2012). As far as the repetition criterion is concerned, it should be used to know the aggressor's intention. When an aggressor sends several messages or posts information repeatedly, it is clear that his/her intention is to harm the target (Baldasare et al. 2012). Nevertheless, students believe that applying the repetition criterion regarding cyberbullying is not always clear because information that is repeated just once can be resent by others and made to go viral (Kota et al. 2014). They also believe that anonymity and the absence of clear legal liabilities promote this kind of behavior, even making people dare to have behaviors they would not have in person (Crosslin and Golman 2014).

3.6.3   Incidence and Differences in Comparison to Other Stages of Education

Many students participating in these studies do not believe cyberbullying is a serious problem in college contexts and assure its incidence is lower in comparison to other stages of education (Baldasare et al. 2012; Crosslin and Golman 2014; Kota et al. 2014). Nevertheless, when asked about specific behaviors, nearly all admit they had some personal experiences at college. In any case, they believe that college students are more mature than those of secondary education, and that maturity has an impact on the importance they give to this problem. For example, they believe college students are more able to distinguish between jokes and actual aggression. They also have more abilities to deal with this kind of behavior; therefore, they do not see it as so problematic (Baldasare et al. 2012; Kota et al. 2014).

In this sense, college students believe that cyberbullying at high school is geared by appearance differences or hierarchy inside peer groups, while cyberbullying at college may originate in issues regarding sexuality, politics, or social problems, which turn aggressive and finally result in cyberbullying (Kota et al. 2014).

3.6.4   Features of Students Involved in Cyberbullying

College students believe they all are vulnerable to cyberbullying, especially considering the wide range of behaviors it can have (Crosslin and Golman 2014, Kota et al. 2014). The variability of the roles that can take place on the Internet have an impact therein because they can be witnesses of these behaviors and turn into victims or aggressors indistinctly all of a sudden (Baldasare et al. 2012). Students believe that cyberbullying is more common among females because the expression of their aggressiveness has been limited to verbal aggression and is, therefore, adapted to these conditions (Baldasare et al. 2012).

Students believe that the victims of these behaviors are generally different somehow—physically, ethnically, and sexually—due to their gender identity, possible disabilities, or on their religious grounds. However, they also believe that those in positions of leaderships, such as athletes or other persons, who are more visible due to their participation in student organizations, may be easy targets. Aggressors are described as coward, impulsive persons that aim at attracting the attention of others, but they can also be good students under serious pressure who release their tension through cyberbullying (Baldasare et al. 2012).

In most cases, victims know their aggressors since cyberbullying is perpetrated by friends, roommates, or former partners. Indeed, the main reason gearing these actions is causing harm to friends, partners, or persons who used to be important to cyberbullies, against whom they seek revenge or feel jealous of. Self-empowerment seems to be a key factor, especially among those persons who suffered any kind of harassment or cyberbullying too.

3.6.5   Consequences of Cyberbullying

Students believe that consequences depend on the central importance of social relationships in their lives since cyberbullying may affect these relationships (Baldasare et al. 2012; Crosslin and Golman 2014). Nevertheless, college students are especially concerned about how cyberbullying can affect their professional career in the long term because any information published on the Internet can be viewed by future employers (Kota et al. 2014).

In the short term, the study where Rivituso (2014) interviewed some victims of cyberbullying in a college context showed that they saw their self-esteem diminished, suffered stress and depression because they do not know how to stop bullying against themselves, and also frustration because college authorities do not take their problem seriously. Victims themselves assure that at this stage, friends play a key role to manage cyberbullying and put an end to it (Rivituso 2014). They also assured that their social lives are more affected when cyberbullying is perpetrated by friends and acquaintances because it originates in their social networks and they cannot ignore it (Baldasare et al. 2012).

3.7   Conclusion

Most of the studies conducted to date have attempted to know the prevalence of cyberbullying behaviors in the university context. Research has demonstrated that college students face similar problems to those face by students in primary and secondary schools. In consequence, research is now analyzing the personal and social factors that make the youth more vulnerable to suffering or exercising cyberbullying. However, the literature investigating the predictors of cyberbullying is deficient in that most studies examine these factors for the entire sample and fail to consider whether predictors could differ by gender. Prevention and intervention programs could use this information to identify males and females at risk of cyberbullying and target these different risk factors.

The data generally demonstrate that cyberbullying is more directed to peers of the same sex; however, there seems to be evidence that males address more cyberbullying to females compared to females using it against males. Different studies have shown that many adolescents face cyberbullying by former friends, ex-classmates and also by boy/girlfriends or ex-boy/girlfriends. In this sense, cyberbullying may be a way to control and harass partners. Research into cyberbullying must analyze to what extent it is practiced in romantic relationships, which gender is more exposed to aggression, and the specific form it takes.

References

Akbulut, Y., & Eristi, B. (2011). Cyberbullying and victimization among Turkish university students. *Australasian Journal of Educational Technology, 27,* 1155–1170.

Alexy, E. M., Burgess, A. W., Baker, T., & Smoyak, S. A. (2005). Perceptions of cyberstalking among college students. *Brief Treatment and Crisis Intervention, 5*(3), 279. doi:10.1093/brief-treatment/mhi020.

Aricak, O. T. (2009). Psychiatric symptomatology as a predictor of cyberbullying among university students. *Eurasian Journal of Educational Research, 34,* 167–184.

Baldasare, A., Bauman, S., Goldman, L., & Robie, A. (2012). Cyberbullying? Voices of college students. *Technologies in Higher Education, 5,* 127–155.

Baroncelli, A., & Ciucci, E. (2014). Unique effects of different components of Trait emotional intelligence in traditional bullying and cyberbullying. *Journal of Adolescence, 37*, 807–815. doi:10.1016/j.adolescence.2014.05.009.

Bauman, S. (2010). Cyberbullying in a rural intermediate school: An exploratory study. *The Journal of Early Adolescence, 30*(6), 803–833. doi:10.1177/0272431609350927.

Burke, S. C., Wallen, M., Vail-Smith, K., & Knox, D. (2011). Using technology to control intimate partners: An exploratory study of college undergraduates. *Computers in Human Behavior, 27*, 1162–1167. doi:10.1016/j.chb.2010.12.010.

Chapell, M. S., Hasselman, S. L., Kitchin, T., Lomon, S. N., MacIver, K. W., & Sarullo, P. L. (2006). Bullying in elementary school, high school, and college. *Adolescence, 41*(164), 633–648.

Crosslin, K. L., & Crosslin, M. B. (2014). Cyberbullying at a Texas university. A mixed-methods approach to examining online aggression. *Texas Public Health Journal, 66*(3), 26–31.

Crosslin, K., & Golman, M. (2014). "Maybe you don't want to face it"–College students' perspectives on cyberbullying. *Computers in Human Behavior, 41*, 14–20. doi:10.1016/j.chb.2014.09.007.

Dilmac, B. (2009). Psychological needs as a predictor of cyber bullying: A preliminary report on college students. *Educational Sciences: Theory and Practice, 9*, 1307–1325.

Durán, M., & Martínez-Pecino, R. (2015). Ciberacoso mediante teléfono móvil e Internet en las relaciones de noviazgo entre jóvenes. *Comunicar, 22*(44), 159–167. doi:10.3916/C44-2015-17.

Eisenberg, D., Gollust, S. E., Golberstein, E., & Hefner, J. L. (2007). Prevalence and correlates of depression, anxiety, and suicidality among university students. *American Journal of Orthopsychiatry, 77*, 534–542. doi:10.1037/0002-9432.77.4.534.

Englander, E., Mills, E., & McCoy, M. (2009). Cyberbullying and information exposure: User-generated content in post-secondary education. *International Journal of Contemporary Sociology, 46*(2), 213–230.

Faucher, C., Jackson, M., & Cassidy, W. (2014). Cyberbullying among university students: Gendered experiences, impacts, and perspectives. *Educational Research International, 2014*, 10. http://dx.doi.org/10.1155/2014/698545.

Finn, J. (2004). A survey of online harassment at a university campus. *Journal of Interpersonal Violence, 19*, 468–483. doi:10.1177/0886260503262083.

Gilroy, M. (2013). Guns, hazing and cyberbullying among top legal issues on campus. *Educational Digest, 78*(8), 45–50.

Hartwell-Walter, M. (2010). *Cyberbullying and teen suicide.* Psych Central. http://psychcentral. con/lib/2010/cyberbullying-and-teen-suicide/.

Hoff, D. L., & Mitchell, S. N. (2009). Cyberbullying: Causes, effects, and remedies. *Journal of Educational Administration, 47*, 652–665. doi:10.1108/09578230910981107.

Holt, M. K., Green, J. G., Reid, G., DiMeo, A., Espelage, D. L., Felix, E. D., Furlong, M. J., Poteat, P., & Sharkey, J. D. (2014). Associations between past bullying experiences and psychosocial and academic functioning among college students. *Journal of American College Health, 62*(8), 552–560. doi:10.1080/07448481.2014.947990.

Jacobs, N. C. L., Dehue, F., Völlink, T., & Lechner, L. (2014). Determinants of adolescents' ineffective and improve coping with cyberbullying: A Delphi study. *Journal of Adolescence, 37*, 373–385. doi:10.1016/j.adolescence.2014.02.011.

Jang, H., Song, J., & Kim, R. (2014). Does the offline bully-victimization influence cyberbullying behavior among youths? Application of general strain theory. *Computers in Human Behavior, 31*, 85–93. doi:10.1016/j.chb.2013.10.007.

Kiriakidis, S. P., & Kavoura, A. (2010). Cyberbullying: A review of the literature on harassment through the internet and other electronic means. *Family and Community Health, 33*(2), 82–93. doi:10.1097/FCH.0b013e3181d593e4.

Kota, R., Schoohs, S., Benson, M., & Moreno, M. A. (2014). Characterizing cyberbullying among college students: Hacking, dirty laundry, and mocking. *Societies, 4*(4), 549–560. doi:10.3390/soc4040549.

Kraft, E., & Wang, J. (2010). An exploratory study of the cyberbullying and cyberstalking experiences and factors related to victimization of students at a public liberal arts college. *International Journal of Technologies, 1,* 74–91. doi:10.4018/jte.2010100106.

Lindsay, M., & Krysik, J. (2012). Online harassment among college students. A replication incorporating new Internet trends. *Information, Communication, & Society, 15,* 703–719. doi:10.10 80/1369118X.2012.674959.

MacDonald, C. D., & Roberts-Pittman, B. (2010). Cyberbullying among college students: Prevalence and demographic differences. *Procedia: Social and behavioral Sciences, 9,* 2003–2009. doi:10.1016/j.sbspro.2010.12.436.

Mateus, S., Veiga, A. M., Costa, P., & das Dores, M. J. (2015). Cyberbullying: The hidden side of college students. *Computers in Human Behavior, 43,* 167–182. doi:10.1016/j.chb.2014.10.045.

Meriläinen, M., Puhakka, H., & Sinkkonen, H. (2015). Students' suggestions for eliminating bullying at a university. *British Journal of Guidance & Counselling, 43,* 202–215. doi:10.1080/0 3069885.2014.950943.

Molluzzo, J. C., & Lawler, J. (2012). A study of the perceptions of college students on cyberbullying. *Information Systems Education Journal, 10*(4), 84–109.

Myers, C. A., & Cowie, H. (2013). University students' views on bullying from the perspective on different participant roles. *Pastoral Care in Education, 31,* 251–267. doi:10.1080/026439 44.2013.811696.

Nocentini, A., Calmaestra, J., Schultze-Krumbholz, A., Scheithauer, H., Ortega, R., & Menesini, E. (2010). Cyberbullying: Labels, behaviours and definition in three European countries. *Australian Journal of Guidance and Counselling, 20*(2), 129–142. doi:10.1375/ajgc.20.2.129.

Palfrey, J., & Gasser, U. (2008). Opening universities in a digital era. *New England Journal of Higher Education, 23*(1), 22–24.

Paullet, K., & Pinchot, J. (2014). Behind the screen where today's bully plays: Perceptions of college students on cyberbullying. *Journal of Information Systems Education, 25*(1), 63–69.

Pellegrini, A. D., & Bartini, J. D. (2002). A longitudinal study of bullying, dominance, and victimization during the transition from primary school through secondary school. *British Journal of Developmental Psychology, 20,* 259–280. doi:10.1348/026151002166442.

Prensky, R. (2001). Digital natives, digital inmigrants. *On the Horizon, 9*(5), 1–6. doi:10.1108/10748120110424816.

Rivituso, J. (2014). Cyberbullying victimization among college students: An interpretive phenomenological analysis. *Journal of Information Systems Education, 25,* 71–75.

Salmivalli, C. (2010). Bullying and peer group: A review. *Aggression and Violent Behavior, 15*(2), 112–120. doi:10.1016/j.avb.2009.08.007.

Schenk, A. M., & Fremouw, W. J. (2012). Prevalence, psychological impact, and coping of cyberbully victims among college students. *Journal of School Violence, 11*(1), 21–37. doi:10.1080/ 15388220.2011.630310.

Schenk, A. M., Fremouw, W. J., & Keelan, C. M. (2013). Characteristics of college cyberbullies. *Computers in Human Behavior, 29,* 2320–2327. doi:10.1016/j.chb.2013.05.013.

Selkie, E. M., Kota, R., Chan, Y., & Moreno, M. (2015). Cyberbullying, depression and problema alcohol use in female college students: A multisite study. *Cyberpsychology, Behavior, and Social Networking, 18*(2), 79–86. doi:10.1089/cyber.2014.0371.

Sevcikova, A., Smahel, D., & Otavova, M. (2012). The perception of cyberbullying in adolescent victims. *Emotional & Behavioural Difficulties, 17*(3–4), 319–328. doi:10.1080/13632752.20 12.704309.

Smith, J. A., & Yoon, J. (2013). Cyberbullying presence, extent, & forms in a midwestern postsecondary institution. *Information Systems Educational Journal, 11,* 52–78.

Smith, P. K., Mahdavi, J., Carvalho, M., Fisher, S., Russell, S., & Tippett, N. (2008). Cyberbullying: Its nature and impact in secondary school pupils. *Journal of Child Psychology and Psychiatry, 49,* 376–385. doi:10.1111/j.1469-7610.2007.01846.x.

Spitzberg, B. H. (2002). The tactical topography of stalking victimization and management. *Trauma Violence Abuse, 3,* 261–288. doi:10.1177/1524838002237330.

Subrahmanyam, K., Smahel, D., & Greenfield, P. (2006). Connecting developmental constructions to the Internet: Identity presentation and sexual exploration in online teen chat rooms. *Developmental Psychology, 42*(3), 395–406. doi:10.1037/0012-1649.42.3.395.

Tokunaga, R. S. (2010). Following you home from school: A critical review and synthesis of research on cyberbullying victimization. *Computers in Human Behavior, 26,* 277–287. doi:10.1016/j.chb.2009.11.014.

Tomsa, R., Jenaro, C., Campbell, M., & Neacsu, D. (2013). Student's experiences with traditional bullying and cyberbullying: Findings from a Romanian simple. *Procedia. Social and Behavioral Sciences, 78,* 586–590. doi:10.1016/j.sbspro.2013.04.356.

Turan, N., Polat, O., Karapirli, M., Uysal, C., & Turan, S. G. (2011). The new violence type of the era: Cyber bullying among university students. Violence among university students. *Neurology Psychiatry & Brain Research, 17,* 21–26. doi:10.1016/j.npbr.2011.02.005.

Vandebosch, H., & Van Cleemput, K. (2009). Cyberbullying among youngsters: Profiles of bullies and victims. *New Media & Society, 11,* 1349–1371. doi:10.1177/1461444809341263.

Walker, C. M., Sockman, B. R., & Koehn, S. (2011). An exploratory study of cyberbullying with undergraduate university students. *TechTrends, 55*(2), 31–38. doi:10.1007/s11528-011-0481-0.

Walrave, M., & Heirman, W. (2011). Cyberbullying: Predicting victimization and perpetration. *Children and Society, 25,* 59–72. doi:10.1111/j.1099-0860.2009.00260.x.

Washington, E. T. (2014). Why did Tweet that? An examination of cyberbullying among undergraduate students at an urban research university. http://umwa.memphis.edu/etd/.

Zacchilli, T. L., & Valerio, C. V. (2011). The knowledge and prevalence of cuberbullying in a college sample. *Journal of Scientific Psychology*, 11–23. http://www.psyencelab.com/images/The_Knowledge_and_Prevalence_of_Cyberbullying_in_a_College_Sample.pdf.

Zalaquett, C. P., & Chatters, S. J. (2014). Cyberbullying in college: Frequency, characteristic, and practical implications. *Sage Open, 4,* 1–8. doi:10.1177/2158244014526721.

Chapter 4
Gender Differences and Cyberbullying Towards Faculty Members in Higher Education

Wanda Cassidy, Margaret Jackson and Chantal Faucher

4.1 Introduction

The ubiquity of information and communication technologies (ICTs) in the personal and professional lives of university faculty members has been valuable; however, these advances have also resulted in an increased opportunity for negative behaviours, such as cyberbullying. The phenomenon of cyberbullying has come to the fore in the past decade, although we typically associate the term with youthful behaviour and not with adults. Cyberbullying research has been aimed at children and youth of middle school and high school age (see Cassidy et al. 2013, for a comprehensive review of this literature). The earlier ostensible consensus definition of cyberbullying suggested it was another form of traditionally defined bullying: 'an aggressive, intentional act carried out by a group or individual, using electronic forms of contact, repeatedly and over time against a victim who cannot easily defend him or herself' (Smith et al. 2008, p. 376). In this rapidly evolving field of inquiry, researchers increasingly are providing nuances with respect to what intent, repetition, and power imbalance signify in the context of cyberbullying as well as evaluating the impacts of anonymity and the hypothetically limitless audience for the bullying (Dooley et al. 2009; Grigg 2010; Kowalski et al. 2012; Menesini 2012;

W. Cassidy (✉)
Faculty of Education, Simon Fraser University, 8888 University Drive,
Burnaby, BC V5A 1S6, Canada
e-mail: cassidy@sfu.ca

M. Jackson
School of Criminology, Simon Fraser University, 8888 University Drive,
Burnaby, BC V5A 1S6, Canada
e-mail: margarej@sfu.ca

C. Faucher
Centre for Education, Law and Society, Simon Fraser University,
250-13450 - 102 Avenue, Surrey, BC V3T 0A3, Canada
e-mail: cfaucher@sfu.ca

© Springer International Publishing Switzerland 2016
R. Navarro et al. (eds.), *Cyberbullying Across the Globe*,
DOI 10.1007/978-3-319-25552-1_4

79

Nocentini et al. 2010; Patchin and Hinduja 2012; Smith 2012; Vandebosch and Van Cleemput 2009; von Marées and Petermann 2012). This understanding has led us to adopt a broader definition of cyberbullying: Through ICT media, cyberbullying uses language or images to defame, threaten, harass, bully, exclude, discriminate, demean, humiliate, stalk, disclose personal information, or contain offensive, vulgar, or derogatory comments with an intent to harm or hurt the recipient.

Cyberbullying at the postsecondary level has not been a priority of this emerging research area. For those who have investigated cyberbullying at universities, the focus primarily has been on undergraduate students' experiences (Beran et al. 2012; Dilmaç 2009; Finn 2004; Molluzzo and Lawler 2012; Schenk and Fremouw 2012; Turan et al. 2011; Walker et al. 2011; Wankel and Wankel 2012; Wensley and Campbell 2012; Zhang et al. 2010). Relatively little attention has been paid to the experiences of university faculty members or other teaching personnel. The emerging scholarship on cyberbullying in the workplace (Baruch 2005; D'Cruz and Noronha 2013; McQuade et al. 2009; Piotrowski 2012; Privitera and Campbell 2009), however, provides some parallels to the cyberbullying of university personnel. Further, some connections have been drawn between cyberbullying in the K-12 sector, universities, workplaces, and beyond (Bauman 2011, 2012; Englander 2008; McKay et al. 2008; McQuade et al. 2009).

We see cyberbullying against faculty members and other teaching personnel in universities along this lifespan continuum. Cyberbullying in universities is distinctively situated as a bridge between bullying in schools and in the workplace (Cowie et al. 2013; McKay et al. 2008). Several continuities have been highlighted, such as the persistence of roles, victim, bully, bully-victim (Bauman 2011; Beran et al. 2012), and the similar impacts reported at both the school and workplace levels (Baruch 2005; Beran et al. 2012; Cassidy et al. 2013).

Individual and contextual factors influence cyberbullying behaviours that take place in schools and workplaces (see Jones and Scott 2012). The theoretical framing of cyberbullying in terms of power is particularly relevant in the context of higher education. Cyberbullying also relates to incivility in the classroom and workplace. It has been pointed out that lower level mistreatments can escalate into more severe forms of harassment and even violence (Cortina et al. 2001; Wildermuth and Davis 2012). Our contextual understanding of incivility and harassment in universities as workplaces is premised on an awareness of the power imbalances that exist between university students and faculty members or other teaching personnel as well as between colleagues.

This chapter examines online survey data from 331 university faculty members and other teaching personnel (including teaching assistants, tutor markers, instructors, lecturers, and student advisors) from four Canadian universities. The purpose of the survey was to determine the nature, extent, and impacts of cyberbullying experienced by faculty members as well as their opinions about the problem and possible solutions.

4.2   Literature Review

4.2.1   Cyberbullying Correlates

The view of cyberbullying in higher education as a part of a behavioural continuum suggests that knowledge regarding cyberbullying in other realms (K-12, workplace) can inform and assist in theoretically framing this study. However, the nature of interpersonal relationships and interactions that exists between faculty and students as well as between colleagues in the specific context of higher education suggests that attention also be given to power imbalances that are at play and how these may present in the form of cyberbullying.

The research literature on the correlates of cyberbullying relate primarily to youth; however, the perspective of cyberbullying throughout the lifespan (Bauman 2012; McKay et al. 2008; McQuade et al. 2009) suggests that an awareness of known correlates may assist us in our examination of cyberbullying towards university faculty members. For example, research on youth indicates that heavy ICT usage may increase risk of exposure to cyberbullying (Smith 2012; Vandebosch and Van Cleemput 2009; von Marées and Petermann 2012; Yilmaz 2011).

Gender is one of the most examined correlates. Some work suggests that females are more likely to experience cyberbullying than traditional face-to-face bullying (Dooley et al. 2009; Jackson et al. 2009; Kowalski et al. 2012; Li 2005). Moreover, the online environment has given rise to new forms of sexual and gender harassment, such as 'sexting', 'morphing', 'virtual rape', and 'revenge porn', to which women are particularly vulnerable (Cassidy et al. 2012; CCSO Cybercrime Working Group 2013; Halder and Jaishankar 2009; Hinduja and Patchin 2012; Shariff and Gouin 2005). Indeed, according to Halder and Jaishankar (2009), women are the second most vulnerable group online, after children.

We have come to understand bullying as stemming from a power and control imbalance between the bully and the victim (Olweus 1993), and the same may be said of cyberbullying. However, the power differential in cyberbullying may be attributable to different sources; for example, ease with technology, number of viewers, potential anonymity of the perpetrator, and 24/7 access to the victim online (Dooley et al. 2009; Nocentini et al. 2010; Shariff and Gouin 2005; Vandebosch and Van Cleemput 2009; von Marées and Petermann, 2012). The hierarchical nature of universities may suggest one straightforward interpretation of power imbalances between senior and junior colleagues and between professors and students. However, in the context of higher education, a number of variables such as status, position, role, authority, gender, ethnicity, and age have an impact in shaping the relative and perceived power of individuals, whether in faculty–student relationships or in relationships between colleagues. The significance of these power differentials allows us to situate the analysis of cyberbullying within the Power and Control Model (Pence and Paymar 1993), where the abuser uses such tactics as intimidation, threats, harmful language, social standing, exclusion, harassment, and technology to exert control over the victim (see also Faucher et al. 2014).

4.2.2 Cyberbullying in Higher Education

The cyberbullying experienced by faculty members has not been well examined within the research literature. To date, we are aware of only three studies specifically documenting cyberbullying against faculty (Blizard 2014; Minor et al. 2013; Vance 2010), two of which were restricted to online learning environments. We also found some research on online misbehaviour, which refers to cyberbullying experienced by faculty members, but within the context of online incivility (Clark et al. 2012; Jones and Scott 2012; Wildermuth and Davis 2012). Cyberbullying in universities appears to be conveyed primarily through e-mail (Martin and Olson 2011; McKay et al. 2008). However, scholarship on workplace bullying suggests: 'bullying on the e-mail system appears to be at the same level as other communication modes used to conduct bullying and negative outcomes of bullying exist irrespectively to the media of communication' (Baruch 2005, p. 366). Websites such as Rate My Professor, YouTube pranks, Facebook, gossip and confession websites, and defamatory online profiles have also received attention as formats for the cyberbullying of professors (see, for example, Binns 2007; Browne 2014; Daniloff 2009; Martin and Olson 2011).

Blizard (2014) surveyed 36 instructors and conducted in-depth interviews with four members from this group at a Canadian university. She found e-mail or faculty polling sites were the main formats employed to target faculty members, many of whom experienced a wide range of negative effects, some of which were severe and long lasting.

Minor and colleagues (2013) surveyed 68 online instructors at a large online American university. About a third of their respondents reported that they had been cyberbullied by students. Of those who were targeted, about a third reported the matter to their direct supervisor. The majority did not know what resources were available or felt that there were no resources available to help them should they encounter cyberbullying from students. Concerns which impeded respondents in reporting instances of cyberbullying included: fear of impacting further teaching opportunities; fear of decreasing student retention rates; embarrassment; fear of not being supported by the supervisor; and time requirements for adequately addressing the issue.

Vance (2010) surveyed 225 students and 56 faculty respondents engaged in online learning environments. Cyber-harassment (the term he uses) in online learning occurred at least once for 12 % of students and 39 % of faculty respondents, and more than once for 2 % of students and 16 % of faculty. Older faculty and students and those who had been involved in more than 20 online courses (primarily faculty members) reported higher rates of cyber-harassment. The most common types of cyber-harassment experienced were e-mail and flaming (online verbal abuse). The majority of those targeted did not report the incident(s), citing reasons such as: doubt that authorities could help, not thinking it was an offence, not knowing where to report, and fear of retaliation.

Jones and Scott (2012) examined factors related to the sociocultural context of the university classroom that may be conducive to incivility and cyberbullying among students. Although the cyberbullying in this case was not against faculty members, it raises a number of relevant issues. Considerations such as perceived power imbalances, perceived lack of consequences to cyberbullying, frustration and dissatisfaction, and motivations such as higher grades were contributors to cyberbullying.

Wildermuth and Davis (2012) reviewed the literature regarding students' uncivil electronic discourse aimed at faculty members. The authors contend that student incivility has increased due to specific aspects of online interactions (such as perceived anonymity, asynchronicity, lack of nonverbal cues, greater potential for misinterpretations), broader trends in declining civility and changing definitions of politeness, and the informal nature of higher education coupled with students' sense of entitlement and consumerist attitudes towards their education. Student incivility, as a result, can lead to faculty stress, decreased morale, cynicism, disengagement, lower standards, and violence.

4.2.3   Academic Entitlement, Incivility, and Harassment in Higher Education

The literature on academic entitlement, classroom incivility, and harassment can also aid in our understanding of the issue of cyberbullying towards faculty members in higher education. Academic entitlement refers to 'expectations of high rewards for modest effort, expectations of special consideration and accommodation by teachers when it comes to grades, and impatience and anger when their expectations and perceived needs are not met' (Greenberger et al. 2008, p. 1194). There is a body of work documenting an increase in academic entitlement among higher education students in recent years (Boswell 2012; Chowning and Campbell 2009; Ciani et al. 2008; Greenberger et al. 2008; Kopp and Finney 2013). Academic entitlement has also been associated with student incivility (Chowning and Campbell 2009; Kopp and Finney 2013). Morrissette (2001, p. 1) has defined incivility as:

> the intentional behaviour of students to disrupt and interfere with the teaching and learning process of others. This behaviour can range from students who dominate and foster tension in the classroom to students who attend classes unprepared, are passively rude, or unwilling to participate in the learning process.

Student incivility towards faculty members is a form of contrapower harassment, which occurs when a person with presumably less power bullies someone with more power (DeSouza 2011; Lampman 2012). This incivility can occur in the classroom, outside of the classroom, as well as online (Bjorklund and Rehling 2011; Boice 1996; DeSouza 2011; Meyers et al. 2006). Young, female, low-status, and minority faculty members appear to face a greater risk of exposure to incivility both in terms of frequency and severity of the behaviours (DeSouza 2011; Knepp 2012; Lampman 2012; Rowland 2009; Twale and De Luca 2008).

Aside from the individualistic traits of perpetrators, we should also consider some broader contextual factors linked to our education system that encourage and perpetuate academic entitlement and incivility in higher education. E-mail access to professors has created, rightly or wrongly, an impression of constant availability to students and has lessened the formality of student–faculty exchanges due to the casual nature of online modes of communication (Greenberger et al. 2008; Wildermuth and Davis 2012). More generally, online communication creates a sense of anonymity, a disconnect with the potential negative consequences of our words and actions, an absence of nonverbal cues available in in-person communication, and asynchronicity in exchanges, all of which play a part in uncivil online exchanges and cyberbullying (DeSouza 2011; Kowalski et al. 2012; Smith and Slonje 2010; Tokunaga 2010; Topcu and Erdur-Baker 2012; Wildermuth and Davis 2012). Furthermore, certain characteristics of the university classroom, such as large class size and impersonal instructor–student relationships may also add to the feeling of anonymity and the behaviours it engenders (Jones and Scott 2012; Knepp 2012). Additionally, students who adopt consumerist attitudes towards education may believe they are entitled to good grades in exchange for paying tuition. Such beliefs then may feed the academic entitlement attitudes related to student incivility (Knepp 2012; Morrissette 2001; Rowland 2009). Academic entitlement and consumerist attitudes may unsettle the perceived power imbalance between students and the faculty members who are seen as exerting control over their grades (see Blizard 2014).

Incivility and cyberbullying are not unidirectional. Less has been said about the misbehaviour of faculty towards students or colleagues than about misbehaviour targeting faculty members. Although faculty cyberbullying of students was not a focus of our study, we did investigate cyberbullying by colleagues and we found no literature directly related to this topic. However, adopting the same theoretical frame as above, we did note some work on faculty incivility and workplace bullying to consider. For example, Twale and De Luca's (2008) work on faculty incivility links university governance structures, committees, hierarchy, and bureaucracy to this problem. They also argued that the entry of previously excluded groups such as women and minorities and the growing corporate culture are precipitating factors of the academic bully culture.

Civility, both online and offline, and countering the problematic behaviours of cyberbullying and incivility are educational as well as societal challenges. However, incivility and workplace bullying also seriously impact the victim as well as the university culture as a whole. A wide array of effects are reported such as: trauma; distress; psychosomatic symptoms; student and/or faculty disengagement; unwarranted negative faculty evaluations and increased fear over job security; lowering of standards, including unwarranted grade inflation; low morale; high stress; cynicism; decreased motivation; and in rare instances the culmination into physical violence, homicide, and suicidal thoughts (Blizard 2014; Boice 1996; Ciani et al. 2008; DeSouza 2011; Lampman 2012; Wildermuth and Davis 2012).

4.3 Methods

This chapter reports on findings from sections of a broader study of cyberbullying at the university level, which includes a policy scan, student and faculty surveys, student focus groups, faculty interviews, and policymaker interviews at four Canadian universities. Two of the universities are in British Columbia, one in the Prairies, and one in Atlantic Canada. Here, we are reporting on the findings from the faculty surveys from the four participating universities. An online survey, using Fluid Surveys, was disseminated through various mailing lists to gain maximum exposure. The survey included 111 items, which included both closed and open-ended questions related to demographics, ICT usage patterns, experiences of cyberbullying from students or colleagues, solutions, and their opinions about the phenomenon. The surveys were anonymous and no identifiers were used. Three hundred and thirty-one faculty members completed the surveys, during the period September 2012 to February 2014.

Cyberbullying was defined at the outset of the survey as: 'Cyberbullying uses language that can defame, threaten, harass, bully, exclude, discriminate, demean, humiliate, stalk, disclose personal information, or contain offensive, vulgar or derogatory comments. Cyberbullying is intended to harm or hurt the recipient'. Respondents were then provided with a list of examples of cyberbullying, including the medium used, and asked to comment about their experiences over the past 12 months; for example, receiving nasty, mean, rude, vulgar, hurtful, or harassing e-mail or text messages; having terrible, derogatory, sexist, racist or homophobic things written about you online; someone posting an embarrassing photo or video of you online; someone pretending to be you online; and being deliberately excluded from an online group or chat.

4.4   Results

4.4.1   Respondents' Profile

Background Professors constituted the largest group of respondents (45%), followed by teaching assistants or tutor markers (18%), instructors (14%), student advisors and others with teaching-related positions (12%), and lecturers (9%). Participants varied in terms of teaching experience, level of employment security, and type of interaction with students and colleagues. Each participant, however, was involved in a teaching role and had a degree of power or control over students at the university. Our analysis of these different groups of teaching personnel indicates that there were no statistically significant quantitative differences between them as far as experiences of cyberbullying by students or by colleagues were concerned; therefore, we have grouped them together in this analysis.

The faculty members who responded to the survey were drawn from many different faculties in each of the universities. Of those who responded, 31% were from Faculties of Arts and Social Sciences, 15% from the Faculty of Education, and 13% each from the Faculties of Science and of Health. The remaining 28% came from Applied Sciences, Business, Kinesiology, Law, Medicine/Dentistry, Preparation and Extension courses, and administrative units. Survey respondents were predominantly female (68%), Caucasian (84%), identified English as their first language (81%), and were born in Canada (70%). Forty-seven percent of respondents had been working at the university for 5 years or less, while 48% of respondents had tenure or a permanent position; these percentages were approximately equally divided between female and male respondents. The age profiles were also similar for male and female respondents.

As the responses came in, it became apparent that gender, however, would be an issue worth examining. Data from the Council of Canadian Academies (2012) indicate that, for the academic year 2008–2009, 32.6% of all faculty members in Canada were women, with the percentage at three of the four participating universities between 32 and 39% (pp. 194–195). Data on our fourth university was not provided in the Council report; however, sources within the institution suggest a higher proportion of female faculty at 54%. Nonetheless, these percentages are much lower than the 68% of female respondents to the survey.

Survey respondents were also asked whether they would volunteer to participate in a one-on-one interview on solutions to the problem of cyberbullying. Almost all volunteers were women. It should also be noted that the female respondents to the online student survey, reported elsewhere (Faucher et al. 2014), outnumbered male respondents three to one. Women appear to have a greater interest in, or willingness to engage with, this topic than do men.

Female respondents also showed a higher level of concern about the problem of cyberbullying at university. On a five-point scale from extremely concerned to not concerned at all, 84% of females indicated that they were extremely concerned or somewhat concerned about the problem compared to only 54% of males. Respondents were also asked to rate the importance of preventing cyberbullying and of encouraging and teaching respectful online communications among the various competing priorities at the university. Here again, gendered perspectives surfaced as 86% of females versus 72% of males felt it was extremely or somewhat important to prevent cyberbullying, while 98% of females versus 84% of males felt it was extremely or somewhat important to encourage and teach respectful online communications. This greater level of concern about the issue may have contributed to the gender discrepancies in response rates noted above.

4.4.2 Faculty Members' Experiences with Cyberbullying

Prevalence and Background Characteristics Table 4.1 provides the rates of cyberbullying victimization by gender as reported by respondents.

Overall, 25% of faculty respondents had experienced cyberbullying either from students (15%) and/or from colleagues (12%) in the last 12 months. A small number, only ten individuals, had experienced cyberbullying from both students and colleagues. Female faculty members were targeted more often by both students and colleagues. While the percentage of female faculty members targeted by students was only slightly higher than their male counterparts (16% vs. 13%), almost twice as many female faculty members than males were targeted by colleagues (14% vs. 8%).

Table 4.1 Prevalence of faculty cyberbullying victimization by gender

Victims of cyberbullying	Males (%)	Females (%)	Total (%)
Overall (in last 12 months)	18	27	25
By students at the university	13	16	15
By a colleague	8	14	12

Table 4.2 identifies some of the background characteristics of those faculty members who had experienced cyberbullying.

As noted in this table, professors and those with tenure or a permanent position experienced more cyberbullying overall from both students and colleagues (31%) compared to sessional instructors (26%), teaching assistants and tutor markers (18%), and those without tenure (19%). Those in less permanent and less senior positions, however, experienced much more cyberbullying from students than from colleagues. Faculty members who self-identified as being from a visible minority experienced slightly more cyberbullying than those who identified as Caucasian (27% vs. 24%), with most of the cyberbullying coming from students (19%) rather than colleagues (12%). Similarly, those for whom English is not a first language were targeted more often by students (17%) than by colleagues (12%).

ICT usage variables bore some relationship to cyberbullying. Faculty members who spent over 6 hours each day online for their professional activities and/or over 6 hours for their personal activities experienced more cyberbullying from students than from colleagues. No correlations, however, could be found between ICT usage and cyberbullying by colleagues. Although 71% of faculty respondents had

Table 4.2 Percentage of respondents with different background variables who have been cyberbullied (CB)

Respondents	CB by student (%)	CB by colleague (%)	CB by either (%)
Overall (in last 12 months)	15	12	25
... who have tenure/a permanent position	18	18	31
... who do not have tenure/a permanent position	12	8	19
... who are teaching assistants or tutor markers	15	5	18
... who are sessional instructors	17	11	26
... who are professors	18	18	31
... for whom English is not 1st language	17	12	23
... who are on Facebook	15	11	24
... who identify as Caucasian	14	13	24
... who identify as part of a visible minority group	19	12	27
... who have their own blog	17	13	28
... who have their own website	18	14	28
... who spend 6+ hours online/day for professional activity	19	11	26
... who spend 3+ hours online/day for personal activity	17	11	26
... who spend 6+ hours online/day for personal activity	32	5	32

a Facebook page, they were no more likely than non-Facebook users to experience cyberbullying by students or by colleagues. Further, having their own blog or their own website also did not appear to be correlated with cyberbullying by students or by colleagues.

Form of Technology Used E-mail was, by far, the most common vehicle used to cyberbully (reported by 74% of those targeted by students and 78% of those targeted by colleagues). Forty-two percent of respondents noted being targeted by students on a professor-rating website, with 28% indicating course-related sites, blogs, forums, or chatrooms. Only 10% of respondents targeted by colleagues indicated that this had occurred on Facebook or other similar social media sites.

Reasons for Being Cyberbullied 'Teaching-related reasons' was noted as the most common reason (78% of the time) for being cyberbullied by students; that is, a grade they assigned a student, their teaching style, something they said to a student or in class, their course content, organization, deadlines, schedule, or assignments. Next was their 'position or role at the university' (36%). Female respondents also identified their gender as a reason for being cyberbullied by students, although none of the male respondents gave this reason. Among those respondents who explained why they had been cyberbullied by students, gender ranked third after the two most common explanations cited above. In most cases, the cyberbullying was carried out by a student or students known by their victims.

Respondents who were cyberbullied by colleagues most often cited 'work-related reasons' for being targeted (80 %): a professional difference of opinion, competition between university colleagues, professional jealousy, their professional status, and an attempt to establish power and control. They also noted their position or role at the university (49%), gender (17%), and age (17%). In all but one of the cases, the cyberbullying was carried out by a colleague or colleagues that the faculty respondent knew.

Perceived Intent and Impacts of Cyberbullying When asked about what they perceived as the intent of students' cyberbullying against them, the most frequently cited descriptors were: insulting (70%), demanding (52%), demeaning, belittling, derogatory (50%), spreading rumours (40%), harassing (36%), and rude or vulgar (30%). In terms of impacts, those reported with the greatest frequency were: It affected their ability to do their work, including productivity, loss of confidence, and concentration problems (64%); it affected their relationships with students and/or university colleagues (62%); feeling that their emotional security or physical safety was threatened (34%); mental health issues, including anxiety, depression, and emotional outbursts (30%); they felt like quitting their job at the university (30%); and physical health issues, including headaches, stomach problems, nausea, heart palpitations or chest pain, and sweating (28%). The majority (64%) did something to try to stop the cyberbullying from students, but less than half of them felt that it had worked.

Respondents described the intent behind the cyberbullying they experienced from colleagues in ways similar to the cyberbullying from students: insulting (73%), demeaning, belittling, derogatory (59%), harassing (46%), spreading rumours (39%), and demanding (37%). They also added other intents: meant to exclude them (29%), threatening (29%), and humiliating or embarrassing (29%). Many felt that it affected their ability to do their work (73%), made them feel like quitting their jobs (49%), affected their relationships with students and/or university colleagues (49%) and/or their relationships outside of the university (39%), and made them feel that their emotional security or physical safety was threatened (46%). Some also experienced mental health issues (39%), and/or physical health issues (29%) as a result. The majority (66.7%) said they tried to do something to stop the cyberbullying by colleagues, but again less than half of them felt that it had worked.

Seeking Help Most targeted faculty members told someone about their experiences, although they were more likely to tell someone if the perpetrator was a colleague (73% told) rather than a student (58% told). Women were much more likely to tell someone than were men. Victims mainly told their colleagues, partners, and/or friends. Few reported the incident to their superiors or to others who might have assisted them in an official capacity (for example, university administration, counselling services, union/faculty association, human rights office, or campus security). Those who did report the cyberbullying to authorities were almost exclusively women.

4.4.3   Opinions About Cyberbullying at University

General Opinions We put a list of statements to the respondents and asked them to rate their agreement with each of them on a scale ranging from: strongly disagree, disagree somewhat, neutral (neither agree nor disagree), agree somewhat, strongly agree, or don't know. For the purposes of simplifying the analysis, the two 'agree' responses were collapsed into a single category, as were the two 'disagree' responses. The strongest level of agreement came from the following two statements: 'I would like to help create a more kind and respectful online world' (66% agree); and 'I would report cyberbullying if I could do it anonymously' (42%).

The strongest disagreement came from the following statements: 'Cyberbullying can't hurt you; it is just words in virtual space' (85% disagree); 'I have the right to say anything I want online because of freedom of expression' (78% disagree); 'Cyberbullying is a normal part of the online world; it can't be stopped' (64% disagree); 'Solutions to cyberbullying lie with youth as they are more techno-savvy' (54% disagree).

Differences in Opinions Between Victims and Non-victims Faculty members who had experienced cyberbullying differed in their responses to some of the opinions posed. For example, victims were less likely than non-victims to disagree with the statement that 'Cyberbullying is a normal part of the online world; it can't be stopped' (51% of victims disagreed compared to 64% overall). Further, those who had been victimized by colleagues were more likely than non-victims to agree with the same statement (22% agreed compared to 12% overall). This disparity may reflect the victims' feelings of frustration when trying to stop the cyberbullying they were experiencing. Faculty members who had been cyberbullied by students were also more inclined to agree with the statement that 'Students are less likely to bully online if they are happy with their university life/course grades' (36% vs. 25% overall).

Relationship Between Opinions and Gender Males and females held similar opinions on many of the non-policy-related opinion questions. For example, both males and females generally agreed that they would like to help create a more kind and respectful online world and had similar responses to the statements that 'it is the university's responsibility to stop or prevent online bullying', and that 'they would report cyberbullying if they could do it anonymously'. Both males and females overwhelmingly disagreed with the statements: 'Cyberbullying can't hurt you; it's just words in virtual space' and 'I have the right to say anything I want online because of freedom of expression'. Male and female respondents generally disagreed with the statement 'Cyberbullying is a normal part of the online world; it can't be stopped', although female respondents were more likely to disagree (69% female, 52% male).

4.4.4 Opinions About University Policies

Statements related to university policies elicited much more ambivalence and uncertainty from the respondents; these included statements about student conduct, harassment, and bullying, as well as awareness of these policies, their clarity, enforcement, and effectiveness.

Table 4.3 illustrates the lack of consensus among faculty respondents on these points.

Table 4.3 Respondents' levels of agreement with opinion statements about cyberbullying

Opinion statements	Disagree (%)	Neutral (%)	Agree (%)	Don't know (%[a])
Faculty members are aware of the university policies and procedures on student conduct, harassment and bullying	40	17	21	11
University policies and procedures on student conduct, harassment and bullying are clear on prohibited behaviour/sanctions	27	22	23	17
Policies and procedures on student conduct, harassment and bullying are enforced at this university	18	25	18	29
Policies and procedures on student conduct, harassment and bullying are effective at this university	20	25	12	31
Faculty members can access support services if they are victims of cyberbullying at this university	10	21	31	28

[a] Row percentages do not total 100% as the missing data are not shown. Approximately 10% of respondents did not answer the opinion section near the end of the survey

Only 23% of respondents said that their university policies and procedures on student conduct, harassment, and bullying were clear, with 27% indicating strong disagreement with this statement and 17% answering that they did not know the answer to this question. Nearly a third of respondents did not know if the policies were enforced or if the policies were effective. Further, in most cases, faculty members chose 'neutral' or 'don't know' rather than agreeing or disagreeing with the statements about the policies. Almost 50% of respondents, for example, chose 'neutral' or 'don't know' when asked about policy enforcement, effectiveness, and accessing support services, if victimized by cyberbullying.

Overall, their responses indicate that many are either unaware of what policies are in place or what support services are provided, or do not believe they are communicated effectively or enforced. Further, since most victims did not report their experiences with cyberbullying to an administrator at the university (discussed above), it is unlikely that they had any direct experience with whether the policies were clear, effective, or enforced, thus contributing to the wide range of responses across the agree/disagree scale.

Policy Responses and Gender Female faculty were more likely than male faculty to disagree that the policies are clear (29% of females disagreed vs. 22% of males), enforced (21% vs. 12%), and effective (24% vs. 11%). About 28% of respondents did not know if victims of cyberbullying at the university would be able to access support services, and of those respondents who believed support would not be accessible, 14% were women and only 2% men.

Relationship Between Policy Opinions and Victimization Experience There were obvious differences in opinions between victims and non-victims in relation to university policies. Table 4.4 compares the responses from the full sample with those who were victimized by students and by colleagues.

Table 4.4 Comparison of disagreement rates on opinion statements based on cyberbullying experience(s)

Opinion statements	Total (% disagree)	Cyberbullied by students (% disagree)	Cyberbullied by colleagues (% disagree)
Faculty members are aware of the university policies and procedures on student conduct, harassment and bullying	40	38	44
University policies and procedures on student conduct, harassment and bullying are clear on prohibited behaviour/sanctions	27	34	39
Policies and procedures on student conduct, harassment and bullying are enforced at this university	18	38	29
Policies and procedures on student conduct, harassment and bullying are effective at this university	20	42	29
Faculty members can access support services if they are victims of cyberbullying at this university	10	28	27

These findings suggested that those who had been victims of cyberbullying had a far more negative view of the university policies and their capacity to adequately address cyberbullying situations. Faculty members who had been victimized by students were particularly concerned that the university policies were not clear, not effective, and not enforced. The questions that were asked of participants in this section only addressed policies relating to student conduct and not conduct by colleagues, as we did not anticipate the relatively high percentage of faculty members who had been cyberbullied by colleagues. Even so, faculty members who had been cyberbullied by colleagues were much more critical of relevant university policies than the total sample of participants. Respondents who had been cyberbullied by students and/or by colleagues also showed a higher level of disagreement regarding access to support services if victimized.

4.4.5 Opinions About Solutions to Cyberbullying at University

Respondents were provided with a list of 15 suggested solutions to cyberbullying at the university level and asked to rank their top five choices. The top three choices overall for faculty respondents were:

1. Develop a more respectful university culture where kind behaviour is modelled by all.
2. Engage the university community in developing a strong university anti-cyberbullying policy.
3. Provide counselling/support services for cyberbullied victims.

Each of these three solutions was ranked among the top five by more than half of the respondents, as were suspending or expelling students who engage in cyberbullying, organizing workshops on cyberbullying and its effects, and creating an anonymous phone-in line for reporting cyberbullying. These rankings were generally agreed upon by both male and female faculty members indicating overall support for a multipronged approach to countering cyberbullying: strengthening policy, modelling respectful behaviour, educating the university community about the problems of cyberbullying, strengthening reporting procedures and victim services, and also dealing strongly with perpetrators.

Gender Differences Some gender differences were evident. Women showed slightly stronger support for dealing harshly with offenders, including involving the police if necessary or expelling students from the university. Male faculty were somewhat more favourable to the provision of counselling/support services to both cyberbullies and their targets, ranking counselling for victims as the top solution overall. Men were less favourable to proactive approaches such as the creation of workshops on cyberbullying or establishing prevention as a priority at the university. Likewise, male faculty were more likely than women to support taking a step back from the problem and employing dispute resolution approaches between concerned parties or letting students take charge of this issue.

4.5   Discussion and Conclusion

These survey findings highlight the pervasiveness of ICT in university life, which has increased the potential of being negatively targeted or cyberbullied. Twenty-five percent of faculty members across four Canadian universities have been victims of cyberbullying at the university in 12 months preceding the administration of the surveys. Fifteen percent were targeted by students and 12% by colleagues. These numbers point to the need for universities to make the prevention and curtailment of cyberbullying a priority, just as it is in schools at the lower levels.

4.5.1   Gender Differences

The gender differences found throughout the survey are the most striking findings to report. This was also the case in our study of student-to-student cyberbullying at the university level (see Faucher et al. 2014). Female faculty, including those in permanent and non-permanent positions, and at both the senior and junior levels, are more likely to be targeted than male faculty members. Both students and colleagues target women faculty more often than they do men.

Female faculty responded to the surveys in far greater numbers than men and almost exclusively women volunteered to be interviewed. Women faculty were more engaged with the problem and expressed a greater level of concern for the potential impacts on them personally as well as professionally. Male respondents tended to have a more hands-off attitude to the problem, as demonstrated by their higher level of agreement with statements such as cyberbullying is normal, it is not the university's responsibility to stop or prevent it, and that students should take charge of the issue and work out their own solutions. Female faculty members, on the other hand, wanted cyberbullying to become more of a priority issue on campus as well as wanting administrators to develop more effective policies and to deal more harshly with offenders, including the possibilities of involvement with the police or expulsion of the offender from the university. Female faculty were less confident than male respondents about the efficacy of current university policies related to cyberbullying as well as the availability of support services for victims.

Female faculty targeted by cyberbullies report a greater range of negative impacts on their professional and personal lives than do men. The fact that nearly three quarters of victims of cyberbullying by students and nearly all of the respondents who reported being cyberbullied by a colleague reported that the cyberbullying came from someone they knew reflects negatively on the work culture of the university. This finding is not specific to these universities, however, as female faculty members have been found to be more vulnerable in other studies as well (DeSouza 2011; Knepp 2012; Lampman 2012; Rowland 2009; Twale and De Luca 2008).

Female victims said the messages they received were insulting, demanding, belittling/demeaning, and/or harassing, and that it affected their ability to work, their mental health, and their relationships inside and/or outside the university, with one quarter wanting to quit. Although women were more likely than men to tell someone about being a target of cyberbullying, they tended to tell a colleague, partner, or friend that they had been targeted rather than an administrator at the university. Of those who did try to stop the cyberbullying, less than half said that their efforts were successful.

4.5.2 Power Imbalances

Many of the findings emerging from the gender differences are consistent with the Power and Control Model explanation mentioned earlier (Pence and Paymar 1993). The Power and Control Model allows us to describe cyberbullying as a form of abuse whereby one party attempts to exert control over the other. Gender is clearly a key factor at play in the Power and Control Model dynamic for cyberbullying at the university level. Female faculty members reported that they were most often targeted for work-related reasons, including professional jealously, status, competitiveness, or to establish power and control. Finally, age was also a factor of significance in cyberbullying between colleagues, one which typically may reflect imbalances in power and control.

There are also indications that racial minority status or speaking English as a second language might make a faculty member more vulnerable to be cyberbullied. These findings, along with gender and age, suggest that a rights-based or *Charter of Rights and Freedoms* lens could be used to analyse the relationship between the marginality a faculty member experiences, and his or her vulnerability to being cyberbullied. It is important to more thoroughly investigate factors such as age, race, ethnicity and language in future studies.

Since tenure and rank did not impact the amount of cyberbullying experienced by faculty members, it may be that a broader understanding of power is needed. Perceived power in the university context may not be uniquely tied to the academic hierarchy. Academic entitlement and consumerist attitudes to education may also lead to power imbalances in favour of the students. The vast majority of faculty who experienced cyberbullying by students attributed the abuse to teaching-related reasons. Academically entitled students may believe they are justified in reacting in a demanding, insulting, or harassing manner when they are dissatisfied with the content or outcomes of their education.

The literature on cyberbullying in the K-12 sector suggests that anonymity may confer power to cyberbullies and leave targets feeling powerless. The same may be true within the higher education context, although anonymity may not wield the same power at this level. Faculty members knew most of the students and all of the colleagues who targeted them. It appears that students still sent harassing, demeaning, and derogatory messages to their instructors, even when their names were attached to the message. Similarly, colleagues did not try to hide their identity when sending a hurtful e-mail to a colleague. There appear to be other factors at work here that need further investigation.

In conclusion, this study raises the issue of cyberbullying of faculty at university and the need for university administrators to develop effective and transparent policies that address the problem and to communicate these policies within the university community. More attention also needs to be given to services for victims. The workplace environment is not a healthy one for those at the receiving end of cyberbullying by students and colleagues. Women faculty members are particularly vulnerable. Much of the cyberbullying is taking place under the radar of administrators since faculty are unlikely to communicate their experiences to those in charge, unless they can be assured that appropriate actions will be taken to help the victim and deal effectively with the perpetrator.

References

Baruch, Y. (2005). Bullying on the net: Adverse behaviour on email and its impact. *Information and Management, 42*, 361–371.

Bauman, S. (2011). *Cyberbullying: What counselors need to know*. Alexandria: American Counseling Association.

Bauman, S. (June 2012). *Research on cyberbullying: A lifespan perspective*. Keynote presentation at International Conference on Cyberbullying: COST IS0801, Paris, France.

Beran, T. N., Rinaldi, C., Bickham, D. S., & Rich, M. (2012). Evidence for the need to support adolescents dealing with harassment and cyber-harassment: Prevalence, progression, and impact. *School Psychology International, 33*(5), 562–576. doi:10.1177/0143034312446976.

Binns, A. (2 March 2007). Staff suffer bullying by students on the web. *Times Higher Education*. www.timeshighereducation.co.uk/208037.article.

Bjorklund, W. L., & Rehling, D. L. (2011). Incivility beyond the classroom. *InSight: A Journal of Scholarly Teaching, 6*, 28–36. www.insightjournal.net.

Blizard, L. M. (2014). *Faculty members' perceived experiences and impact of cyberbullying from students at a Canadian university: A mixed methods study* (Doctoral dissertation, Simon Fraser University, Burnaby, BC). http://summit.sfu.ca/item/13897.

Boice, B. (1996). Classroom incivilities. *Research in Higher Education, 37*(4), 453–486. doi:10.1007/BF01730110.

Boswell, S. S. (2012). "I *deserve* success": Academic entitlement attitudes and their relationships with course self-efficacy, social networking, and demographic variables. *Social Psychology of Education, 15*, 353–365. doi:10.1007/s11218-012-9184-4.

Browne, R. (9 September 2014). Students aren't the only cyberbullying victims. *Maclean's*. http://www.macleans.ca/society/technology/students-arent-the-only-cyberbullying-victims/.

Cassidy, W., Brown, K., & Jackson, M. (2012). 'Under the radar': Educators and cyberbullying in schools. *School Psychology International, 33*(5), 520–532. doi:10.1177/0143034312445245.

Cassidy, W., Faucher, C., & Jackson, M. (2013). Cyberbullying among youth: A comprehensive review of current international research and its implications and application to policy and practice. *School Psychology International, 34*(6), 575–612. doi:10.1177/0143034313479697.

CCSO Cybercrime Working Group. (2013). *Cyberbullying and the non-consensual distribution of intimate images*. (Report to the Federal/Provincial/Territorial Ministers Responsible for Justice and Public Safety). Ottawa, ON: Department of Justice, Canada. www.justice.gc.ca/eng/rp-pr/other-autre/cndii-cdncii/pdf/cndii-cdncii-eng.pdf.

Chowning, K., & Campbell, N. J. (2009). Development and validation of a measure of academic entitlement: Individual differences in students' externalized responsibility and entitled expectations. *Journal of Educational Psychology, 101*(4), 982–997. doi:10.1037/a0016351.

Ciani, K. D., Summers, J. J., & Easter, M. A. (2008). Gender differences in academic entitlement among college students. *The Journal of Genetic Psychology, 169*(4), 332–344. doi:10.3200/GNTP.169.4.332-344.

Clark, C. M., Werth, L., & Ahten, S. (2012). Cyber-bullying and incivility in the online learning environment, part 1: Addressing faculty and student perceptions. *Nurse Educator, 37*(4), 150–156.

Cortina, L. M., Magley, V. J., Williams, J. H., & Langout, R. D. (2001). Incivility in the workplace: Incidence and impact. *Journal of Occupational Health Psychology, 6*(1), 64–80. doi:10.1037//1076-8998.6.1.64.

Council of Canadian Academies. (2012). *Strengthening Canada's research rapacity: The gender dimension—The expert panel on women in university research*. Ottawa: Council of Canadian Academies.

Cowie, H., Bauman, S., Coyne, I., Myers, C., Pörhölä, M., & Almeida, A. (2013). Cyberbullying amongst university students: An emergent cause for concern? In P. K. Smith & G. Steffgen (Eds.), *Cyberbullying through the new media: Findings from an international network* (pp. 165–177). London: Psychology Press.

D'Cruz, P., & Noronha, E. (2013). Navigating the extended reach: Target experiences of cyberbullying at work. *Information and Organization, 23*, 324–343. doi:10.1016/j.infoandorg.2013.09.001.

Daniloff, D. (2009). Cyberbullying goes to college. *Bostonia*. www.bu.edu/bostonia/spring09.

DeSouza, E. R. (2011). Frequency rates and correlates of contrapower harassment in higher education. *Journal of Interpersonal Violence, 26*(1), 158–188. doi:10.1177/0886260510362878.

Dilmaç, B. (2009). Psychological needs as a predictor of cyber bullying: A preliminary report on college students. *Educational Sciences: Theory & Practice, 9*(3), 1307–1325. www.edam.com.tr/kuyeb/en/default.asp.

Dooley, J. J., Pyżalski, J., & Cross, D. (2009). Cyberbullying versus face-to-face bullying: A theoretical and conceptual review. *Journal of Psychology, 217*(4), 182–188. doi:10.1027/0044-3409.217.4.182.

Englander, E. K. (2008). Cyberbullying and information exposure: User-generated content in post-secondary education. In Massachusetts Aggression Research Center (MARC) Publications, Paper 11. http://vc.bridgew.edu/marc_pubs/11.

Faucher, C., Jackson, M., & Cassidy, W. (2014). Cyberbullying among university students: Gendered experiences, impacts, and perspectives. *Education Research International*. doi:10.1155/2014/698545.

Finn, J. (2004). A survey of online harassment at a university campus. *Journal of Interpersonal Violence, 19*, 468–483. doi:10.1177/0886260503262083.

Greenberger, E., Lessard, J., Chen, C., & Farruggia, S. P. (2008). Self-entitled college students: Contributions of personality, parenting, and motivational factors. *Journal of Youth and Adolescence, 37*, 1193–1204. doi:10.1007/S10964-008-9284-9.

Grigg, D. W. (2010). Cyber-aggression: Definition and concept of cyberbullying. *Australian Journal of Guidance and Counselling, 20*(2), 143–156. doi:10.1375/ajgc.20.2.143.

Halder, D., & Jaishankar, K. (2009). Cyber socializing and victimization of women. *Temida, 5*–26. doi:10.2298/TEM0903005H.

Hinduja, S., & Patchin, J. W. (2012). *School climate 2.0: Preventing cyberbullying and sexting one classroom at a time*. Thousand Oaks: Corwin.

Jackson, M., Cassidy, W., & Brown, K. (2009). *"you were born ugly and youl die ugly too": Cyber-bullying as relational aggression. In Education: Special Issue on Technology and Social Media, Part, 1,* 15(2), 68–82. http://www.ineducation.ca/article/you-were-born-ugly-and-youl-die-ugly-too-cyber-bullying-relational-aggression.

Jones, J. C., & Scott, S. (2012). Cyberbullying in the university classroom: A multiplicity of issues. In L. A. Wankel & C. Wankel (Eds.), *Misbehavior online in higher education: Cutting-edge technologies in higher education* (pp. 157–182). Bingley: Emerald.

Knepp, K. A. F. (2012). Understanding student and faculty incivility in higher education. *The Journal of Effective Teaching, 12*(1), 33–46. www.uncw.edu/cte/et/.

Kopp, J. P., & Finney, S. J. (2013). Linking academic entitlement and student incivility using latent means modeling. *Journal of Experimental Education, 81*(3), 322–336. doi:10.1080/00220973. 2012.727887.

Kowalski, R. M., Limber, S. P., & Agatston, P. W. (2012). *Cyberbullying: Bullying in the digital age* (2nd ed.). Malden: Wiley-Blackwell.

Lampman, C. (2012). Women faculty at risk: U.S. professors report on their experiences with student incivility, bullying, aggression, and sexual attention. *NASPA Journal About Women in Higher Education, 5*(2), 184–208. doi:10.1515/njawhe-2012-1108.

Li, Q. (2005). New bottle but old wine: A research of cyberbullying in schools. *Computers in Human Behavior, 23*(4), 1777–1791. doi:10.1016/j.chb.2005.10.005.

Martin, Q., & Olson, D. (2011). College cyberbullying: The virtual bathroom wall. *The Journal of Technology in Student Affairs, Summer*. [online edition].

McKay, R., Arnold, D. H., Fratzl, J., & Thomas, R. (2008). Workplace bullying in academia: A Canadian study. *Employee Responsibility and Rights Journal, 20*, 77–100. doi:10.1007/s10672-008-9073-3.

McQuade, S. C., Colt, J. P., & Meyer, N. B. B. (2009). *Cyber bullying: Protecting kids and adults from online bullies*. Westport: Praeger.

Menesini, E. (2012). Cyberbullying: The right value of the phenomenon. Comments on the paper "Cyberbullying: An overrated phenomenon?". *European Journal of Developmental Psychology, 9*(5), 544–552. doi:10.1080/17405629.2012.706449.

Meyers, S. A., Bender, J., Hill, E. K., & Thomas, S. Y. (2006). How do faculty experience and respond to classroom conflict? *International Journal of Teaching and Learning in Higher Education, 18*(3), 180–187. http://isetl.org/ijtlhe/.

Minor, M. A., Smith, G. S., & Brashen, H. (2013). Cyberbullying in higher education. *Journal of Educational Research and Practice, 3*(1), 15–29. doi:10.5590/JERAP.2013.03.1.02.

Molluzzo, J. C., & Lawler, J. P. (2012). A study of the perceptions of college students on cyberbullying. *Information Systems Education Journal, 10*(4), 84–109. http://isedj.org/2012-10/.

Morrissette, P. J. (2001). *Reducing incivility in the university/college classroom. International Electronic Journal for Leadership in Education, 5*(4), 1–13. http://www.ucalgary.ca/iejll/morrissette.

Nocentini, A., Calmaestra, J., Schultze-Krumboltz, A., Scheithauer, H., Ortega, R., & Menesini, E. (2010). Cyberbullying: Labels, behaviours and definition in three European countries. *Australian Journal of Guidance and Counselling, 20*(2), 129–142. doi:10.1375/ajgc.20.2.129.

Olweus, D. (1993). *Bullying at school: What we know and what we can do*. New York: Blackwell.

Patchin, J. W., & Hinduja, S. (2012). Cyberbullying: An update and synthesis of the research. In J. W. Patchin & S. Hinduja (Eds.), *Cyberbullying prevention and response: Expert perspectives* (pp. 13–35). New York: Routledge.

Pence, E., & Paymar, M. (1993). *Education groups for men who batter: The Duluth model*. New York: Springer Publishing.

Piotrowski, C. (2012). From workplace bullying to cyberbullying: The enigma of e-harassment in modern organizations. *Organization Development Journal, 30*(4), 44–53.

Privitera, C., & Campbell, M. A. (2009). Cyberbullying: The new face of workplace bullying? *CyberPsychology and Behaviour, 12*, 395–400. doi:10.1089/cpb.2009.0025.

Rowland, M. L. (2009). *Faculty experiences with incivility in adult higher education*. Paper presented at the Midwest Research-to-Practice Conference. Chicago, IL.

Schenk, A. M., & Fremouw, W. J. (2012). Prevalence, psychological impact, and coping of cyberbully victims among college students. *Journal of School Violence, 11*(1), 21–37. doi:10.1080/15388220.2011.630310.

Shariff, S., & Gouin, R. (September 2005). *CYBER-DILEMMAS: Gendered hierarchies, free expression and cyber-safety in schools*. Paper presented at Oxford Internet Institute International conference Safety and Security in a Networked World. Oxford, UK. www.oii.ox.ac.uk/cyber-safety.

Smith, P. K. (2012). Cyberbullying and cyber aggression. In S. R. Jimerson, A. B. Nickerson, M. J. Mayer, & M. J. Furlong (Eds.), *Handbook of school violence and school safety: International research and practice* (2nd ed., pp. 93–103). New York: Routledge.

Smith, P. K., & Slonje, R. (2010). Cyberbullying: The nature and extent of a new kind of bullying, in and out of school. In S. R. Jimerson, S. M. Swearer, & D. L. Espelage (Eds.), *Handbook of bullying in schools: An international perspective* (pp. 249–262). New York: Routledge.

Smith, P. K., Mahdavi, J., Carvalho, M., Fisher, S., Russell, S., & Tippett, N. (2008). Cyberbullying: Its nature and impact in secondary school pupils. *Journal of Child Psychology and Psychiatry, 49*(4), 376–385. doi:10.1111/j.1469-7610.2007.01846.x.

Tokunaga, R. S. (2010). Following you home from school: A critical review and synthesis of research on cyberbullying victimization. *Computers in Human Behavior, 26*(3), 277–287. doi:10.1016/j.chb.2009.11.014.

Topcu, Ç., & Erdur-Baker, Ö (2012). Affective and cognitive empathy as mediators of gender differences in cyber and traditional bullying. *School Psychology International, 33*(5), 550–561. doi:10.1177/0143034312446882.

Turan, N., Polat, O., Karapirli, M., Uysal, C., & Turan, S. G. (2011). The new violence type of the era: Cyber bullying among university students—Violence among university students. *Neurology, Psychiatry and Brain Research, 17*, 21–26. doi:10.1016/j.npbr.2011.02.005.

Twale, D. J., & De Luca, B. M. (2008). *Faculty incivility: The rise of the academic bully culture and what to do about it.* San Francisco: Jossey-Bass.

Vance, J. W. (2010). *Cyber-harassment in higher education: Online learning environments* (Ed.D. dissertation). University of Southern California, Los Angeles, CA. http://digitallibrary.usc.edu/cdm/ref/collection/p15799coll127/id/309077.

Vandebosch, H., & Van Cleemput, K. (2009). Cyber bullying among youngsters: Prevalence and profile of bullies and victims. *New Media & Society, 11*, 1349–1371. doi:10.1177/1461444809341263.

von Marées, N., & Petermann, F. (2012). Cyberbullying: An increasing challenge for schools. *School Psychology International, 33*(5), 467–476. doi:10.1177/0143034312445241.

Walker, C. M., Sockman, B. R., & Koehn, S. (2011). An exploratory study of cyberbullying with undergraduate university students. *TechTrends, 55*(2), 31–38. doi:10.1007/S1152-011-0481-0.

Wankel, L. A., & Wankel, C. (2012). Misbehavior online, a new frontier in higher education: Introduction. In L. A. Wankel & C. Wankel (Eds.), *Misbehavior online in higher education: Cutting-edge technologies in higher education* (pp. 1–10). Bingley: Emerald.

Wensley, K., & Campbell, M. (2012). Heterosexual and nonheterosexual young university students' involvement in traditional and cyber forms of bullying. *Cyberpsychology, Behavior, and Social Networking, 15*(12), 649–654. doi:10.1089/cyber.2012.0132.

Wildermuth, S., & Davis, C. B. (2012). Flaming the faculty: Exploring root causes, consequences, and potential remedies to the problem of instructor-focused uncivil online student discourse in higher education. In L. A. Wankel & C. Wankel (Eds.), *Misbehavior online in higher education: Cutting-edge technologies in higher education* (pp. 379–404). Bingley: Emerald.

Yilmaz, H. (2011). Cyberbullying in Turkish middle schools: An exploratory study. *School Psychology International, 32*(6), 645–654. doi:10.1177/0143034311410262.

Zhang, A. T., Land, L. P. W., & Dick, G. (2010). Key influences of cyberbullying for university students. *PACIS 2010 Proceedings.* Paper 83. http://aisel.aisnet.org/pacis2010/83.

Chapter 5
Family Relationships and Cyberbullying

Sofía Buelga, Belén Martínez-Ferrer and Gonzalo Musitu

Research about existing relations between family relationships and cyberbullying (CB), as a form of harassment among peers that differs from traditional bullying, is still relatively new. As Low and Espelage (2013) indicate, just as when research into traditional bullying began, scientific literature on this harassment involving use of new technologies has firstly centered on knowing the prevalence and incidence of this behavior among adolescents to the detriment of analyzing the underlying risk and protection factors. This chapter analyzes the family setting in relation to CB, and particularly it will be focused on the following variables: parent–children (family) communication, socialization, and parental monitoring by underlining the communalities that exist with bullying in adolescence.

5.1 Family Functioning, Bullying, and Cyberbullying

Family functioning refers to the set of characteristics that define a family as a group and explains its regular features and how it behaves (McCubbin and McCubbin 2013; McCubbin and Thompson 1987). In families with adolescents, their psychosocial adaptation will depend on the family group balance to which they belong to a great extent, that is, on family functioning. This, in turn, depends on the family group's capacity to adapt to the changes, which emerge in the family, for example, when one family member reaches adolescence, the emotional and affective link,

S. Buelga (✉)
Department of Social Psychology, University of Valencia, 46010 Valencia, Spain
e-mail: sofia.buelga@uv.es

B. Martínez-Ferrer
Department of Education and Social Psychology, Pablo de Olavide University, Seville, Spain

G. Musitu
Department of Psychology, Pablo de Olavide University, Seville, Spain

© Springer International Publishing Switzerland 2016
R. Navarro et al. (eds.), *Cyberbullying Across the Globe,*
DOI 10.1007/978-3-319-25552-1_5

and the quality of communication, among family members. At the same time, it is also well known that the degree of adolescents' adaptation can also have an influence on the family group. For example, adolescents' participation in risk or unhealthy behaviors (e.g., criminal conducts, violence, taking certain substances, or unsuitable use of new technologies) can become a serious stressor for the family and affect its balance or even make its imbalance more acute.

One particularly critical stage for family balance is when one of the family members reaches adolescence. In a family with adolescent members, it is necessary to renegotiate the degree of independence and control at all levels. We quite often perceive that development-type changes and adolescents' requirements disrupt good family functioning, so it is also necessary to reorganize the rules of interaction between parents and children (Keijsers and Poulin 2013; Minuchin 1974). Therefore, in this stage, growing flexibility for family limits must exist to accept children's independence, and to manage a whole of changes that allow adolescents to move inside and outside the family system. One particular task the family faces is to synchronize two antagonistic movements: the system moves toward the family group unit, maintaining affective links and a feeling of belonging; a shift toward differentiation and singular members' autonomy (Díaz-Morales et al. 2014).

During this period, it is necessary to transform family relationships in order to replace the unilateral paternal–maternal authority by using a more participative and cooperative communication style with children. The family should increase the level of reciprocity and equality in the parent–children interaction, especially considering that adolescents start questioning parental authority during adolescence and demanding a certain degree of autonomy, which is a relevant part for them to form their identity.

This autonomy does not mean family relationships breakup but will change and become more equal and reciprocal. Autonomy is not merely external but is also internal so that adolescents have the chance to make decisions that affect their own life without feeling guilty and having to judge their own actions according to the criteria attributed to their parents. In line with this, Steinberg (1985, 2000) points out in his classic studies that the search for the typical autonomy of adolescence comprises three types of independence: emotional autonomy, behavioral autonomy, and autonomy of values.

Furthermore, this emancipation process is not linear, it is influenced by personal traits and parents' behavior. Therefore, we must place the definitions of self that were valid in childhood to one side and shape a self that adapts to experience. It is also necessary for adolescents to maintain their link with parents to receive their approval and agreement; in other words, adolescents not only wish parents to recognize that they are no longer children but also expect them to approve the new changes that come into play that form their identity.

Indeed conflicts between parents and children are often merely a consequence associated with adolescents' search for more freedom to make their own decisions, based on their perception, but their parents threaten this freedom. Therefore, one of the main causes of family conflict in adolescence is precisely the degree of control that parents have on certain aspects of adolecents' life. Adolescents claim freedom in an increasing number of areas that were previously under their parents' control.

In adolescence, youths start to consider that certain matters depend on personal decision-making, a view that parents do not always share. Thus when parents wish to control their offspring's more personal areas, for example, their use of social networks, conflicts arise. Yet these conflicts can sometimes be an excellent chance for parents to assess and review their own beliefs to make the relationship with their children more flexible. Conflicts also allow to amend, if necessary, the rules of interaction among family members so that everyone involved can demonstate their understanding, respect, and approval of other people's opinions (Longmore et al. 2013; Wray-Lake et al. 2010). The following sections analyze essential aspects of family functioning, such as family climate, parent–child communication, and socialization in the family in relation to CB.

Empirical evidence for behavior problems in adolescence, which includes violence among peers, has consistently shown the importance of the family to explain such behaviors. The research by Ybarra and Mitchell (2004) is one of the first studies to link CB with family variables. These authors found that poor family relationships, evaluated by poor monitoring, lack an emotional link and that frequent severe discipline relates with more frequent cyberaggression and victimization. As David-Ferdon and Hertz (2009) state, the fact that cyberbullies appear more willing to participate in other forms of aggression with peers suggests underlying risk factors that are common to different violent expressions. CB and bullying, especially verbal and relational forms, appear to be the expression of challenging or transgressor behavior that is tolerated more than physical bullying (Low and Espelage 2013). It doubtlessly seems that both harassment expressions between peers must respond to a similar family reality. This might be because the environments, where such virtual and non-virtual behaviors take place, interrelate and affect each other (Kowalski et al. 2014; Subrahmanyam and Šmahel 2011). Table 5.1 summarizes the family variables related with bullying and CB.

Nonetheless, the relationship between both harassment expressions among peers seems more complex than it initially appeared because being a perpetrator or a victim in a given setting does not necessarily entail playing an identical role in other contexts. A previous study affirmed a positive relation between being an aggressive victim in traditional bullying situations and participating as a cyberbully on the Internet (Taiariol 2010). Other authors have also stated that a low percentage of youths are victims or perpetrators of CB but not involved in school bullying (Kowalski et al. 2014; Olweus 2012).

Table 5.1 Family predictor factors of bullying and cyberbullying

Aoyama et al. 2012; Buelga 2013; Hinduja and Patchin 2013; Kowalski et al. 2014; Makri-Botsari and Karagianni 2014; Navarro et al. 2013; Rosen et al. 2008; Wade and Beran 2011; Wang et al. 2009	Authoritarian parental style and excessive use of punishment
	Permissiveness and tolerance of offspring's aggressive behavior
	Inconsistent, ineffective discipline, which can be too slack or too severe
	Lack of parental affection, support, and implication
	Family communication problems
	Conflicts between partners or between parents and children
	Use of violence at home to solve family conflicts

5.1.1 Family Climate

Family climate, as a closely linked dimension to family functioning, is one of the most widely studied variables in the onset and explanation of nonadaptive behaviors and violent behaviors among offspring (Becvar 2013; Musitu 2013; Rueger et al. 2010). This concept alludes to the climate perceived and constructed by family members and includes three dimensions: cohesion, expressiveness, and conflict (Moos and Moos 1981; Musitu et al. 2001; Tippett et al. 2013).

We can define cohesion as the emotional link perceived by family members, which suggests an affective dimension of family climate (Olson 1986; Scabini and Manzi 2011). Many studies have demonstrated that cohesion is an important factor to protect children getting involved in violent behaviors (Moreno 2013; Sijtsema et al. 2013). Former studies have found an association of cohesion with fewer children participating as perpetrators and victims for CB (Ortega-Barón 2013; Taiariol 2010). These findings corroborate the importance of cohesion as a protector factor of violent behavior, and in a virtual setting, as it promotes a greater feeling of security and reinforces the parent–children emotional connection (Sijtsema et al. 2013; Solecki et al. 2014).

Family conflict also presents major implications in children's adaptation. The usual arguments and fights between parents and between parents and children, above all prevalence of violent and nonfunctional conflict-solving strategies, can predict violent attitudes and behaviors in children (Martínez-Ferrer et al. 2011b; Moreno 2013). A two-way relation exists between a high rate of dispute in the family and behavior problems in adolescents. Family conflicts can generate nonadaptive behaviors in children. Normally these behaviors imply more family stress, which for families with poor family functioning, aggravates the existing family climate with new arguments. When the family takes no functional measures to solve this, the negative family interaction pattern worsens, hence the level of family conflictiveness rises (Becvar 2013; Martínez-Ferrer et al. 2009).

Consequently, violent behavior becomes worse and generalizes to other relevant settings for adolescents, for example, schools, the community, the virtual setting (Buelga and Chóliz 2013; Kiriakidis and Kavoura 2010; Schenk et al. 2013). Therefore, cohesion and conflict dimensions of family climate are related with a greater implication in violent behaviors in different contexts and evidently with less promotion of children's social and personal resources. This implies a greater predisposition to becoming a perpetrator (Buist et al. 2004; Martínez-Ferrer et al. 2011a), while not having enough psychosocial resources predisposes to being a victim of violence (Buelga et al. 2014).

5.1.2 Parent–Children Communication

One of the most relevant variables in research on the family and adolescence is family communication. In his classic studies on family functioning, David H. Olson

(1985, 1991) underlines that a quality family climate depends on the type of family communication. Family communication is the facilitating dimension upon which to construct parents–children relationships, the emotional link, and the way to confront and solve problems and conflicts in the family context (Olson 1986, 1991).

Hence positive, fluent, and open communication with clear, respectful, and empathetic exchanges of viewpoints between parents and children reinforces family cohesion, reduces conflict and favors psychosocial adaptation in family members (Branje et al. 2013; Longmore et al. 2013; Solecki et al. 2014). Positive and inductive parent–children communication relates with less implication in aggressive behaviors, in the online and offline settings (Appel et al. 2014). In bullying studies it has been observed that victims who positively appreciate communication with their parents have reported lower levels of depression symptoms, perceived stress and solitude compared with victims who have family communication problems (Cava 2011; Estévez et al. 2006; Proctor and Linley 2014). Otherwise, negative, cutting or challenging communication among family members can be a very important factor in the onset of children's violent and criminal conduct (Estévez and Emler 2010; Moral and Ovejero 2013).

This connection between family communication and violence is also evident in CB. In a study by Ortega-Baron (2013), cyberbullies showed inappropriate patterns of family communication, characterized by offensive communication filled with critical and unclear messages. As with traditional bullying, negative family communication strongly relates with the perception of poor parental support, which relates, in turn, with high levels of CB (Wang et al. 2009; Solecki et al. 2014). It would seem that negative communication and insufficient parental support relate with not only less self-control in children but also with more frequent participation in aggressive behavior and CB. Likewise, cybervictims, normally of the aggressive type, frequently perceive family communication as a problem and something to avoid. They feel they do not have the necessary opening to share this problem with their parents. The negative climate increases persistence in cybervictimization dynamics, which ends up settling in children's interior world and transforming family processes into circularities (Makri-Botsari and Karagianni 2014). Children frequently attempt to break these circularities by resorting to the people they feel closer to, normally peers. However, they do not often find the help they expected because peers lack the resources needed to solve this situation (Brooks et al. 2012; Martínez-Ferrer 2013).

The immediate diffusion of CB and loss of control of this diffusion make it extremely hard for cybervictims to solve the CB problem, even with peers' help. For example, eliminating a victim's false profile or a forum created to insult or to humiliate victims requires parents' active participation because removing such content normally entails resorting to professionals and legal measures. When family communication is poor and conflictive, children avoid sharing such distressing situations, so parents are unaware of not only the CB problem their children suffer, but also the emotional distress they endure. Along these lines, González-Prada et al. (2014) state that in 10 of every 13 suicide cases among adolescent CB victims, the family had no idea that their child was a victim of online violence.

5.2   Parental Styles and Cyberbullying

Darling and Steinberg (1993) and Musitu (2002) defined parental styles as a collection of attitudes toward one's offspring, which collectively create an "emotional
climate" in which to express parents' behaviors. These behaviors include those that
help achieve a socialization objective and those that do not, such as gesture, tone of
voice, body language, and spontaneous expression of emotions.

Based on two dimensions, implication/acceptance and control/imposition,
Musitu and García (2004) developed a proposal of four types of parental socialization styles. Implication and acceptance refer to the affective dimension. Parents appear to be affectionate and loving toward their children when they behave suitably
but attempt to reason and dialog with them about the unsuitability of their behavior
when they behave incorrectly. If, however, parents' level of implication/acceptance
is low when their children's behaviors are suitable, parents show indifference, and
when these behaviors are not suitable, parents do not dialog or attempt to reason
with them and are completely indifferent to their children's behaviors, regardless of
them being suitable or not.

The above authors observed that the control/imposition dimension is independent of the implication/acceptance dimension. Parents employing high levels of
control/imposition when their children do not behave as they wish, and irrespectively of them reasoning with them or not, they attempt to impose their criterion so
that their children do not repeat such behavior. This control can be physical, verbal,
or can consist in depriving their children of something that they positively appreciate, for example, meeting up with friends, watching TV or using the Internet.

Different researchers have been observed that parental styles, also known as educational styles, have an influence on behavior problems that children develop, such
as implication in violent behaviors and harassing peers (Kokkinos 2013; Manuel
et al. 2014). Likewise, parental styles influence online behavior in adolescents
(Rosen et al. 2008), possibly because, as former studies have confirmed, using the
Internet is an activity performed mainly at home (Valcke et al. 2010).

The relation between parental styles and CB appears to follow the same pattern
as in traditional bullying and in other violent expressions. Styles that are emotionally inadequate, poorly democratic and too much punishment can be associated
with adolescents getting more involved in violent behaviors (Longmore et al. 2013;
Moral and Ovejero 2013). In particular, there is a link between authoritarian and
careless styles, characterized by low implication/acceptance, and children participating more in CB behaviors as perpetrators (Makri-Botsari and Karagianni 2014;
Rosen et al. 2008). Also as in traditional bullying, adolescents from authoritarian-
type families, characterized by rejection and little communication, employ more
aggressive forms of CB (Makri-Botsari and Karagianni 2014). There is also a relation between careless/authoritarian styles and greater cybervictimization (Kokkinos
2013; Ybarra and Mitchell 2004). Both careless/authoritarian styles share poor affection, and little implication/acceptance by children, and this aspect relates closely
with both CB and cybervictimization (Accordino and Accordino 2011; Kowalski
et al. 2014, Ybarra and Mitchell 2004).

Conversely, authoritative and permissive styles, which share many similarities with indulgence style based on affection and implication, relate with less cyber-victimization. Moreover when adolescents come from families where styles are predominantly authoritative and permissive, children express more trust in their parents–children relationships, so they share such problems with their parents much more easily when they are the object of CB than adolescents whose parents use authoritarian/careless styles more frequently (Makri-Botsari and Karagianni 2014). Children who perceive that family relationships are close and feel a strong emotional link with their parents are less likely to get involved in CB. Moreover, if these children are vicitims of negative behavior, they approach their parents more asking for help, which relates with a positive perception of parental support. As pointed out by Musitu and Cava (2001), parental styles that evoke affection and parents' implication are more efficacious than styles that evoke imposition to achieve. For example, adolescents with affective parental styles internalized a feeling of responsibility for their own actions and better accepted rules.

Therefore, parental implication, the existence of an emotional link and dialog between parents and children are very important aspects to learn functional forms of social interaction, which evidently include interactions over new technologies. These findings suggest continuity between offline and online contexts that goes beyond areas of attitudes, preferences and social relationships. According to Makri-Botsari and Karagianni (2014), adolescents transfer the challenges they face to the cyberspace and the emotions they feel to the real (offline) setting. Therefore, those adolescents who perceive their family relationships as poorly expressive in emotional terms, who have difficulties communicating with their parents, and whose relationships with their parents involve indifference or rejection are more likely to get involved in aggressive behaviors over the Internet.

It is also interesting to underline that parental socialization styles are stable in all aspects related with adolescents' life and their family climate. Therefore, it is interesting to add the proposal of Valcke et al. (2010) about parental styles on the Internet *(Internet Parenting Styles)* based on two dimensions: control and parental implication on the Internet. Parental control reflects, on the one hand, the degree to which parents are present and are, on the other hand, a guide for children when they browse the Internet and establish rules of its use and when certain actions are forbidden that parents regard as negative. Parental implication and warmth allude to communication with and support of children in matters in the settings they participate in, which include security in new technologies, for the purpose of creating a supporting and respectful climate where children can express their concerns and doubts about using the information and communications technology (ICT). Implication and warmth also refer to parents' attitude of understanding and respect when they find out that their children have browsed non-recommended Internet sites of risk. This dimension also alludes to parents and children jointly using the Internet and sharing websites to visit and dialog on. If we bear both dimensions in mind, these authors establish four parental styles on the Internet that present major communalities with the aforementioned parental styles:

- Permissive style: high degree of implication and poor control, as reflected in lack of explicit limits in children's online performance that provides fondness and warmth but barely guides them in their cybernetic behavior. These parents avoid confrontations with their children, give them whatever they ask, and respect their ideas and wishes.
- The laissez-faire style: poor implication/control, careless style in classic formulations, characterized by lack of support, poor communication about aspects of new technologies, and no rules about and restrictions of Internet use.
- Authoritative style: high level of implication/control, evidenced in behaviors that imply clear rules and practices about, for instance, the time that children can spend using the Internet. These parents talk to their children about Internet-related aspects and expect their children to be responsible and behave on the Internet in a self-adjusting manner.
- Authoritarian style: low level of implication and high level of control, characterized by a search for inconditional obedience and by accepting their ideas about Internet use. There is very little talk about Internet-related subjects, and they show no inclination to dialog about or negotiate Internet access.

5.3   Parental Monitoring of Internet Use and CB Prevention

One of the most widely studied themes has been parental monitoring of Internet use and its relation with inappropriate online behaviors, considering that behaviors such as CB are done from home, irrespectively of using a mobile device or not. Nevertheless, most parents are unaware of the interactions that take place on the Internet and whether their children are cyberbullies or cybervictims (Gasior 2010; Taiariol 2010; Valcke et al. 2010). The influence that parental monitoring has on CB must be stronger than the impact on other violent behaviors like verbal and relational bullying because most CB occurs when children are at home and alone in their own rooms (Buelga 2013; Low and Espelage 2013).

Parental monitoring of online use comprises controlling the time that children spend using the Internet and involves monitoring the websites they visit, the contacts they establish in the social networks, and the activities they carry out. To go about this, parents establish rules and adopt other mechanisms to control their children's online activities that allow the transmission of attitudes and values in relation to the behavior shown in virtual settings. Parental monitoring of online use enables a surer feeling of security and self-adjustment with online behavior (Sasson and Mesch 2014; Vandebosch 2014).

Many studies have underlined that parental monitoring of children's online use is a protection factor for the involvement in risk behaviors on the Internet, especially in childhood and at the beginning of adolescence, since parental monitoring lowers the participation in behaviors like CB, exposure to pornography, and revealing personal data (Lwin et al. 2008; Navarro et al. 2013). Conversely, several studies have found a relation between poor parental monitoring of the online activities and a higher risk of participating in CB behaviors as either a cyberbully (Buelga et al. 2015; Kowalski et al. 2014) and a cybervictim (Aoyama et al. 2012; Low and Espelage 2013; Taiariol 2010).

The parental monitoring strategies adopted to control children's online behavior are called *parental mediation* (Navarro et al. 2013; Sasson and Mesch 2014) which, according to Livingstone and Helsper (2008), we can group into the following types: active co-use, restrictions in interaction, technical restrictions, monitoring. *Active co-use* includes all the strategies used to limit user-system interactivity, such as sharing personal data, online shopping, filling in forms and questionnaires, or downloading applications when children are alone. Therefore, these activities must take place only when parents and children browse the Internet together. Parents can also establish social rules (forbidding or restricting activities) and technical restrictions (filtering or blocking certain activities). *Restrictions in the interaction* center on forbidding social or peer-to-peer activities, for example, using e-mail, chat, instant messaging, online games, and illegal downloading. Using *technical restrictions* is one of the exclusive mediation strategies for Internet-related risk behaviors. Finally, *open or hidden control of an adolescent's online activity* alludes to monitoring the behaviors that take place after using the Internet. This strategy has received much criticism as it can infringe children's privacy.

Another possible classification of parental monitoring on the Internet entails adopting three strategies: restrictive mediation, evaluative mediation, and co-use. As indicated by Navarro et al. (2013), *restrictive mediation* includes parental strategies that enable parents to control the websites visited, the software installed or the electronic devices employed. *Evaluative mediation* refers to establishing rules and norms about the information that adolescents must not share or the time they spend on the Internet. Finally, *co-use* implies that parents actively participate with their children when they access the Internet, and they recommend, help, and guide them when they browse the Internet.

There are many studies which suggest that using different parental mediation strategies lowers the likelihood of adolescents getting involved in online risk behaviors. For example, the perspective of parents studying a possible punishment seems to dissuade adolescents from participating in CB behaviors (Hinduja and Patchin 2013). There is also an association that links strict rules about Internet use, intervention and parental mediation with less likelihood of being a cybervictim of different forms of CB (Leung and Lee 2012). It would seem that the time an adolescent spends on the Internet is an important predictor of cybervictimization (Hinduja and Patchin 2008, 2013; Sasson et al. 2011).

Nonetheless, parental mediation is not exempt of some controversy and major restrictions. It is important to stress that although parents wish to actively participate in this type of monitoring, they frequently do not know how to carry it out because many parents possess less knowledge of the Internet than their children (Buelga 2013; Buelga and Chóliz 2013). Children and adolescents are *digital natives* (Prensky 2001) who have been born and bred with the development of a highly advanced technological society. Consequently, they have more technological knowledge than their parents, the so-called *digital immigrant generations*. This digital gap means that suitable parental monitoring of their children's cybernetic activity is difficult.

Some authors have found a relation between parents having better knowledge of new technologies and less participation of their children in CB behaviors (Mesch 2009; Navarro et al. 2013; Vandebosch 2014). Thus, many CB prevention programs include training and resources for parents and teachers that allow them to use new technologies securely and jointly with their children/students and which provide them with information about dangers on the Internet.

Parental knowledge about new technologies and trusting parents–children relationships plays a key role in the appearance, maintenance, and prevention of CB (Makri-Botsari and Karagianni 2014).

5.3.1 Parental Monitoring of Internet Use or Family Communication?

As mentioned earlier, one of the most well-studied family variables to prevent CB is parental monitoring, also known as parental mediation. Most research coincides in highlighting the role played by parental mediation in preventing CB and stresses that active monitoring, restriction, and supervision to less occurrence of cyber-victimization and CB. Yet much controversy about these statements still exists, which, despite their objective being safe Internet use, neither are always efficient nor promote self-adjustment in online behavior.

The parental control of online activities shows no similar effectiveness throughout life cycle; indeed the opposite is true as this strategy does not seem to offer the desired success in mid- or late adolescence. In fact, Law et al. (2010) pointed out that monitoring practices, such as controlling children's Internet access, relate with cyberaggression behaviors. Conversely, maintaining open communication with children about Internet use has proved a relevant resource because it alerts adolescents about the chances, risks, and scope of their behaviors on the Internet (Appel et al. 2014; Sasson et al. 2011; Solecki et al. 2014). Adolescents who talk more with their parents spontaneously about their Internet activities are less likely to participate in CB behaviors (Law et al. 2010; Stattin and Kerr 2000). When adolescents face potentially harmful Internet contents, the individuals who positively appreciate communication with their parents normally talk about these experiences (Appel et al. 2014). The answer to the question posed in this section is that family communication is more effective for controlling children's behavior in the specific use of new technologies, especially with adolescents.

5.4 Preventing CB in the Family: The Importance of Family Communication

As we previously stressed, family relationships can increase the risk of adolescents getting involved in CB as perpetrators or victims. Yet, the family can also protect adolescents from participating in forms of bullying using new technologies, as formerly observed with traditional bullying and other behavior problems. There are studies that have reported a close link between a negative family context and adolescents having fewer social and individual resources (Buist et al. 2004; Longmore et al. 2013; Proctor and Linley 2014), and this close link relates to a higher degree of vulnerability to victimization (Buelga et al. 2014; Van Dijk et al. 2014). Indeed those adolescents who positively value the family climate and family communication make better use of their personal resources and are, therefore, less vulnerable to peer victimization at school (Povedano et al. 2012). As one of the main sources of support, the family plays a central role in preventing the many dangers presented in the cyberspace for children: access to pornographic material, sexual blackmail (e.g., grooming), or aggressive behaviors with peers caused by CB situations (Navarro et al. 2013; Subrahmanyam and Šmahel 2011).

Undoubtedly, parent–children communication is the central point through which a positive climate emerges, socialization styles come into play and it helps prevent risk behaviors in children. Parents need to talk with their children to know what worries and motivates them when they browse the Internet. It is true that adolescents' virtual world, particularly risk behaviors like CB, is barely visible in an adults world, especially their parents' world, and not only for controlling privacy in social networks, but also because adolescents can build their virtual world as an area protected from parental monitoring.

For parent–children dialog to be efficient and constructive, it is important that parents have a more realistic view about the interactions that take place among adolescents on social networks. As we have seen, researchers have observed a link between parents' real knowledge and awareness about CB and less implication in these behaviors in children (Buelga and Chóliz 2013; Navarro et al. 2013) because this allows parents to teach how to interact more safely in the cyberspace and to warn children about its potential dangers (Gasior 2010; Law et al. 2010). Educating parents about using new technologies not only reduces the opportunities children have of getting involved in risk behaviors on the Internet but also promotes dialog on themes that interest their children, which makes family communication stronger (Buelga 2013; Longmore et al. 2013; Taiariol 2010).

Fluent communication about the nature, content, and potential risks of the Internet is certainly one of the most successful strategies to prevent addiction or excessive use of ICT and to avoid their potential risks (Holtz and Appel 2011; Valcke et al. 2011). So, it is very important to transmit the idea of continuing with codes and rules between virtual and non-virtual contexts and to, therefore, underline any risk behaviors in a given setting (e.g., inviting strangers home) nor must offspring take such risks on the Internet. It is important to warn about the dangers of accepting invitations of friendship and files from strangers. We should also make children and adolescents aware about possible negative consequences of CB behaviors, such as sexting, grooming, etc.

Previous research has pointed that conversing about the beneficial aspects and risks of the Internet in a positive climate when CB situations occur stimulate parents' capacity to support their children emotionally and psychologically and to start taking actions to stop this intimidation (Kowalski et al. 2012). Doubtlessly, this is one of the most challenging aspects that parents face as adolescents quite often dodge talking with their parents about negative online experiences, even when they have been cybervictims (González-Prada et al. 2014). Kowalski et al. (2012) attribute this tendency to remain silent about CB to three reasons, which adolescents consider to be undesirable consequences: (1) fear that parents worry about them becoming victims again, so they forbid them to use the Internet, (2) deny admitting that parents were right about the dangers on the Internet, (3) fear that parents' intervention will make the situation worse rather than improve it. There are certainly good reasons for these fears, for instance, parents' most usual reaction when their children are the target of CB is to forbid them access to the Internet, which children perceive as a very negative way to act (Strom and Strom 2005).

Other generally recommended prevention measures include parental mediation techniques for Internet use. For example in children, it is possible to combine communication and Internet co-use with installing a parental control program in computers. Parental control allows them to set a timetable to access the Internet, to stop children from starting a session at certain times, and does not allow access to certain programs and websites, thus denying children access to blocked contents. Placing a computer in a place shared by everyone at home can encourage parent–children communication and can stimulate children to share their knowedge about the Internet, for example, techniques and ways to access it (Buelga and Chóliz 2013; Taiariol 2010).

In short, information, awareness, and education of responsible new technologies use in a family climate are the supports upon which we can build the prevention of online harassment. In a world where the interconnection between new technologies and the real world becomes increasingly closer, parents play a vital role in guiding and controlling the use and abuse of new technologies and in defining the limits and risks of going too far in negotiation terms.

Acknowledgments This study forms part of Research Project PSI2012-33464 "school violence, dating violence, and parent–children violence in adolescence from the ecological perspective," subsidized by the Spanish Ministry of Economy and Competitiveness and Project SM-I-16/2014 "Preventing suicide and depression in adolescent victims of CB in the Valencian Community," subsidized by the Regional Valencian Ministry of Health (Spain).

References

Accordino, D. B., & Accordino, M. P. (2011). An exploratory study of face-to-face and cyberbullying in sixth grade students. *American Secondary Education, 40*(1), 14–30.

Aoyama, I., Utsumi, S., & Hasegawa, M. (2012). Cyberbullying in Japan: Cases, government reports, adolescent relational aggression and parental monitoring roles. In Q. Li, D. Cross & P.K. Smith (Eds.), *Cyberbullying in the global playground: Research from international perspectives,* (183–201). Oxford: iley-Blackwell. doi:10.1002/9781119954484.ch9.

Appel, M., Stiglbauer, B., Batinic, B., & Holtz, P. (2014). Internet use and verbal aggression: The moderating role of parents and peers. *Computers in Human Behavior, 33,* 235–241.

Becvar, D. S. (2013). *Handbook of family resilience.* New York: Springer. doi:11.1007/978-1-4614-3917-2.

Branje, S., Laursen, B., & Collins, W. A. (2013). Parent-child communication during adolescence. In A. L. Vangelisti (Ed.), *The Routledge handbook of family communication*, (pp. 271–286) New York: Routledge.

Brooks, F. M., Magnusson, J., Spencer, N., & Morgan, A. (2012). Adolescent multiple risk behaviour: an asset approach to the role of family, school and community. *Journal of Public Health, 34*(Suppl 1), 148–156. doi:10.1093/pubmed/fds001.

Buelga, S. (2013). El cyberbullying: Cuando la red no es un lugar seguro. In E. Estévez (Ed.), *Los problemas en la adolescencia: Repuestas y sugerencias para padres y profesionales* (pp. 121–140). Madrid: Síntesis.

Buelga, S., & Chóliz, M. (2013). El adolescente frente a las nuevas tecnologías de la información y de la comunicación. In G. Musitu (Ed.), *Adolescencia y familia: Nuevos retos en el Siglo XXI* (pp. 209–228). México: Trillas.

Buelga, S., Cava, M. J., & Torralba, E. (2014). *Influence of family environment in victims of cyberbullying*. Paper presented at the meeting of the XII National Congress of Social Psychology. Seville: Spain.

Buelga, S., Iranzo, B., Cava, M. J., & Torralba, E. (2015). Cyberbullying aggressor adolescent's psychosocial profile. *International Journal of Social Psychology, 30*(2), 382–406. doi:10.108 0/21711976.2015.1016754.

Buist, K. L., Deković, M., Meeus, W., & van Aken, M. A. (2004). The reciprocal relationship between early adolescent attachment and internalizing and externalizing problem behaviour. *Journal of Adolescence, 27*(3), 251–266. doi:10.1016/j.adolescence.2003.11.012.

Cava, M. J. (2011). Family, teachers, and peers: Keys for supporting victims of bullying. *Psychosocial Intervention, 20*(2), 183–192.

Darling, N., & Steinberg, L. (1993). Parenting style as context: An integrative model. *Psychological Bulletin, 113*, 487–496. doi:10.1037//0033-2909.113.3.487.

David-Ferdon, C., & Hertz, M. F. (2009). *Electronic media and youth violence: A CDC issue brief for researchers*. Atlanta: Centers for Disease Control.

Díaz-Morales, J. F., Escribano, C., Jankowski, K. S., Vollmer, C., & Randler, C. (2014). Evening adolescents: The role of family relationships and pubertal development. *Journal of Adolescence, 37*(4), 425–432. doi:10.1016/j.adolescence.2014.03.001.

Estévez, E., & Emler, N. (2010). A structural modelling approach to predict adolescent offending behaviour from family, school and community factors. *European Journal on Criminal Policy and Research, 16*, 201–220.

Estévez, E., Martínez-Ferrer, B., Moreno, D., & Musitu, G. (2006). Relaciones familiares, rechazo entre iguales y violencia escolar. *Cultura y Educación, 18*(3–4), 335–344. doi:10.1174/113564006779173046.

Gasior, R. M. (2010). *Parental awareness of cyberbullying* (Doctoral dissertation). B.A., California State University. Chico.

González-Prada, M., Buelga, S., & Ortega-Barón (2014). Suicides in cyberbullying victims. Paper presented at the meeting of the I International Congress of Criminonoly. Valencia: Spain.

Hinduja, S., & Patchin, J. W. (2008). Personal information of adolescents on the Internet: A quantitative content analysis of MySpace. *Journal of Adolescence, 31*(1), 125–146. doi:10.1016/j. adolescence.2007.05.004.

Hinduja, S., & Patchin, J. (2013). Social influences on cyberbullying behaviors among middle and high school students. *Journal of Youth and Adolescence, 42*, 711–722. doi:10.1007/s10964-012-9902-4.

Holtz, P., & Appel, M. (2011). Internet use and video gaming predict problem behavior in early adolescence. *Journal of Adolescence, 34*(1), 49–58. doi:10.1016/j.adolescence.2010.02.004.

Keijsers, L., & Poulin, F. (2013). Developmental changes in parent–child communication throughout adolescence. *Developmental Psychology, 49*(12), 2301. doi:10.1037/a0032217.

Kiriakidis, S. P., & Kavoura, A. (2010). Cyberbullying: A review of the literature on harassment through the internet and other electronic means. *Family & Community Health, 33*(2), 82–93. doi:10.1097/FCH.0b013e3181d593e4.

Kokkinos, C. M. (2013). Bullying and victimization in early adolescence: Associations with attachment style and perceived parenting. *Journal of School Violence, 12*(2), 174–192. doi:10.1 080/15388220.2013.766134.

Kowalski, R. M., Limber, S., Limber, S. P., & Agatston, P. W. (2012). *Cyberbullying: Bullying in the digital age.* Chichester, West Sussex: Wiley.

Kowalski, R. M., Giumetti, G. W., Schroeder, A. N., & Lattanner, M. R. (2014). Bullying in the digital age: A critical review and meta-analysis of cyberbullying research among youth. *Psychological Bulletin, 140*(4), 1073–1137. doi:10.1037/a0035618.

Law, D. M., Shapka, J. D., & Olson, B. F. (2010). To control or not to control? Parenting behaviours and adolescent online aggression. *Computers in Human Behavior, 26*(6), 1651–1656. doi:10.1016/j.chb.2010.06.013.

Leung, L., & Lee, P. S. (2012). The influences of information literacy, internet addiction and parenting styles on internet risks. *New Media & Society, 14*(1), 117–136. doi:10.1177/1461444811410406.

Livingstone, S., & Helsper, E. J. (2008). Parental mediation of children's internet use. *Journal of Broadcasting & Electronic Media, 52*(4), 581–599. doi:10.1080/08838150802437396.

Longmore, M. A., Manning, W. D., & Giordano, P. C. (2013). Parent-child relationships in adolescence. In M. A. Fine & F. D. Fincham (Eds.), *Handbook of family theories: A content-based approach* (pp. 28–50). New York: Routledge. doi:10.4324/9780203075180.ch3.

Low, S., & Espelage, D. (2013). Differentiating cyber bullying perpetration from non-physical bullying: Commonalities across race, individual, and family predictors. *Psychology of Violence, 3*(1), 39. doi:10.1037/a0030308.

Lwin, M. O., Stanaland, A. J., & Miyazaki, A. D. (2008). Protecting children's privacy online: How parental mediation strategies affect website safeguard effectiveness. *Journal of Retailing, 84*(2), 205–217. doi:10.1016/j.jretai.2008.04.004.

Makri-Botsari, E., & Karagianni, G. (2014). Cyberbullying in Greek adolescents: The role of parents. *Social and Behavioral Sciences, 116,* 3241–3253. doi:10.1016/j.sbspro.2014.01.742.

Manuel, J., García-Linares, M. C., & Casanova-Arias, P. F. (2014). Relaciones entre estilos educativos parentales y agresividad en adolescentes. *Electronic Journal of Research in Educational Psychology, 12*(32), 147–170.

Martínez-Ferrer, B. (2013). El mundo social del adolescente: Amistades y pareja. In E. Estévez (Ed.), *Los problemas en la adolescencia: Respuestas y sugerencias para padres y educadores* (pp. 71–96). Madrid: Síntesis.

Martínez-Ferrer, B., Murgui, S., Musitu, G., & Monreal, M. C. (2009). El rol del apoyo parental, las actitudes hacia la escuela y la autoestima en la violencia escolar en adolescente. *International Journal of Clinical and Health Psychology, 8,* 679–692.

Martínez-Ferrer, B., Amador, L. V., Moreno, D., & Musitu, G. (2011a). Implicación y participación comunitaria y ajuste psicosocial en adolescentes. *Psicología y Salud, 21*(2), 205–214.

Martínez-Ferrer, B., Moreno, D., Amador, L., & Orford, J. (2011b). School victimization among adolescents. An analysis from an ecological perspective. *Psychosocial Intervention, 20*(2), 149–160. doi:10.5093/in2011v20n2a3.

McCubbin, H. I., & Thompson, A. I. (1987). Family typologies and family assessment. In H.I. McCubbin & A. I. Thompson (Eds.), *Family Assessment Inventories for Research and Practice,* (pp. 35–49). Madison: University of Wisconsin-Madison.

McCubbin, L. D., & McCubbin, H. I. (2013). Resilience in ethnic family systems: A relational theory for research and practice. In D.S. Becvar (Ed.), *Handbook of family resilience* (pp. 175–195). New York: Springer. doi:10.1007/978-1-4614-3917-2_11.

Mesch, G. S. (2009). Parental mediation, online activities, and cyberbullying. *CyberPsychology & Behavior, 12*(4), 387–393. doi:10.1089/cpb.2009.0068.

Minuchin, S. (1974). *Families and family therapy.* Boston: Harward University Press.

Moos, R. H., & Moos, B. S. (1981). *Family environment scale manual.* Palo Alto: Consulting Psychologist Press.

Moral, M. V., & Ovejero, A. (2013). Perception of family social climate and attitudes towards bullying in adolescents. *European Journal of Investigation in Health, Psychology and Education, 3*(2), 149–160.

Moreno, D. (2013). Delincuencia y Adolescencia. In G. Musitu (Ed.), *Adolescencia y familia: Nuevos retos en el Siglo XXI* (pp. 156–177). México: Trillas.

Musitu, G. (2002). Las conductas violentas de los adolescentes en la escuela: El rol de la familia. *Aula abierta, 79,* 109–138.

Musitu, G. (2013). *Mujer y migración. Los nuevos desafíos en América Latina.* México: Editorial Trillas.

Musitu, G., & Cava, M. J. (2001). *La familia y la educación.* Barcelona: Octaedro.

Musitu, G., & García, J. F. (2004). Consecuencias de la socialización familiar en la cultura española. *Psicothema, 16*(2), 288–293.

Musitu, G., Buelga, S., Lila, M., & Cava, M. J. (2001). *Familia y adolescencia.* Madrid: Síntesis.

Navarro, R., Serna, C., Martínez, V., & Ruiz-Oliva, R. (2013). The role of Internet use and parental mediation on cyberbullying victimization among Spanish children from rural public schools. *European Journal of Psychology of Education, 28*(3), 725–745. doi: 10.1007/s10212-012-0137-2.

Olson, D. H. (1986). Circumplex Model VII: Validation Studies and FACES III. *Family Social Science.* University of Minnesota 25(3), (pp. 337–351). doi: 10.1111/j.1545-5300.1986.00337.x.

Olson, D. H. (1991). Commentary: Three-dimensional (3-D) circumplex model and revised scoring of FACES III. *Family Process, 30*(1), 74–79. doi:10.1111/j.1545-5300.1991.00074.x.

Olweus, D. (2012). Comments on cyberbullying article: A rejoinder. *European Journal of Developmental Psychology, 9*(5), 559–568. doi:10.1080/17405629.2012.705086.

Ortega-Barón, J. (2013). *Influencia del clima escolar y del clima familiar en víctimas de cyberbullying.* Trabajo final de Master. Universidad de Valencia, Valencia.

Povedano, A., Jiménez, T. I., Moreno, D., Amador, L. V., & Musitu, G. (2012). Relación del conflicto y la expresividad familiar con la victimización en la escuela: El rol de la autoestima, la sintomatología depresiva y el género de los adolescentes. *Infancia y Aprendizaje, 35*(4), 421–432. doi:10.1174/021037012803495285.

Prensky, M. (2001). Digital natives, digital immigrants part 1. *On the Horizon, 9*(5), 1–6. doi:10.1108/10748120110424816.

Proctor, C., & Linley, P. A. (2014). Life satisfaction in youth. In G. A. Fava & C. Ruini (Eds.), *Increasing psychological well-being in clinical and educational settings* (pp. 199–215). Netherlands: Springer. doi:10.1007/978-94-017-8669-0_13.

Rosen, L. D., Cheever, N. A., & Carrier, L. M. (2008). The association of parenting style and child age with parental limit setting and adolescent MySpace behavior. *Journal of Applied Developmental Psychology, 29,* 459–471. doi:10.1016/j.appdev.2008.07.005.

Rueger, S. Y., Malecki, C. K., & Demaray, M. K. (2010). Relationship between multiple sources of perceived social support and psychological and academic adjustment in early adolescence: Comparisons across gender. *Journal of Youth and Adolescence, 39*(1), 47–61. doi:10.1007/s10964-008-9368-6.

Sasson, H., & Mesch, G. (2014). Parental mediation, peer norms and risky online behavior among adolescents. *Computers in Human Behavior, 33,* 32–38. doi:10.1016/j.chb.2013.12.025.

Sasson, H., Erez, R., & Elgali, Z. (2011). Risks on the web: Adolescents' perceptions and coping mechanisms. *The 4th Knowledge Cities World Summit,* 350.

Scabini, E., & Manzi, C. (2011). Family processes and identity. In S.J. Schwartz, K. Luyckx, & V.L. Vignoles (Eds.), *Handbook of identity theory and research* (pp. 565–584). New York: Springer.

Schenk, A. M., Fremouw, W. J., & Keelan, C. M. (2013). Characteristics of college cyberbullies. *Computers in Human Behavior, 29*(6), 2320–2327. doi:10.1016/j.chb.2013.05.013.

Sijtsema, J. J., Nederhof, E., Veenstra, R., Ormel, J., Oldehinkel, A. J., & Ellis, B. J. (2013). Effects of family cohesion and heart rate reactivity on aggressive/rule-breaking behavior and prosocial behavior in adolescence: The tracking adolescents' individual lives survey study. *Development and Psychopathology, 25*(03), 699–712. doi:10.1017/S0954579413000114.

Solecki, S., McLaughlin, K., & Goldschmidt, K. (2014). Promoting positive offline relationships to reduce negative online experiences. *Journal of Pediatric Nursing, 29*(5), 482–484. doi:10.1016/j.pedn.2014.07.001.

Stattin, H., & Kerr, M. (2000). Parental monitoring: A reinterpretation. *Child Development, 71*(4), 1072–1085. doi:10.1111/1467-8624.00210.

Steinberg, L. (1985). *Adolescence*. New York: Knopf.

Steinberg, L. (2000). The family at adolescence: Transition and transformation. *Journal of Adolescent Health, 27*(3), 170–178. doi:10.1016/S1054-139X(99)00115-9.

Strom, P. S., & Strom, R. D. (2005). When teens turn cyberbullies. *Education Digest: Essential Readings Condensed for Quick Review, 71*(4), 35–41.

Subrahmanyam, K., & Šmahel, D. (2011). The darker sides of the internet: Violence, cyber bullying and victimization. In K. Subrahmanyam & D. Šmahel (Eds.), *Digital youth: The role of media in development* (pp. 179–199). New York: Springer. doi:10.1007/978-1-4419-6278-2_10.

Taiariol, J. (2010). Cyberbullying. The Role of family and school. Wayne State University Dissertations, Paper 118, January 2010, Detroit, Michigan (retrieved october, 30, 2014 from http://digitalcommons.wayne.edu./oa_dissertations/118).

Tippett, N., Wolke, D., & Platt, L. (2013). Ethnicity and bullying involvement in a national UK youth sample. *Journal of Adolescence, 36*(4), 639–649. doi:10.1016/j.adolescence.2013.03.013.

Valcke, M., Bonte, S., De Wever, B., & Rots, I. (2010). Internet parenting styles and the impact on internet use of primary school children. *Computers & Education, 55*(2), 454–464. doi:10.1016/j.compedu.2010.02.009.

Valcke, M., De Wever, B., Van Keer, H., & Schellens, T. (2011). Long-term study of safe internet use of young children. *Computers & Education, 57*(1), 1292–1305. doi:10.1016/j.compedu.2011.01.010.

Van Dijk, M. P., Branje, S., Keijsers, L., Hawk, S. T., Hale, W. W., & Meeus, W. (2014). Self-concept clarity across adolescence: Longitudinal associations with open communication with parents and internalizing symptoms. *Journal of Youth and Adolescence, 43*(11), 1861–1876. doi:10.1007/s10964-013-0055-x.

Vandebosch, H. (2014). Addressing cyberbullying using a multi-stakeholder approach: The Flemish case. In S.Van der Hof, B.Van den Berg & B. Schermer (Eds.) *Minding Minors Wandering the Web: Regulating Online Child Safety* (pp. 245–262). TMC Asser Press. doi:10.1007/978-94-6265-005-3_14.

Wade, A., & Beran, T. (2011). Cyberbullying: The new era of bullying. *Canadian Journal of School Psychology, 26*, 44–61. doi:10.1177/0829573510396318.

Wang, J., Iannotti, R. J., & Nansel, T. R. (2009). School bullying among adolescents in the United States: Physical, verbal, relational, and cyber. *Journal of Adolescent Health, 45*(4), 368–375. doi:10.1016/j.jadohealth.2009.03.021.

Wray-Lake, L., Crouter, A. C., & McHale, S. M. (2010). Developmental patterns in decision-making autonomy across middle childhood and adolescence: European American parents' perspectives. *Child Development, 81*(2), 636–651. doi:10.1111/j.1467-8624.2009.01420.x.

Ybarra, M. L., & Mitchell, K. J. (2004). Youth engaging in online harassment: Associations with caregiver–child relationships, Internet use, and personal characteristics. *Journal of adolescence, 27*(3), 319–336. doi:10.1016/j.adolescence.2004.03.007.

Part II
Global Research

Chapter 6
Cyberbullying Matters: Examining the Incremental Impact of Cyberbullying On Outcomes Over and Above Traditional Bullying in North America

Gary W. Giumetti and Robin M. Kowalski

Since 1992, there have been decreases in most measures of school violence (Robers et al. 2014). At the same time, however, there has been a dramatic increase (post-Columbine) in the public's attention to bullying. One place where this is evident is in news articles in the popular press. While there were fewer than 150 articles that contained the term bullying pre-Columbine (pre-1999), this number now far surpasses 1000. Another indicator is in state laws passed in relation to bullying. Prior to Columbine, no states had laws regulating bullying. Currently, 49 states (excluding Montana) have laws pertaining to bullying. The statutes in 20 of these states include "cyberbullying," with 48 states referencing "electronic harassment" (Hinduja and Patchin 2014). A final indicator of the increased attention given to bullying is in the research literature. A search of the psychological search engine PsycINFO reveals that in 1990, only five articles had been published containing the word "bully" or "bullying." Within the first 9 months of the current year, that number exceeds 470.

One might speculate that the increased attention given to bullying denotes an increase in the prevalence rate of the phenomenon. This does not appear to be the case, however (Robers et al. 2014). Rather, it seems to reflect an increased awareness and recognition of bullying and the forms it can take. Additionally, during the time frame in which public attention, state laws, and increased research have emerged, a new form of bullying has developed known as cyberbullying or electronic bullying. Under consideration in the current chapter is the degree to which cyberbullying is both similar to and different from traditional bullying and the extent to which cyberbullying contributes unique variance to the negative consequences that follow involvement in bullying above and beyond those associated with traditional bullying. After defining bullying and cyberbullying, we will examine their prevalence rates and consequences. The chapter will then focus on similarities and differences

G. W. Giumetti (✉)
Department of Psychology, Quinnipiac University, Hamden, CT 06518, USA
e-mail: gary.giumetti@quinnipiac.edu

R. M. Kowalski
Department of Psychology, Clemson University, Clemson, SC, USA

© Springer International Publishing Switzerland 2016
R. Navarro et al. (eds.), *Cyberbullying Across the Globe,*
DOI 10.1007/978-3-319-25552-1_6

between traditional bullying and cyberbullying followed by a statistical analysis of the predictive utility of cyberbullying in accounting for unique variance in adverse effects above and beyond that accounted for by traditional bullying.

6.1 Defining Bullying

Researchers have shown more agreement in their conceptualizations of traditional bullying than cyberbullying. Traditional bullying has most often been defined as an aggressive act that is intended to cause harm or distress, that is typically repeated over time, and that reflects a power imbalance between the victim(s) and perpetrator(s) (Olweus 1993, 2013). With traditional bullying, this power imbalance can reflect differences in physical strength, size, or social standing. Traditional bullying can be either direct (e.g., physical, verbal) or indirect (e.g., spreading rumors, gossiping, excluding). The most common forms of bullying for both males and females are verbally being made fun of or teased, followed by having rumors spread (Robers et al. 2014).

Cyberbullying refers to the use of electronic communication technologies to bully others (Kowalski et al. 2012a, 2014; Kowalski and Limber 2007, 2013). Like traditional bullying, cyberbullying is frequently defined as an aggressive act that is often repeated over time (e.g., a single e-mail sent to hundreds of people) and that reflects an imbalance of power between the parties involved. With cyberbullying, however, the power imbalance may also reflect differences in technological expertise.

Although researchers agree on a general level regarding how to define cyberbullying, they frequently differ from one another in the specifics of how to best conceptualize the phenomenon. Cyberbullying can assume any of a number of different forms and be perpetrated through a host of different media. For example, Willard (2007) has created a taxonomy of cyberbullying behaviors that includes flaming, harassment, outing and trickery, exclusion, impersonation, cyberstalking, and sexting. Pyżalski (2012) also categorized cyberbullying according to the nature of the target: cyberbullying against celebrities, the vulnerable, groups, random people known only online, and school staff. Cyberbullying via any of these forms or against any of these targets can be perpetrated through a number of different venues including: social media, e-mail, instant messaging, chat rooms, web sites, text messages, or online games.

One of the issues surrounding the definition and conceptualization of cyberbullying is whether it should be viewed as simply a new form of bullying, and, thus, an extension of traditional bullying, or whether it represents a unique type of aggression, and thus, a construct independent of traditional bullying. Researchers are mixed in their opinions on this issue. Data from several studies show that involvement in traditional bullying is correlated with involvement in cyberbullying (e.g., Gradinger et al. 2009; Hinduja and Patchin 2009; Kowalski et al. 2012b; Menesini et al. 2012).

However, the co-occurrence of the two types of bullying does not resolve the issue. Mehari et al. (2014, p. 1) stated that it is best to view cyberbullying "as a new dimension on which aggression can be classified, rather than cyberbullying as a distinct counterpart to existing forms of aggression." They emphasized that both the form (physical, verbal, relational) and media (face-to-face, cyber) are important in identifying aggressive behaviors. As additional evidence for their perspective, they suggest that cyberbullying shares in common many of the predictors of other forms of aggression. This perspective is shared by Olweus (2013; see also, Smith et al. 2008), who stated that "to be cyber bullied or to cyber bully other students seems to a large extent to be part of a general pattern of bullying, where use of the electronic media is only one possible form and, in addition, is a form with a quite low prevalence" (p. 767).

Alternatively, Menesini et al. (2012) found evidence for the additive effects of both traditional bullying and cyberbullying. Specifically, they found that both types of bullying explained variance in internalizing and externalizing symptoms (e.g., anxiety, depression, aggressive behavior) after accounting for the other type of bullying. In their meta-analysis, Kowalski et al. (2014) found evidence that cyberbullying may be an extension of traditional bullying but noted that "traditional bullying explained only 20 % of variance in reports of cyberbullying...suggesting that not all individuals who report being bullied in traditional ways also report being cyberbullied" (p. 1124).

6.2   Prevalence of Bullying

The first systematic study of traditional bullying was conducted by Dan Olweus in Norway and Sweden (Olweus 1993). In a sample of over 150,000 elementary and middle school-aged youth, Olweus found that 9 % were victims of traditional bullying, 7 % perpetrated bullying, and 2 % were bully/victims (both victims and perpetrators). The first study in the USA that used a nationally representative sample found somewhat higher rates of bullying. In a sample of over 15,000 youth in grades 6 through 10, Nansel and her colleagues (2001) observed that 17 % of the respondents reported being victimized "sometimes" or more often, 19 % reported perpetrating bullying "sometimes" or more often, and 6 % were bully/victims "sometimes" or more often. More recently, Olweus and Limber (2010) surveyed over 500,000 children. Among youth in grades 3 through 12, 17 % reported being bullied two to three times a month or more and 10 % indicated they had perpetrated bullying against their peers two to three times a month or more. According to Olweus and Limber (2010), using these prevalence rates, approximately 11 million school-age children are involved with bullying regularly.

Reported prevalence rates of traditional bullying vary with the sex of the respondents. Across most studies, boys report perpetrating traditional bullying more than girls (Cook et al. 2010; Olweus 1993; Olweus and Limber 2010). Cook et al. (2010) conducted a meta-analysis of 153 studies examining sex differences in bullying since 1970 and found that boys are more likely than girls to be both perpetrators of traditional bullying and bully/victims. Sex differences in victimization are a bit less clear, however. The meta-analysis conducted by Cook et al. found that boys were slightly more likely than girls to be victims of traditional bullying. However, consistency across studies regarding this finding is lacking.

Prevalence rates of cyberbullying are highly variable across studies (Kowalski et al. 2014; Livingstone and Smith 2014). This variability stems from a number of different factors, including different definitions used to conceptualize and, therefore, operationalize cyberbullying, whether cyberbullying is assessed with a single item ("Have you ever been cyberbullied") or multiple items ("Have you been cyberbullied via text message," "....email," etc.), the time parameter within which the cyberbullying occurred (e.g., previous 2 months, 6 months, 1 year, lifetime), and the criteria used to establish involvement with bullying (e.g., at least once, two to three times a month or more; Kowalski et al. 2014; Modecki et al. 2014). Due in part to this variability, researchers have debated the static nature of cyberbullying, arguing over whether prevalence rates of cyberbullying are increasing, decreasing, or remaining constant (Olweus 2013; Slonje and Smith 2008).

In a survey of middle school students, Hinduja and Patchin (2009) found that 9% had been cyberbullied within the previous 30 days, 17% in their lifetime. In terms of perpetration, 8% had perpetrated cyberbullying in the previous 30 days, 18% in their lifetime. Kowalski and Limber (2007) observed that 18% of middle school students in their sample reported being victims of cyberbullying within the previous 2 months, 11% had perpetrated cyberbullying during the same time period. Reports from the National Crime Victimization Survey of youth ages 12–18 showed victimization rates of 9% (Robers et al. 2014). Across studies, victimization rates range from approximately 10–40% (Lenhart 2010; see, however, Juvonen and Gross 2008). A recent meta-analysis of prevalence rates of both traditional bullying and cyberbullying across 80 studies found that rates of traditional bullying are double that of cyberbullying (Modecki et al. 2014). Specifically, researchers found average prevalence rates of 35% for traditional bullying and 15% for cyberbullying. In spite of individual variability across studies, the prevalence rates of cyberbullying, while lower than those of traditional bullying, highlight a problem that warrants attention.

As with traditional bullying, reported prevalence rates of cyberbullying vary with the sex of the respondent. Kowalski and Limber (2007) found that girls were about twice as likely as boys to be victims of cyberbullying (see also Messias et al. 2014). However, other studies have found no sex differences in cyberbullying victimization or perpetration (Williams and Guerra 2007). A recent meta-analysis by Bartlett (2014) found that males were more likely than females to perpetrate cyberbullying but that this effect was moderated by age. At younger ages, females reported perpetrating cyberbullying more than males. By late adolescence, however, males outnumbered females in the frequency of perpetrating cyberbullying.

6.3 Consequences of Bullying

In examining the consequences associated with involvement in bullying, a couple of points are noteworthy. First, because few longitudinal studies of bullying have been conducted, it is difficult to discern the temporal order of bullying involvement and the consequences attached to bullying. In other words, are variables such as depression and anxiety effects of bullying, precursors to bullying, or both? While few would doubt that repeated victimization leads to negative physical and psychological consequences, low self-esteem, anxiety, and depression are characteristics that may also invite bullying from others.

In addition, a number of variables determine the impact that bullying in whatever form will have on the individuals involved. "Themes related to publicity, anonymity of perpetrators, features of the medium, presence of bystanders, and individual level factors [are]...potential influences upon impact severity" (Dredge et al. 2014, p. 287). The manner in which individuals appraise the situation also determines its severity. People who perceive the situation to be harmful and threatening and who view themselves as having few resources to cope with the situation at hand will likely experience more negative consequences than those who appraise the situation as more manageable (Lazarus and Folkman 1984).

Individual-level factors aside, involvement in bullying as victim, perpetrator, or both (i.e., bully/victims) can result in both short- and long-term consequences. These consequences can be physical, psychological, social, and/or academic (Anthony et al. 2010; Arseneault et al. 2010; Gini and Pozzoli 2009; Kowalski and Limber 2013). Victims of traditional bullying are more likely than those not involved in bullying to be anxious (Fekkes et al. 2004; Garnefski and Kraaij 2014), depressed (Hawker and Boulton 2000), and to have lower self-esteem (Egan and Perry 1998; Rigby and Slee 1993). Suicidal ideation is also higher among children who have been bullied (Rigby 1997). Compared to children who are not bullied, those who report victimization also report lower academic achievement (Arseneault et al. 2006; Wang et al. 2014) and a desire to avoid school (Rigby 1997). Bullies, victims, and bully/victims are also more likely to carry a weapon than individuals not involved with bullying (van Geel et al. 2014a).

Similar to traditional bullying, cyberbullying is also associated with a host of short- and long-term negative consequences. Indeed, the list mirrors that accompanying traditional bullying: anxiety, depression, low self-esteem, higher suicidal ideation, and poor academic performance (Didden et al. 2009; Hinduja and Patchin 2010; Kowalski and Limber 2013; Livingstone and Smith 2014; Nixon 2014; Perren et al. 2010; Vazsonyi et al. 2012). In addition, cyberbullying victimization and perpetration are associated with increased tobacco, alcohol, and drug use (Ybarra and Mitchell 2004).

Limited research has found that the effects of bullying are moderated by the sex of the victim. In their meta-analysis, Kowalski et al. (2014), for example, found that sex moderated the relationship between cybervictimization and depression. The relationship between cybervictimization and depression was stronger for samples that contained more females. Similar research by Brown et al. (2014) noted that girls experienced more negative effects from bullying victimization than boys.

Research has shown that multiple sources of victimization are particularly problematic for victims. This has implications for bullying in that victims of cyberbullying are more likely than individuals not involved with cyberbullying to also be victims of traditional bullying (Kowalski et al. 2014; Kowalski et al. 2012b).

A few studies have directly addressed the joint contributions of involvement in traditional bullying and cyberbullying to the experience of negative physical and psychological consequences. Wigderson and Lynch (2013), for example, stated that victims of cyberbullying experienced adverse effects of their victimization above and beyond those associated with their experience as a victim of traditional bullying. Similarly, van Geel et al. (2014b) observed that suicidal ideation was highest among individuals who had experienced both traditional bullying and cyberbullying, followed by those who had experienced only cyberbullying, and then by those who were victims of only traditional bullying.

6.4   Overlap of Traditional Bullying and Cyberbullying

As suggested by their definitions, traditional bullying and cyberbullying share certain features in common. Both involve acts of aggression that are intended to cause harm or distress, that are typically repeated over time, and that reflect a power imbalance between the parties involved. Beyond that, however, each has unique features that distinguish the two types of bullying. One key feature of cyberbullying is perceived anonymity. While people are never as anonymous online as they believe themselves to be, some use the umbrella of anonymity to perpetrate acts of aggression online that they would never consider perpetrating face-to-face, perhaps as retaliation for traditional bullying victimization. Indeed, Kowalski and Limber (2007) found that just under 50% of the victims of cyberbullying in their sample did not know the identity of the perpetrator. Additionally, the punitive fears associated with disclosing traditional bullying and cyberbullying victimization differ. Victims of traditional bullying fear that they will be revictimized if they disclose their bullying status. Victims of cyberbullying, on the other hand, fear that their technology will be taken away.

Many bullying researchers have noted that traditional bullying and cyberbullying overlap to a great extent (Kowalski et al. 2014; Modecki et al. 2014; Riebel et al. 2009), with as many as 88% of victims (or perpetrators) of traditional bullying also being cyberbullying victims (or perpetrators; Olweus 2013). This leaves a relatively small group of individuals who are uniquely engaging in cyberbullying perpetration or experiencing cyber victimization ($\sim$10% in Olweus 2012, $\sim$17% in Landstedt and Persson 2014). We agree with Olweus (2013) that, in order to understand the effects of cyberbullying, one must also take into consideration the extent to which individuals are also experiencing traditional bullying. As noted in Kowalski et al. (2014), the best way to examine the unique effects of cyberbullying over and above traditional bullying is to conduct an hierarchical regression analysis with traditional bullying entered in step 1 and cyberbullying entered in step 2 as predictors of outcomes.

Existing research on this issue has begun to document the unique effects of cyberbullying over traditional bullying. Findings from numerous research studies have already suggested that cyberbullying does indeed contribute unique variance to negative outcomes, while controlling for traditional bullying (e.g., Dempsey et al. 2009; Fredstrom et al. 2011; Machmutow et al. 2012; Menesini et al. 2012; Perren et al. 2010; Perren and Gutzwiller-Helfenfinger 2012; Sakellariou et al. 2012). For example, in Fredstrom et al. (2011), the authors found that cybervictimization predicted unique variance in self-esteem, social stress, anxiety, depressive symptoms, and self-efficacy, while controlling for traditional victimization. Additionally, Menesini et al. (2012) compared an additive model (cybervictimization over traditional victimization) to a multiplicative model (interaction of cybervictimization and traditional victimization) and mainly found support for the additive model, with cybervictimization explaining unique variance in somatic symptoms as well as anxious and depressive symptoms, while controlling for traditional victimization.

The current study adds to this literature by examining the unique effects of cyberbullying and cybervictimization over and above traditional bullying and victimization on outcomes. We report the results of secondary data analyses on two large-scale cyberbullying datasets (Kowalski and Limber 2013; Kowalski et al. 2012b), which included the following outcome variables: self-esteem, anxiety, depression, grades in school, health, absenteeism, and leaving school early due to sickness.

6.4.1 Method

6.4.1.1 Participants

Data for the current study were drawn from two large-scale studies from North America (Kowalski and Limber 2013; Kowalski et al. 2012b). The first sample contained 931 students (433 females, 485 males; M age = 15.16 years, standard deviation (SD) = 1.76 years) from 6–12th grades drawn from two schools in Pennsylvania (Kowalski and Limber 2013). The second sample contained 4720 students (2273 females, 2237 males, M age = 15.2 years, SD = 1.8 years) from 6–12th grades from eight schools across North America (Kowalski et al. 2012b). All participants volunteered to participate, passive consent was obtained from parents, and the studies were approved by the university's institutional review board.

6.4.1.2 Materials

Traditional Bullying and Cyberbullying Across both studies, traditional bullying and traditional victimization were measured using one item for each construct that were drawn from the Olweus Bully/Victim Questionnaire (Olweus 1996/2004). Cyberbullying perpetration and victimization were similarly assessed using a single item each drawn from the Electronic Bullying Questionnaire (Kowalski and Limber 2007). Specifically, participants were given a definition of bullying/cyberbullying and then asked to indicate how often they experienced bullying/cyberbullying or traditional victimization/cyber victimization in the past couple of months using a 5-point response scale (1 = never, 5 = several times per week).

Outcomes Participants in both samples also completed a measure of self-esteem using the Rosenberg self-esteem scale (Rosenberg 1965). The Rosenberg Self-

Esteem Scale contained 10 items ($\alpha_{K\&L} = .85$, $\alpha_{K,M,\&L} = .86$) with a 5-point response format (1 = strongly disagree, 5 = strongly agree), and a sample item is "I take a positive attitude toward myself."

Other measures in the first sample (Kowalski and Limber 2013) include anxiety, school performance, physical health, and depression. Anxiety was measured using the Beck Youth Anxiety Scale (Beck et al. 2005). The Beck Youth Anxiety Scale contained 20 items ($\alpha_{K\&L} = .94$) related to anxiety, including "I worry," and respondents used a 4-point scale (1 = never, 4 = always). The measures of school performance assessed absenteeism, leaving school early due to sickness, and grades in school. For the absenteeism and leaving school early measures, participants indicated how often in the last couple of months (since winter break) they were absent from school or left school early because they were sick. To measure grades, participants were asked to indicate the grades that they *usually* get in school from a list of nine choices ranging from "mostly A's" to "mostly F's." Physical health outcomes were measured by asking participants to indicate how often they had experienced ten symptoms (e.g., problems sleeping, $\alpha = .85$; Fekkes et al. 2004) in the past 4 weeks. Finally, depression was measured using the Beck Youth Depression Scale (Beck et al. 2005), which contained 20 items ($\alpha = .96$) related to depression (e.g., "I feel lonely"), and participants responded on a 4-point scale (1 = never, 4 = always).

Social anxiety was assessed in the second sample (Kowalski et al. 2012b) using the Interaction Anxiousness Scale (Leary 1983), a 15-item measure of the dispositional tendency to experience social anxiety ($\alpha_{K,M,\&L} = .79$). Participants indicated how characteristic each item was of them using a 5-point response format (1 = not at all, 5 = extremely).

6.4.1.3 Procedure

Participants in both samples were given surveys to complete while in school. The surveys were completed using paper and pencil. All students who were asked agreed to participate.

6.4.1.4 Analysis

In order to determine the unique additive effects of cyberbullying, we conducted hierarchical linear regression with traditional bullying or victimization in step 1 and cyberbullying or cybervictimization in step 2. We then looked at the significance of the change in R^2 between the two models.

6.4.2 Results

Results from hierarchical linear regression are reported in Table 6.1. Analyses of the Kowalski and Limber (2013) data indicate that cyberbullying perpetration pre-

Table 6.1 Standardized regression coefficients and explained variance (R^2) from hierarchical linear regression results

Sample	Outcome	TB	CB	ΔR^2	TV	CV	ΔR^2
K and L	Absenteeism	0.06	0.12*	.01*	−.01	.13*	.01*
	Anxiety	0.03	0.20*	.03*	.26*	.17*	.02*
	Depression	0.14*	0.14*	.02*	.20*	.21*	.04*
	Grades	−0.09*	−0.11*	.01*	−.03	−.15*	.02*
	Health	0.12*	0.12*	.01*	.22*	.14*	.02*
	Leaving school early due to sickness	0.05	0.11*	.01*	.10*	0.07	0.004
	Self-esteem	0.15*	0.11*	.01*	.09*	.20*	.03*
K, M, and L	Social anxiety	0.13*	0.08*	.01*	.06*	.05*	.002*
	Self-esteem	0.15*	0.11*	.01*	0.20*	0.18*	.03*

Values beneath TB, CB, TV, and CV represent standardized regression coefficients from model 2 of the hierarchical linear regression. *K and L* Kowalski and Limber (2013) study, *K, M, and L* Kowalski et al. (2012b) study
TB traditional bullying perpetration, *CB* cyberbullying perpetration, *TV* traditional bullying victimization, *CV* cyberbullying victimization
*$p < .05$

dicted significant ($p < .01$) incremental variance in all outcome variables tested over and above traditional bullying perpetration. Specifically, cyberbullying perpetration (CB) predicted unique variance in absenteeism ($\Delta R^2 = .01$, $p = .004$), anxiety ($\Delta R^2 = .03$, $p < .001$), depression ($\Delta R^2 = .02$, $p < .001$), grades in school ($\Delta R^2 = .01$, $p = .004$), physical health ($\Delta R^2 = .01$, $p = .003$), leaving school early due to sickness ($\Delta R^2 = .01$, $p = .007$), and self-esteem ($\Delta R^2 = .01$, $p = .003$), while controlling for traditional bullying perpetration. When traditional victimization was entered in step 1 of regression, cybervictimization predicted significant incremental variance in all outcomes tested, except leaving school early due to sickness. Specifically, cybervictimization predicted unique variance in absenteeism ($\Delta R^2 = .01$, $p = .001$), anxiety ($\Delta R^2 = .02$, $p < .001$), depression ($\Delta R^2 = .04$, $p < .001$), grades in school ($\Delta R^2 = .02$, $p < .001$), physical health ($\Delta R^2 = .02$, $p < .001$), and self-esteem ($\Delta R^2 = .03$, $p < .001$), while controlling for traditional bullying victimization.

Analyses of the Kowalski et al.'s (2012b) data are also presented in Table 6.1 and reveal that cyberbullying perpetration predicted significant incremental variance in social anxiety ($\Delta R^2 = .01$, $p < .001$) and self-esteem ($\Delta R^2 = .01$, $p < .001$) when controlling for traditional bullying perpetration. Additionally, cybervictimization predicted significant incremental variance in social anxiety ($\Delta R^2 = .002$, $p = .004$) and self-esteem ($\Delta R^2 = .03$, $p < .001$), while controlling for traditional victimization.

6.4.3 Discussion

Researchers have called for a more contextualized examination of the effects of cyberbullying on youth by putting it within the context of traditional forms of bullying (Olweus 2013). The results of the current study add to the existing literature by showing that cyberbullying perpetration and victimization predict several important individual-level outcomes while controlling for traditional bullying and victimization. These outcomes include absenteeism from school, anxiety, depression, grades in school, physical health, leaving school early due to sickness, and self-esteem. The amount of variance in these outcomes explained is small, ranging from 1 to 4%, but, in all but one analysis, the results were statistically significant.

It is also interesting to note that in three of the analyses for perpetration, traditional bullying was not a significant predictor of absenteeism, anxiety, nor leaving school early due to sickness when cyberbullying was added to the model. Additionally, for two of the analyses for victimization, traditional victimization was not a significant predictor of absenteeism or grades in school when cybervictimization was added to the model. These findings suggest that there may be a unique set of variables that are predicted by cyberbullying and cybervictimization but not by traditional bullying and traditional victimization. This adds to the divergent validity argument made by others (e.g., Dempsey et al. 2009), suggesting that cyberbullying may indeed be a unique construct from traditional bullying.

These results have practical implications. Given that cyberbullying perpetration and cybervictimization had unique relationships with many individual-level outcomes over and above traditional bullying and victimization, respectively, this has implications for prevention and intervention programs. Specifically, programs should not only be aimed at reducing the incidence of traditional bullying but also at reducing cyberbullying. Also, education should be aimed at increasing parental awareness of their child's involvement in traditional bullying as well as cyberbullying. Additionally, these results highlight the necessity of studying cyberbullying within the context of traditional bullying. Without examining cyberbullying within the context of traditional bullying, results may only tell part of the story and are likely to be inflated (Kowalski et al. 2014). Therefore, future researchers should be sure to measure both traditional bullying and cyberbullying in their studies. Further, analyses should include both forms of bullying in the model to enable researchers to determine the unique effects of cyberbullying versus traditional bullying.

Of course, the current study is not without limitations. First, the data for the current studies included in the analysis were collected at single time points, thus limiting causal inferences. That is, we cannot be certain that cyberbullying victimization is causing an increase in anxiety or depressive symptoms or decreases in self-esteem. It could be the case that students with these traits may be more likely to be the target of cyberbullying behavior from others. Given the difficulty of manipulating cyberbullying and traditional bullying, future research should attempt to gather longitudinal data from youth over several measurement occasions to help add to our understanding of the causal linkages with these outcome variables. Another limitation of the current study is that the data were all collected via self-report from a single-source, which raises the potential for mono-method bias (Podsakoff et al. 2003) or inflated correlations among variables since they were all gathered from the same source using the same method (i.e., self-report). Future research should, therefore, gather data using multiple sources, such as from peers, teachers, school counselors, or parents.

6.5 Conclusion

Bullying among youth represents a significant threat to child and adolescent well-being. Years of research have indicated that, on average, 35 % of youth experience traditional bullying and 15 % experience cyberbullying (Modecki et al. 2014). Researchers have begun to tease apart the unique effects of the medium of experiencing bullying on individual outcomes (e.g., Menesini et al. 2012), and the current study adds to this literature by demonstrating that cyberbullying explains a significant amount of unique variance over traditional bullying in several important individual outcomes, including self-esteem, anxiety, depression, absenteeism, grades in school, physical health, and leaving school early due to sickness. Future researchers are encouraged to measure both cyberbullying and traditional bullying in their studies to best understand the impact of the medium (traditional vs. cyber) through which bullying is occurring on youth. Additionally, prevention and intervention efforts should be targeted at mitigating both traditional bullying and cyberbullying among youth in an integrated way.

References

Anthony, B. J., Wessler, S. L., & Sebian, J. K. (2010). Commentary: Guiding a public health approach to bullying. *Journal of Pediatric Psychology, 35,* 1113–1115. doi:10.1093/jpepsy/jsq083.

Arseneault, L., Walsh, E., Trzesniewski, K., Newcombe, R., Caspi, A., & Moffitt, T. E. (2006). Bullying victimization uniquely contributes to adjustment problems in young children: A nationally representative cohort study. *Pediatrics, 118,* 130–138. doi:10.1542/peds.2005-2388.

Arseneault, L., Bowes, L., & Shakoor, S. (2010). Bullying victimization in youths and mental health problems: Much ado about nothing? *Psychological Medicine, 40,* 717–729. doi:10.1017/S0033291709991383.

Bartlett, C. (2014). A meta-analysis of sex differences in cyber-bullying behavior: The moderating role of age. *Aggressive Behavior, 40,* 474–488. doi:10.1002/ab.21555.

Beck, J. S., Beck, A. T., Jolly, J. B., & Steer, R. A. (2005). *Beck youth inventories for children and adolescents* (2nd edn.). San Antonio: Harcourt Assessment.

Brown, C. F., Demaray, M., & Secord, S. M. (2014). Cyber victimization in middle school and relations to social emotional outcomes. *Computers in Human Behavior, 35,* 12–21. doi:10.1016/j.chb.2014.02.014.

Cook, C. R., Williams, K. R., Guerra, N. G., Kim, T. E., & Sadek, S. (2010). Predictors of bullying and victimization in childhood and adolescence: A meta-analytic investigation. *School Psychology Quarterly, 25*(2), 65–83. doi:10.1037/a0020149.

Dempsey, A. G., Sulkowski, M. L., Nichols, R., & Storch, E. A. (2009). Differences between peer victimization in cyber and physical settings and associated psychosocial adjustment in early adolescence. *Psychology in the Schools, 46*(10), 962–972. doi:10.1002/pits.20437.

Didden, R., Scholte, R. H. J., Korzilius, H., de Moor, J. M. H., Vermeulen, A., O'Reilly, M., Lang, R., & Lancioni, G. E. (2009). Cyberbullying among students with intellectual and developmental disability in special education settings. *Developmental Neurorehabilitation, 12,* 146–151. doi:10.1080/17518420902971356.

Dredge, R., Gleeson, J., & de la Piedad Garcia, X. (2014). Risk factors associated with impact severity of cyberbullying victimization: A qualitative study of adolescent online social networking. *Cyberpsychology, Behavior and Social Networking, 17*(5), 287–291. doi:10.1089/cyber.2013.0541.

Egan, S. K., & Perry, D. G. (1998). Does low self-regard invite victimization? *Developmental Psychology, 34,* 299–309. doi:10.1037//0012-1649.34.2.299.

Fekkes, M., Pijpers, F. I. M., & Verloove-VanHorick, S. P. (2004). Bullying behavior and associations with psychosomatic complaints and depression in victims. *Journal of Pediatrics, 144,* 17–22. doi:10.1016/j.jpeds.2003.09.025.

Fredstrom, B. K., Adams, R. E., & Gilman, R. (2011). Electronic and school-based victimization: Unique contexts for adjustment difficulties during adolescence. *Journal of Youth & Adolescence, 40*(4), 405–415. doi:10.1007/s10964-010-9569-7.

Garnefski, N., & Kraaij, V. (2014). Bully victimization and emotional problems in adolescents: Moderation by specific cognitive coping strategies? *Journal of Adolescence, 37*(7), 1153–1160. doi:10.1016/j.adolescence.2014.07.005.

Gini, G., & Pozzoli, T. (2009). Association between bullying and psychosomatic problems: A meta-analysis. *Pediatrics, 123*(3), 1059–1065. doi:10.1542/peds.2008-1215.

Gradinger, P., Strohmeier, D., & Spiel, C. (2009). Traditional bullying and cyberbullying: Identification of risk groups for adjustment problems. *Zeitschrift Für Psychologie/Journal of Psychology, 217*(4), 205–213. doi:10.1027/0044-3409.217.4.205.

Hawker, D. S. J., & Boulton, M. J. (2000). Twenty years' research on peer victimization and psychosocial maladjustment: A meta-analytic review of cross-sectional studies. *Journal of Child Psychology and Psychiatry, 41,* 441–455.

Hinduja, S., & Patchin, J. W. (2009). *Bullying beyond the schoolyard: Preventing and responding to cyberbullying.* Thousand Oaks: Corwin Press.

Hinduja, S., & Patchin, J. W. (2010). Bullying, cyberbullying, and suicide. *Archives of Suicide Research, 14*(3), 206–221. doi:10.1080/13811118.2010.494133.

Hinduja, S., & Patchin, J. W. (2014). State cyberbullying laws: A brief review of state cyberbullying laws and policies. http://www.cyberbullying.us/Bullying_and_Cyberbullying_Laws.pdf.

Juvonen, J., & Gross, E. F. (2008). Extending the school grounds? Bullying experiences in cyberspace. *Journal of School Health, 78,* 496–505. doi:10.1111/j.1746-1561.2008.00335.x.

Kowalski, R. M., & Limber, S. P. (2007). Electronic bullying among middle school students. *Journal of Adolescent Health, 41*(6 Suppl), S22–S30. doi:10.1016/j.jadohealth.2007.08.017.

Kowalski, R. M., & Limber, S. P. (2013). Psychological, physical, and academic correlates of cyberbullying and traditional bullying. *Journal of Adolescent Health, 53,* S13–S20. doi:10.1016/j.jadohealth.2012.09.018.

Kowalski, R. M., Limber, S. E., & Agatston, P. W. (2012a). *Cyberbullying: Bullying in the digital age* (2nd edn.). Malden: Wiley-Blackwell.

Kowalski, R. M., Morgan, C. A., & Limber, S. E. (2012b). Traditional bullying as a potential warning sign of cyberbullying. *School Psychology International, 33,* 505–519. doi:10.1177/0143034312445244.

Kowalski, R. M., Giumetti, G. W., Schroeder, A. N., & Lattanner, M. R. (2014). Bullying in the digital age: A critical review and meta-analysis of cyberbullying research among youth. *Psychological Bulletin, 140*(4), 1073–1137. doi:10.1037/a0035618.

Landstedt, E., & Persson, S. (2014). Bullying, cyberbullying, and mental health in young people. *Scandinavian Journal of Public Health, 42*(4), 393–399. doi:10.1177/1403494814525004.

Lazarus, R. S., & Folkman, S. (1984). *Stress, appraisal and coping.* New York: Springer.

Leary, M. R. (1983). Social anxiousness: The construct and its measurement. *Journal of Personality Assessment, 47,* 66–75. doi:10.1207/s15327752jpa4701_8.

Lenhart, A. (6 May 2010). Cyberbullying: What the research is telling us. http://www.pewinternet.org/Presentations/2010/May/Cyberbullying-2010.aspx.

Livingstone, S., & Smith, P. K. (2014). Annual research review: Harms experienced by child users of online and mobile technologies: The nature, prevalence and management of sexual and aggressive risks in the digital age. *Journal of Child Psychology and Psychiatry, 55,* 635–654. doi:10.1111/jcpp.12197.

Machmutow, K., Perren, S., Sticca, F., & Alsaker, F. D. (2012). Peer victimisation and depressive symptoms: Can specific coping strategies buffer the negative impact of cybervictimisation? *Emotional & Behavioural Difficulties, 17,* 403–420. doi:10.1080/13632752.2012.704310.

Mehari, K. R., Farrell, A. D., & Le, A. H. (2014). Cyberbullying among adolescents: Measures in search of a construct. *Psychology of Violence, 4*(4), 399–415. doi:10.1037/a0037521.

Menesini, E., Calussi, P., & Nocentini, A. (2012). Cyberbullying and traditional bullying: Unique, additive, and synergistic effects on psychological health symptoms. In Q. Li, D. Cross, & P. K. Smith (Eds.), *Cyberbullying in the global playground: Research on international perspectives* (pp. 245–262). Malden: Blackwell.

Messias, E., Kindrick, K., & Castro, J. (2014). School bullying, cyberbullying, or both: Correlates of teen suicidality in the 2011 CDC youth risk behavior survey. *Comprehensive Psychiatry, 55*(5), 1063–1068. doi:10.1016/j.comppsych.2014.02.005.

Modecki, K. L., Minchin, J., Harbaugh, A. G., Guerra, N. G., & Runions, K. C. (2014). Bullying prevalence across contexts: A meta-analysis measuring cyber and traditional bullying. *Journal of Adolescent Health.* doi:10.1016/j.jadohealth.2014.06.007.

Nansel, T., Overpeck, M., Pilla, R., Ruan, W., Simons-Morton, B., & Scheidt, P. (2001). Bullying behaviors among US youth: Prevalence and association with psychosocial adjustment. *Journal of the American Medical Association, 285,* 2094–2100. doi:10.1001/jama.285.16.2094.

Nixon, C. (2014). Current perspectives: The impact of cyberbullying on adolescent health. *Adolescent Health, Medicine and Therapeutics, 5,* 143–158. doi:10.2147/AHMT.S36456.

Olweus, D. (1993). *Bullying at school: What we know and what we can do.* New York: Blackwell.

Olweus, D. (1996/2004). *The revised Olweus bully/victim questionnaire.* Bergen: Research Centre for Health Promotion (HEMIL).

Olweus, D. (2012). Cyberbullying: An overrated phenomenon? *European Journal of Developmental Psychology, 9,* 520–538. doi:10.1080/17405629.2012.682358.

Olweus, D. (2013). School bullying: Development and some important challenges. *Annual Review of Clinical Psychology, 9,* 1–14. doi:10.1146/annurev-clinpsy-050212-185516.

Olweus, D., & Limber, S. P. (November 2010). *What do we know about bullying: Information from the Olweus bullying questionnaire.* Paper presented at the annual meeting of the International Bullying Prevention Association, Seattle, WA.

Perren, S., & Gutzwiller-Helfenfinger, E. (2012). Cyberbullying and traditional bullying in adolescence: Differential roles of moral disengagement, moral emotions, and moral values. *European Journal of Developmental Psychology, 9,* 195–209. doi:10.1080/17405629.2011.643168.

Perren, S., Dooley, J., Shaw, T., & Cross, D. (2010). Bullying in school and cyberspace: Associations with depressive symptoms in Swiss and Australian adolescents. *Child and Adolescent Psychiatry and Mental Health, 4,* 28. doi:10.1186/1753-2000-4-28.

Podsakoff, P. M., MacKenzie, S. B., Lee, J., & Podsakoff, N. P. (2003). Common method biases in behavioral research: A critical review of the literature and recommended remedies. *Journal of Applied Psychology, 88*(5), 879–903. doi:10.1037/0021-9010.88.5.879.

Pyżalski, J. (2012). From cyberbullying to electronic aggression: Typology of the phenomenon. *Emotional & Behavioural Difficulties, 17*(3–4), 305–317. doi:10.1080/13632752.2012.704319.

Riebel, J., Jäger, R. S., & Fischer, U. C. (2009). Cyberbullying in Germany—An exploration of prevalence, overlapping with real life bullying and coping strategies. *Psychology Science Quarterly, 51*(3), 298–314.

Rigby, K. (1997). *Bullying in schools: And what to do about it.* London: Jessica Kingsley Publishers.

Rigby, K., & Slee, P. T. (1993). Dimensions of interpersonal relations among Australian school children and their implications for psychological well-being. *Journal of Social Psychology, 133,* 33–42. doi:10.1080/00224545.1993.9712116.

Robers, S., Kemp, J., Rathbun, A., & Morgan, R. E. (2014). Indicators of school crime and safety: 2013 (NCES 2014-042/NCJ 243299). National Center for Education Statistics, U.S. Department of Education, and Bureau of Justice Statistics, Office of Justice Programs, U.S. Department of Justice. Washington, DC.

Rosenberg, M. (1965). *Society and the adolescent self-image.* Princeton: Princeton University Press.

Sakellariou, T., Carroll, A., & Houghton, S. (2012). Rates of cyber victimization and bullying among male Australian primary and high school students. *School Psychology International, 33,* 533–549. doi:10.1177/0143034311430374.

Slonje, R., & Smith, P. K. (2008). Cyberbullying: Another main type of bullying? *Scandinavian Journal of Psychology, 49,* 147–154. doi:10.1111/j.1467-9450.2007.00611.x.

Smith, P. K., Mahdavi, J., Carvalho, M., Fisher, S., Russell, S., & Tippett, N. (2008). Cyberbullying: Its nature and impact in secondary school pupils. *Journal of Child Psychology and Psychiatry, 49*(4), 376–385. doi:10.1111/j.1469-7610.2007.01846.x.

van Geel, M., Vedder, P., & Tanilon, J. (2014a). Bullying and weapon carrying: A meta-analysis. *JAMA Pediatrics, 168*(8), 714–720. doi:10.1001/jamapediatrics.2014.213.

van Geel, M., Vedder, P., & Tanilon, J. (2014b). Relationship between peer victimization, cyberbullying, and suicide in children and adolescents: A meta-analysis. *JAMA Pediatrics, 168*(5), 435–442. doi:10.1001/jamapediatrics.2013.4143.

Vazsonyi, A. T., Machackova, H., Sevcikova, A., Smahel, D., & Cerna, A. (2012). Cyberbullying in context: Direct and indirect effects by low self-control across 25 European countries. *European Journal of Developmental Psychology, 9*(2), 210–227. doi:10.1080/17405629.2011.644919.

Wang, W., Vaillancourt, T., Brittain, H. L., McDougall, P., Krygsman, A., Smith, D., Cunningham, C. E., Haltigan, J. D., & Hymel, S. (2014). School climate, peer victimization, and academic achievement: Results from a multi-informant study. *School Psychology Quarterly, 29*(3), 360–377. doi:10.1037/spq0000084.

Wigderson, S., & Lynch, M. (2013). Cyber- and traditional peer victimization: Unique relationships with adolescent well-being. *Psychology of Violence, 3*(4), 297–309. doi:10.1037/a0033657.

Willard, N. E. (2007). *Cyberbullying and cyberthreats: Responding to the challenge of online social aggression, threats, and distress.* Champaign: Research Press.

Williams, K. R., & Guerra, N. G. (2007). Prevalence and predictors of internet bullying. *Journal of Adolescent Health, 41,* 14–21. doi:10.1016/j.jadohealth.2007.08.018.

Ybarra, M. L., & Mitchell, K. J. (2004). Youth engaging in online harassment: Associations with caregiver—child relationships, internet use, and personal characteristics. *Journal of Adolescence, 27,* 319–336. doi:10.1016/j.adolescence.2004.03.007.

Chapter 7
Cyberbullying and Education: A Review of Emergent Issues in Latin America Research

Fabiola Cabra Torres and Gloria Marciales Vivas

7.1 Improper Use of the Internet: A Poorly Understood Problem

In knowledge societies, the multiple uses of the Internet and social networks by children and young people generate different types of statements and initiatives (political, legal, and educational) aimed at counteracting actual and potential risks that cause moral panic to different audiences. People have such reactions in part because of the digital divide between those who have access to new technologies and due to the various situations to which infants and adolescents are exposed which may affect their safety, welfare, and development (Livingstone 2007).

Despite the risks emerging from the new spaces of social exchange in the network, it is undeniable that the Internet has a transformative potential in different areas of human life. Duart (2010) states that something that should concern us is the ability we have to understand and use the Internet, because the inequality between people who have the opportunity to access the educational, social, and economic potential of these social media and people who do not have these opportunities is evident.

The author notes that "There is, therefore, a new digital divide between those people who have a vision and a certain use of the Internet and those who don't. And that gap tends to grow among particular social groups as well as between certain generations of people. And, it is clear that the conceptual gap related to the use of the network determines its use and the ability of individuals and groups to grow and influence socially" (Duart 2010, p. 1). The digital divide is associated with

F. Cabra Torres (✉)
Facultad de Educación, Pontificia Universidad Javeriana,
Edificio 25, Piso 4°Carrera 7 N° 40-62, Bogotá, Colombia
e-mail: f.cabra@javeriana.edu.co

G. Marciales Vivas
Department of Psychology, Pontificia Universidad Javeriana, Bogotá, Colombia

© Springer International Publishing Switzerland 2016
R. Navarro et al. (eds.), *Cyberbullying Across the Globe*,
DOI 10.1007/978-3-319-25552-1_7

both the opportunity to access technologies and the conceptions built around them. Therefore, actions aimed at identifying explanatory factors of problematic use of technologies, such as cyberbullying which ignores fundamental conceptions, may lead to somewhat limited and partial views and promote myths and prohibitions without support in research.

That is why Shariff and Churchill (2010) analyze the complexity of moral, ethical, legal, and pedagogical aspects inherent to cyberbullying and draw attention to the myths that have been built around this social phenomenon. These narratives have contributed to objectify the problem and to look for mechanisms to control it through legal devices which are justified based on statistics.

Cyberbullying—when approached from the myths built around it—can lead to the naive belief that controlling the use of technologies by young people will result in proper handling of the behaviors of harassment and abuse.

Research has demonstrated the relationship between traditional bullying and cyberbullying with homophobic, sexist, racist, and discriminatory attitudes (Shariff 2005 and 2009); however, most studies have ignored the systemic relationships of the phenomenon with attitudes that are rooted, reinforced, and modeled by the adult society (Shariff 2009). Therefore, labeling children as aggressors or victims is not enough if we neglect the fact that these new generations are social actors that respond to a complex variety of influences that affect their lives (Shariff and Churchill 2010).

Statistics contribute to maintaining myths about cyberbullying; when they are magnified or put out of context, for example, they could stimulate fear derived from parents' and teachers' perceptions that something is out of control. Besides, this could promote the idea that adults cannot do anything to protect children and young people from the risk of technology exposure. Accordingly, non-tolerance is proposed as an alternative of control which, as a consequence, justifies punishment as well as disciplinary and punitive actions. These concomitant perceptions and behaviors seem to ignore more comprehensive explanations. Shariff and Churchill (2010) draw attention to:

- The significant influence of teachers' attitudes, given that some of them usually tend in a tacit way to ignore certain verbal harassment expressions or value them as acceptable and inoffensive.
- Parental influence, specially the lack of care, and the way in which adults can be a model of harassment and of discriminatory treatment to others, for example, excluding marginalized groups of society.
- Outdated school curriculum, which does not favor the reflexive dialog about negative behaviors and does not include contents that contribute to facing aggressive ways of social interaction and communication in the classrooms. Similarly, there are curricula that do not stimulate the ethical and responsible use of technologies and the Internet either.
- The common belief that the making of policies or codes of behavior at school is enough to face cyberbullying and to have safe schools. Nonetheless, evidence suggests that the dysfunctional relationship between school management and teachers is associated with harassment of teachers by students.

The previous issues justify the need of taking into account the complexities of the improper use of technologies and questioning all those approaches centered to exert control. Because they are based on partial visions of the phenomenon, they promote merely policing interventions. These views have been demonstrated to be difficult to be put into practice (Campbell 2005).

7.2 Cyberbullying: Concept and Paradigmatic Perspectives

While some authors claim that cyberbullying is just a continuation of the forms of peer-to-peer aggression, which starts in face-to-face relationships (Kowalski et al. 2008), others say that it is a different phenomenon which should be configured as a new field of research, particularly because of its peculiar characteristics, such as the anonymity of perpetrators and the ability to go beyond the time and space boundaries that frame face-to-face human relationships (Jäger et al. 2010).

The differences between traditional bullying and cyberbullying stem from the frequent exchanges in technologies and the potential of electronic communication, characterized by a type of violence much more aggressive than that emerging in face-to-face interactions (Del Río et al. 2010). Some of the characteristics are:

- The all-along mobility and connectivity of new technologies that makes cyberbullying something that transcends all places and reaches numerous recipients. It is not limited to school or home.
- The bullies' invisibility or anonymity, which becomes relevant as a facilitator of new technologies, so as to allow people to act or use false identities and pseudonyms that hinder the chances of being identified.
- The distance between the stalker and the victim of bullying decreases any feelings of guilt and empathy and the awareness of the consequences resulting from aggressions.
- The fact that the digital content used to bully others is stored and difficult to erase or eliminate makes it seem everlasting.
- The ease and speed with which verbal or visual messages are sent using the communication technologies make cyberbullying an effortless practice.
- Finally, cyberbullying has no relationship with the aggressor's or victim's physical strength, size, or age or with the marginal status of the aggressors.

Although cyberbullying does not have an accepted general definition yet, it is considered as any behavior oriented to and repeated over time in order to inflict damage, either through phone, e-mail, or instant messages, or to defame using Web pages (Baruch 2005; Nocentini et al. 2010). The elements which are part of this definition must be clarified:

- Intention: it is one of the most difficult aspects to establish when cyberbullying situations are analyzed (Menesini and Nocentini 2009)

- Repetition: posting a message on the Internet constitutes an act of repetition because these media make it possible (Kowalski et al. 2008; Menesini and Nocentini 2009)
- Imbalance of power in relationships: the victim's inability to get the contents deleted, the lack of skills to manage technologies, or the high social status of the perpetrator within a virtual community can lead to the perception of imbalance and asymmetry in the exercise of power

The complexity of cyberbullying as a phenomenon has led analysts and researchers to broaden their understanding of it and of the intervention spectrum toward overarching perspectives in which social and cultural factors become essential. For this reason, prevention and intervention initiatives begin to embody the cultural dimensions of the problem in its design and evaluation (Li 2008).

Cyberbullying has been approached from paradigmatic perspectives, which guide research and intervention by many routes. On the basis of Pimienta's analysis (2008), three paradigmatic perspectives are identified as follows:

- Technology-based approach: this approach emphasizes on the means rather than the end use of technologies. Research and intervention are directed toward the use of information and communication technologies (ICT) regulation in public and private spaces and the different forms of controlling the occurrence of bullying situations through cyber-surveillance.
- Content- and applications-based approach: this approach emphasizes on the construction of criteria to classify content on the network and pedagogical strategies that may be useful for parents and teachers to prevent cyberbullying situations.
- Approach toward the paradigm shift: this approach incorporates research-based knowledge to foster conditions under which social forms of interaction can be transformed, starting from a complex view of the factors associated with cyberbullying. This phenomenon is approached as an expression of social dynamics that affects individuals' quality of life in a competitive society crossed by market logic.

We consider the latter perspective as one of the bases of the research that we are conducting in the research group *Learning and Information Society* (Pontificia Universidad Javeriana, Bogotá-Colombia). In this perspective, technological tools, whatever they may be, are understood as tools that extend people's capabilities to build new forms of organization and regulation; these are cultural devices which are appropriated and revisited based on the social interaction processes that take place in situated social and cultural contexts. Therefore, in cyberbullying situations, technological devices are instruments which depend on specific contexts and on their users' cultural background as well as on the validated and naturalized forms of interaction in the history of the subjects.

7.2.1   Cyberbullying and the Risk Society

Latin America is the region where the Internet audience has grown the most worldwide. A ComScore report (2013) on digital trends shows some characteristics of user behavior: The Latin American Internet audience, which only accounts for 9% of the global Internet audience, grew by 12% between 2012 and 2013; Facebook is the most used social network in Latin America. Regarding the distribution of users surfing the Internet, 42% of Internet users are in Brazil, followed by Mexico, Argentina, Colombia, Venezuela, Chile, Peru, and Puerto Rico, with a large number of relatively young users.

In this context, the most striking cultural transformations are related to the forms of access to information, communication through new media, and the emergence of new competencies for digital citizenship or civic behavior in digital media. However, these typical social skills of the digital world are not developed properly in school, nor the family helps develop them.

The interest in analyzing children and youth empathy to the Internet and to the new digital media has focused mostly on highlighting risks that emerge from the exchanges and electronic communication. Two types of risks are distinguished: passive and active risks (Del Río et al. 2010). The first one arises from the simple fact of being connected to the Internet or owning a mobile phone and does not require the user's will—for example, when they are victims of virtual harassment or receive obscene messages. The second one refers to situations where the single access to technology facilitates negative action on others.

Moreover, the review of publications in scientific journals related to this line of research has identified three thematic areas which have been mainly targeted (Cabra-Torres and Marciales-Vivas 2011): risk factors (Twyman et al. 2010; Mesch 2009; Dehue et al. 2008), the emotional aspects involved in risk situations (Ortega et al. 2009; Price and Delgleish 2010), and intervention strategies to prevent or overcome bullying situations once they have happened (Mesch 2009; Agatston et al. 2007).

Much of the research on cyberbullying has emphasized the relationship that such behavior has with variables such as gender, age subgroups, social class, Internet activity and its frequency (Cabra-Torres and Marciales-Vivas 2011). Many of these studies are reports based on statistics, and a few of them are barely beginning to include the children and adolescent participation variable to explore the nature of this phenomenon from their experiences.

A review of the investigation shows that cyberbullying measurement requires greater scrutiny as it makes everyday experience invisible and responds to generalizations that are easy to establish with statistics. In this sense, Lankshear and Knobel (2010) argue that surveys measure different variables and produce various results that hinder an accurate and multidimensional analysis; moreover, some figures are often used to support or justify authoritarian policies of greater surveillance. What they consider most damaging is the logic that encompasses studies based on a process of reification-measurement-treatment, where the phenomenon is simplified by means of indicators in order to control it. They warn that figures are not required to take action because each case, by its human nature and consequences, is reprehensible and unacceptable.

In addition, the difficulty in determining cyberbullying incidence through surveys is that it varies from country to country, and it depends on when it has been applied and on the samples used and the different cyberbullying definitions such studies are based on (Campbell et al. 2008).

Regarding the participation of different actors who experience cyberbullying situations, it is worth considering the different perspectives that schools, students, and teachers in the educational context manifest. In addition, schools are asked to generate safe learning environments, students defend their right to free expression and greater privacy for their online conversations, and some parents ask the school not to prohibit mobile phone use or establish penalties (Shariff 2005).

The Argentine Observatory on Violence in Schools, in a recent paper (Campelo and Lerner 2014), criticizes the early studies of bullying which used to assume an explanation based on the pathologic traits of individuals who adopt the role of perpetrators or of potential victims. This approach defines profiles that secure identity, impose labels on subjects, and offer predictions that are associated with their future behaviors such as criminal behavior or suicide acts (see Olweus 2011).

The central problem that the previous approach can bring is the emphasis on pathological subjects and, in children and young people, medicalization or the search for the guilty without addressing the structural dimension of this issue. It is necessary to transcend the problematic dichotomous variable model such as bully victims in order to understand the systemic nature of relations between groups that are affected by various forms of harassment (Campbell 2005).

It is noteworthy that the prevailing conceptions of bullying and cyberbullying have had much influence on institutional and classroom practices as well as on macro policy educational decisions resulting in simplistic solutions (Campelo and Lerner 2014).

Therefore, it requires a systemic view of cyberbullying that incorporates the perspectives of its main actors, as this is an unprecedented problem for many adults, including teachers and families who are not unaware of the many conflicts that begin at school and then extend to social networks and to any virtual space where the intermediation of the school becomes practically impossible.

7.3 Overview of Emergent Issues in Latin American Research

The term "cyberbullying" and its definition are still under construction. The word "bullying" can be defined in many different ways and it is not easily translated in different languages, neither in its purely technical use nor in its daily meanings (Gorostiaga and Paladino 2013). It is less popular within Latin America and has been focused on the use of expressions such as online bullying, cybernetic bullying, and cyberstalking, among others.

Owing to the fact that cyberbullying is an arising global issue within the educational agenda of countries in the Latin American region, three topics are presented here to provide an overview of the phenomenon: the first one is the identification of some illustrative studies undertaken by researchers, the second one is an analysis of some of the regulatory norms that make cyberbullying become a crime and a legal problem, and the third one refers to the efforts made to prevent it in order to enhance society involvement. On this basis, cyberbullying is assumed as a form of violence that goes beyond school, mainly related to interventions through citizenship education. In this chapter, we are mostly concerned with the latter.

7.3.1 Cyberbullying Research

A review of cyberbullying research and its prevalence among the most vulnerable populations in Latin America showed that research is insufficient in this field, and as a consequence, it is very difficult to diagnose the seriousness of this phenomenon in the region. Some studies undertaken in Latin America are presented in Table 7.1.

As is shown in Table 7.1, of the cyberbullying research literature, some articles focus on the differences between traditional bullying and cyberbullying, which constitutes the early stage of studies in this field of inquiry. Similarly, the different forms that cyberbullying takes through social networking Web sites and electronic devices are analyzed as a mean to characterize the types of violence through electronic technology and to establish comparisons.

Without doubt, this is an issue of remarkable importance to clinical psychology and psychiatry because of its impact on children and young people's mental health. Surprisingly, there are a few studies aimed at analyzing the educational and pedagogical dimensions of the problem. Most of early cyberbullying studies focus on adolescents and use survey methodology as a primary strategy.

Spain is the country with the largest number of studies within Iberoamerica (Giménez-Gualdo et al. 2014; León et al. 2012; Álvarez et al. 2011). Most of these

Table 7.1 Some research in Latin America on cyberbullying. (Source: Authors)

Authors	Country	Objective of the study
Del Río et al. (2009)	Comparative analysis of Latin American countries	Describe cyberbullying among students in Argentina, Brazil, Chile, Colombia, Mexico, Peru, and Venezuela
García et al. (2010)	Perú	Identify the prevalence of cyberbullying associated with gender, grade level, and academic performance
García et al. (2011)	México	Establish the differences between bullying and cyberbullying
Matilde (2012)	Uruguay	Analyze the impact of bullying and cyberbullying on public health
Lanzilloti and Korman (2014)	Argentina	Describe the different types of bullying using technologies
Varela et al. (2014)	Chile	Identify the prevalence and manifestation of different forms of cyberbullying (through msn, Internet, and phone with photos), associated with gender, grade, and type of establishment

studies have identified teenagers between the ages of 13 and 16 years as the most vulnerable group, together with women who are the most victimized group (Calmaestra et al. 2008).

Mexico is one of the Latin American countries that give special importance to cyberbullying and cyberstalking as a social problem. Among Mexican researchers who have conducted studies, a recent project in public schools by Vega-López et al. (2013) found that the prevalence of cyberbullying in adolescents between the ages of 14 and 15 years was 14%, and use of text messages and insulting images via mobile phones were identified as the most used methods in peer harassment.

The research results obtained by Vega-López et al. (2013) are consistent with studies conducted in other contexts: In about half of the situations, the bullies are classmates, and despite the suffering this causes to victims, in about 80% of the reported cases bullied children and adolescents do not ask for help from teachers or significant adults. Notwithstanding the aforementioned, family are the fundamental niche to provide containment and support to adolescents when other mechanisms of protection fail to help (approximately 48% of cases). Shame or fear of prohibitions on using the mobile phone are some of the reasons given as an explanation of not reporting the harassment situation to which they are subjected.

In addition, these studies show that there are vulnerability factors that fall into cyberbullying situations such as the involvement of students with low academic achievement, or those having to attend night schools at an early age when they are expected to attend a day school.

In Latin America, the aforementioned results can be taken into account to draw attention to the adolescents' vulnerability and the need to give them the protection required according to their social condition and age, without falling into the trap of treating them as purely victims (Pavez 2013).

The ongoing interest in this issue in the region aims to preserve young people's status as subjects of rights and to teach them strategies to self-monitor contents and platforms they access. One of the main challenges in this context is to maintain a balance between protection and empowerment of this population group in virtual environments.

In contrast with approaches that understand cyberbullying as a public health problem or as a behavior that should be handled with exemplifying sanctions, as we have explained previously, there should be other perspectives and new views that allow us to capture the social dimensions of the phenomenon—to be understood as an expression of social interactions with peers. Adela Cortina (1998), Spanish philosopher, broadens the views on this and other phenomena that arise in social spaces, supposedly protected. According to Cortina, these [negative] social behaviors are closely related to the formation of citizens and the role that education plays in this process.

Although cyberbullying arises as a conflict between individuals (bullies and bullied), schools play a key role in its handling; putting much emphasis on these aspects entails the risk of ignoring the fact that it has become a social problem which requires a twofold effort: to recover a sense of humanity in peer social interactions among peers and to seek fair solutions for those involved in these kinds of situations.

In this context, the concept of "obligation" is particularly relevant because being "obliged" to respect other's dignity has nothing to do with the world of legal mandates and prescriptive norms but with the fact that people are linked to others and that to be linked constitutes an unavoidable form of being a person (Cortina 1998).

In accordance with the aforementioned, any action oriented to the transformation of a phenomenon such as cyberbullying involves creating conditions to recover the connecting links that exist between human beings. This requires promoting education that contributes to the formation of values through the involvement of young people in situations in which values such as freedom, equality, solidarity, respect, and dialog can be experienced (Cortina 2005), overcoming normative views of violence.

7.3.2 Cyberbullying As a Crime: From the Clinical Focus to the Legal Approach

School violence is a very complex phenomenon that takes place in different ways in educational institutions. It includes, among other manifestations, peer harassment, aggressions and abuse by teachers of students and vice versa, teenager abuse by parents, other family members, caregivers, friends, or other individuals living in the house, affecting school life, and situations in which students are exposed to community violence, perpetrated by individuals such as gangs, and so forth (Martínez Rojas 2013). Students may be adversely affected regardless of whether they are victims or witnesses of violent acts. Therefore, bullying or cyberbullying is a particular type of school violence that has begun to receive attention recently.

It is of significance that school violence had never before been an object of policies. Until recently, some countries have advanced in regulations aimed to control and prevent violence—including bullying and cyberbullying actions—based on legal approaches that have influenced school policies and intervention. As we shall see, an analysis of this normative vision, far from providing definitive solutions, opens up a range of new educational and public debates.

Campelo and Lerner (2014) point out that in some anti-bullying policies, harassment is often equated with crime, and consequently, this view promotes denouncing of actions in schools. In serious cases, children are punished by law so that the minimum age has been reduced to make minors legally responsible; in other policies, such as the laws enacted in Chile and Colombia, the school authorities are sanctioned if they fail to adopt the preventive, educational, or disciplinary procedures as indicated in the mandates.

Although there is no policy to give particular treatment to and typify cyberbullying, some of the recent policies that have been enacted are closely related to this problem—for example, topics such as pacific coexistence, social conflict and peace, safety in schools, the practice of human rights, citizen education, confirm the growing visibility and attention given to this issue in schools in Latin America during the last 5 years (Table 7.2).

Table 7.2 School violence prevention in some Latin American countries. (Source: Synthesis based on laws)

Laws enacted by countries	Purpose
Ley de Seguridad Integral Escolar para el Estado Libre y Soberano de Puebla, (2011a) México (a)	Promote the establishment of permanent links between the various elements that interact in the school community and society itself
Ley contra el Acoso Escolar para el Estado de Veracruz de Ignacio de la Llave (2011b) México (b)	Prevent and eliminate bullying in public and private educational institutions of state on the basis of respect for human rights, democracy, equality, and nondiscrimination
Ley N° 20.536 (2011) Sobre violencia escolar o bullying. Chile (c)	Promote a good school life and prevent all forms of physical or mental violence, aggression, or harassment
Ley para la Promoción de la Convivencia Libre de Violencia en el Entorno Escolar del Distrito Federal (2012d) México (d)	Prevent existing school abuse in basic and higher education in the federal district
Ley 26.892, de 2013 Ley para la promoción de la convivencia y el abordaje de la conflictividad social en las instituciones educativas. Argentina (e)	Establish the basis for promotion, institutional intervention, and research and compilation of experiences on living as well as addressing social unrest in educational institutions at all levels and modalities of the national education system
Ley 1620, de 2013 por la cual se crea el Sistema Nacional de Convivencia Escolar y Formación para el Ejercicio de los Derechos Humanos, la Educación para la Sexualidad y la Prevención y Mitigación de la Violencia Escolar. Colombia (f)	Promote and strengthen civic education and strengthening human rights concepts and healthy living as well as minimize rates of bullying and cyberbullying

In relation to laws enacted in Mexico (a, b, d), the multidimensionality and complexity of school violence is highlighted, and a variety of governmental actors and not just the school community enter the play. According to Zurita Rivera (2012), the principles and guidelines could eventually transform the everyday functioning of schools, their dynamics, and institutional culture and also generate changes in conceptions considering this social phenomenon as a cross-cutting issue, which should involve governmental and nongovernmental actors (for instance, the Law of Puebla 2011a).

Within these laws, bullying and cyberbullying actions are explicitly considered. A stereotyped way of referring to roles of aggressor–victim–accomplice is still utilized (for instance, the law of Veracruz). Specifically, the law of the federal district refers to a culture of peace perspective, the gender approach, and human rights of children and young people, and it emphasizes the rights of people exposed to any type of abuse as well as of those generating violence (Zurita Rivera 2012, p. 8).

The law enacted in Argentina (e) draws attention to the need for recognition and reparation for harm or offense to persons who have suffered any type of aggression—a rarely included aspect in other regulations. So, instead of focusing on the individual as a victim or perpetrator unilaterally, it emphasizes the context in which social interactions generate aggressions. This new law points out the formative significance of the potential penalties so that children and adolescents become progressively more responsible for their actions.

The Argentinean law also includes a series of initiatives that address prevention, namely strengthening specialized teams to intervene in violence situations, providing orientation guides to schools to develop their own coexistence rules and encourage students' ownership of them, and a free national hotline to help schools when violence situations arise; another aspect worth highlighting is that it promotes and supports research projects and communication campaigns. All these initiatives go beyond the simple sanctions and contribute to the understanding of the phenomenon by civil society.

In Chile (c), the so called anti-bullying law—consisting of an amendment to the education law—aims to establish a mechanism to regulate and prevent improper and abusive behavior in school life. The law focuses on parents' role and responsibility when their children have generated any aggression, including the use of all corrective means (psychological or medical) to stop their abusive behavior.

In Colombia (f), the enactment of Law 1620 of 2013 adopts a radical position to eradicate school violence based on the adverse impact that the Colombian armed conflict has had on coexistence and well-being at schools. However, the law may have a reductionist approach because it gives much centrality to bullying without considering that school life problems should not be confined to this (Martínez Rojas 2013).

The application of this law has led to changes in the guides of pacific coexistence at schools (called *Manuales de convivencia*) and also to the creation of committees with the participation of entities whose purpose is rights protection, law monitoring, and promotion of denouncing procedures in order to protect the minor's integrity.

Taking together the above country regulations, we can say that some early conceptions that led to simplistic and deterministic solutions are gradually being overcome. Instead, bullying and cyberbullying phenomena are better understood in the complex network of relationships in which the diverse forms of aggression occur in social interactions inside and outside schools.

Thus, the predominant conceptions of bullying and cyberbullying have had their counterparts not only in institutional practices but also in education policy-making and policy-makers. There is a shift from strictly clinical views based on a victimology approach to a legal perspective of human coexistence, which entails implications and consequences in school life and produces community social representations. It is important to note that the profusion of policies and regulations could have an adverse effect. Instead of promoting comprehensive and coordinated actions among diverse actors regarding violence in schools, it could accentuate the inefficiency and lack of coordination, because the legal treatment of these situations can lead to the bureaucratization of educational processes and overemphasis on surveillance policies.

7.3.3 Cyberbullying Prevention: Some Citizen Initiatives

Among the diverse cyberbullying prevention programs in Latin America, the Colombian citizen initiatives become relevant because of the difficult social, economic, and political problems that this country faces. Some of the programs have been created with the hope of strengthening the role of citizens in the solutions. Besides, there has been an increasing awareness of the need for civic education and citizenship participation not only in Colombia but in all of Latin America (Jaramillo and Mesa 2009).

Red Papaz is a parent's network founded in 2002 to foster solidarity between families affected by cyberbullying aggressions. This independent civil organization witnessed the lack of parents' knowledge about the unreliable information their children are accessing and being exposed to through the Internet and decided to take action.

Using the rights-based approach, Red Papaz seeks to make all factors affecting the social and cultural environment of children and adolescents visible, create links among the state, the media, and public and private organizations that are responsible for ensuring a life with dignity for childhood.

The following three programs led by this parents' network deserve to be mentioned: *Aprendiendo a ser Papaz, Escudos para el Alma, and Angel Protector*. A brief description of each one is below:

Aprendiendo a ser Papaz (Learning to be Papaz) This program provides a useful guide for parents to the accompaniment of their children in new experiences as part of their socialization process. Frequently, parents experience complex unexpected situations in which they might not feel prepared and decide they cannot take actions.

Escudos para el Alma (Shields for the Soul) Red Papaz organizes activities in which public and private institutions together with schools share dialogs to explore the visualization of new ideas and initiatives aimed at promoting the protection and defense of children and adolescents in the family, school, and community.

The *Angel Protector* program seeks to raise awareness about risks to which children and adolescents are exposed—such as alcohol and cigarette consumption—and calls for common action not only from government agencies but also from those who sell these products, in order to facilitate protection networks.

One of the valuable actions of this parents' network consists of providing families with a didactic tool called "Kit Papaz," designed to address situations that might affect their children, such as child and youth suicide and bullying, among others.

To some extent, these citizen initiatives contribute to the moral education of families. Following Cortina's view, the moral dimension is understood as the ability to face life against the demoralization of society. Because cyberbullying affects the family environment deeply, they feel vulnerable, alone, and powerless to stop the aggressions.

In the aforementioned initiatives, there is an intervention model that transcends the individualistic aspects: Its main underlying idea is to highlight citizenship education that in this broader sense means educating the individual as a complete social human being able to coexist pacifically with others, as Cortina remarks. The emphasis of the intervention is on the development of competencies such as:

a. *Personal autonomy*: it refers to developing family capacities so that they can build alternatives to the circumstances that afflict them.
b. *Awareness of rights*: it refers to building networks with state institutions and identifying their responsibilities to prevent and stop cybernetic bullying.
c. *Civic links among citizens*: it refers to fostering links between people experiencing this particular situation and others who are able to find solutions.
d. *Responsible participation*: it refers to promoting citizenship participation in order to protect children and adolescent rights.

Another outstanding initiative is *Aulas en Paz* (Classrooms in Peace), a multicomponent program to develop students citizenship competencies in school from an early age (Chaux 2009). It promotes harmonious relationships among students and prevents all types of violent behavior toward others, like cyberbullying. With the support of the Ministry of Education, *Aulas en Paz* has been introduced in areas of Colombia with high levels of armed conflict and seeks to contribute to breaking the cycle of violence and reducing the negative effects of exposure to violent environments.

Therefore, according to the above, cyberbullying prevention would be based on actions guided by responsibility awareness. Here, responsibility supposes that someone is responsible for something or someone who is entrusted for some reason. This consciousness only makes sense in a relational world of coexistence, not in a fragmented one. It is expected that this moral sensibility would be promoted through networking citizens facing cyberbullying.

7.4 Conclusion

Cyberbullying research in Latin America is incipient. Some of the little research focuses on bullying–cyberbullying differences. Other studies, based on the clinical perspective, characterize cyberbullying as a pathologic phenomenon and neglect the educational dimension involved within any intervention.

Hence, some of the intervention programs that have been implemented in Latin America deviate from the medical model and intend to approach the problem from a rights perspective, which contributes to maintain the balance between protection and children and adolescent empowerment in society. How the educational system can help prepare young people to sustain a new democratic way of life has become a fundamental question for many countries (Chaux 2009).

Nowadays, cyberbullying prevalence in Latin America is significant, as are other forms of abuse among peers and school violence. A deeper knowledge of causes and consequences of these behaviors and interactions is crucial, both from the point of view of the people abused and from individuals who passively observe these phenomena without the intention to intervene in such situations; these two aspects are usually ignored in most of the research in the region.

This chapter seeks to widen horizons on cyberbullying in Latin America taking into account two closely interrelated aspects: on the one hand, the need to develop digital citizenship competencies at school and family—considered both as primary mediators of the children and youth socialization process—it implies helping to prepare them to have respectful, democratic, and ethical interactions in virtual environments and become responsible consumers in the digital world (Echeverria 2000), and on the other hand, the importance of implementing educational programs centered on digital skills development and self-regulation strategies in order to empower children as users of ICT, aware of their rights (CEPAL-UNICEF 2014).

The above perspective introduces a broader look that intends to transcend the individual analysis and helps to focus on the analysis of all factors and their interrelationships that may affect cyberbullying prevalence. This view can significantly contribute to its prevention to the extent that accounts for the structural aspects of the phenomenon. As studies have shown, children living in vulnerability conditions whose parents and/or teachers have poor digital skills, and moreover, do not receive any educational support, have higher risk and fewer opportunities to cope with aggression or prevent it.

A fact that has been an obstacle for gaining a comprehensive understanding of cyberbullying has been the narrow views of ICT as simple technological tools. From a more complex and cultural perspective, ICT constitutes dynamic spaces for social and cultural interactions for building capacities and deploying new rights. However,

> the discourses available to children currently focus almost exclusively on risk and protection, and this is potentially undermining their capacity to imagine, and articulate, the benefits digital media offers them in realizing their rights. (Third et al. 2014, p. 29)

Citizenship education in the new digital environment is an emerging issue that must be deepened in terms of new forms of early socialization in virtual scenarios. Providing orientation guidelines and other resources to families and schools is essential so that they contribute to educating their children to establish good social relationships based on tolerance, solidarity, and respect for others and to facilitate ownership of their rights in digital scenarios, for instance,

> 5. Right to personal development and education, to benefit from all the potentials that new technologies offer to improve their learning.
> 8. Parents have the right and the responsibility to guide and agree with their children responsible ICT uses.
> 10. Right to benefit and use new technologies to advance towards a healthier, more peaceful, fairer world respectful with the environment, in which the rights of all children are respected. (CEPAL-UNICEF 2014, p. 8)

Education for citizenship should promote children and youth digital literacy through a combination of formal and informal learning, as citizenship education is not only acquired in the school and family. It is not only learned in the streets and through the media but also in the relationships between the state and civil society and in relationships within the community (Chaux 2009). Because of this complexity, it is necessary to take into account both aspects, risks, and potentials of social contexts, overcoming popular visions of moral panic that distract from the educational function of the school and families in their role as educators of future generations.

References

Agatston, P. W., Kowalski, R., & Limber, S. (2007). Students' perspectives on cyber bullying. *Journal of Adolescent Health, 41*(Suppl 6), 59–60. doi:10.1016/j.jadohealth.2007.09.003.

Álvarez, D., Núñez, J. C., Álvarez, L., Dobarro, A., Rodríguez, C., & y González, P. (2011). Violencia a través de las tecnologías de la información y la comunicación en estudiantes de secundaria. *Anales de Psicología, 27*, 221–231.

Asamblea Legislativa del Distrito Federal. (2012d). Ley para la promoción de la convivencia libre de violencia en el entorno escolar del Distrito Federal. Gaceta Oficial del Distrito Federal, pp. 3–19. http://www.consejeria.df.gob.mx/uploads/gacetas/4f277518c1680.pdf.

Baruch, Y. (2005). Bullying on the Net: Adverse behavior one-mail and its impact. *Information and Management, 42*, 361–371. doi:10.1016/j.im.2004.02.001.

Cabra-Torres, F., & Marciales-Vivas, G. (2011). Internet y pánico moral: revisión de la investigación sobre la interacción de niños y jóvenes con los nuevos medios. *Universitas Psychologica, 10*(3), 855–865.

Calmaestra, J., Ortega, R., & Mora-Merchán, J. A. (2008). Las TIC y la convivencia. Un estudio sobre formas de acoso en el ciberespacio. *Investigación en la Escuela, 64*, 93–103.

Campbell, M. (2005). Cyberbullying: An old problem in a new guise? *Australian Journal of Guidance and Couselling, 15*(1), 68–76. doi:10.1375/ajgc.15.1.68.

Campbell, M., Butler, D., & Kift, S. (2008). A school's duty to provide safe learning environment: Does this include cyberbullyng? *Australia and New Zeland Journal of Law and Education, 13*(2), 21–32.

Campelo, A., & Lerner, M. (2014). *Acoso entre pares: orientación para actuar desde la escuela.* Ciudad Autónoma de Buenos Aires: Ministerio de Educación de la Nación.

CEPAL-UNICEF. (2014). Derechos de la infancia en la era digital. *Boletín de la infancia y adolescencia sobre el avance de los Objetivos de Desarrollo del Milenio, 18*, 4–9.

Chaux, E. (2009). Citizenship competencies in the midst of a violent political conflict: The Colombian educational response. *Harvard Educational Review, 79*(1), 84–93.

ComScore. (2013). El estado actual de la industria digital y las tendencias que están modelando el Futuro. http://www.comscore.com/Insights/Presentations-and-Whitepapers/2013/2013-Latin-America-Digital-Future-in-Focus.

Congreso del Estado de Puebla, LVII Legislatura. (2011a). Ley de Seguridad Integral Escolar para el Estado Libre y Soberano de Puebla. *Gaceta Legislativa*, año1, febrero de 2011.

Congreso del Estado de Veracruz, LXII Legislatura. (2011b). Ley Contra el Acoso Escolar para el Estado de Veracruz de Ignacio de la Llave. *Gaceta Legislativa, 59*, 37–46 (año 1). http://www.legisver.gob.mx/gaceta/gacetaLXII/GACETA59E.pdf.

Cortina, A. (1998). *Hasta un pueblo de demonios.* Madrid: Taurus.

Cortina, A. (2005). *Educación en valores y responsabilidad cívica.* Bogotá: Editorial el Búho Ltda.

Dehue, F., Bolman, C., & Völlink, T. (2008). Cyberbullying: Youngsters' experiences and parental perception. *Cyberpsychology and Behaviour, 11*(2), 217–223. doi:10.1089/cpb.2007.0008.

Del Río, J., Bringue, X., Sadaba, Ch, & González, D. (2009). *Cyberbullying: un análisis comparativo en estudiantes de Argentina, Brasil, Chile, Colombia, México, Perú y Venezuela.* V Congrés Internacional de Comunicació i Realitat. Barcelona. UniversitatRamonLlull.

Del Río, J., Sádaba, Ch, & Bringué, X. (2010). Menores y redes ¿sociales?: de la amistad al cyberbullying. *Revista de estudios de juventud, 88*, 115–129.

Duart, J. (2010). Editorial. Nuevas brechas digitales en la educación superior. *Revista de Universidad y sociedad del conocimiento, 7*(1), 1–2. http://rusc.uoc.edu.

Echeverria, J. (2000). Educación y tecnologías telemáticas. *Revista Iberoamericana de Educación, 24*, 17–36.

García, L., Orellana, O., Pomalay, R., Yanac, E., Sotelo, L., Herrera, E., Sotelo, N., Chávez, H., García, N., Macazana, D., Orellana, D., & Fernandini, P. (2010). Cyberbullying en escolares de educación secundaria de Lima metropolitana. *Revista IIPSI, 3*(12), 83–92.

García, G., Joffre, V., Martínez, G., & Llanes, A. (2011). Ciberbullying: Forma virtual de intimidación escolar. *Revista Colombiana de Psiquiatría, 40*(1), 115–130.

Giménez-Gualdo, A. M., Maquilón-Sánchez, J. J., & Sánchez, P. A. (2014). Acceso a las tecnologías, rendimiento académico y cyberbullying en escolares de secundaria. *Revista Iberoamericana de Psicología y Salud, 5*(2), 119–133.

Gorostiaga, D., & Paladino, C. (2013). Los chicos y las chicas hablan de molestar: un estudio cualitativo de los nombres del bullying. *V Congreso Internacional de Investigación y Práctica Profesional en Psicología XX Jornadas de InvestigaciónNoveno Encuentro de Investigadores en Psicología del MERCOSUR.* Facultad de Psicología—Universidad de Buenos Aires, Buenos Aires.

Jäger, T., Amado, J., Matos, T., & Pessoa, A. (2010). Analysis of experts' and trainers' viewer of cyberbullying. *Australian Journal of Guidance and Counseling, 20*(2), 169–181.

Jaramillo, R., & Mesa, J. A. (2009). Citizenship education as a response to Colombia's social and political context. *Journal of Moral Education, 38*(4), 467–487. doi:10.1080/03057240903321931.

Kowalski, R. M., Limber, S. P., & Agaston, P. (2008). *Cyberbullying.* Malden: Blackwell.

Lankshear, C., & Knobel, M. (2010). Foreword (or beyond 'reify, measure, and treat'). In S. Shariff & A. Churchill (Eds.), *Truths and myths of cyberbullying. International perspectives on stakeholders, responsibility and children's safety* (pp. XI–XVII). New York: Peter Lang Publishing, Inc.

Lanzilloti, A., & Korman, G. (2014). Cyberbullying, características y repercusiones de una nueva modalidad de maltrato escolar. *ActaPsiquiatrica y Psicológica de América Latina, 60*(1), 36–42.

León, B., Felipe, E., Fajardo, F., & Gómez, T. (2012). Cyberbullying en una muestra de estudiantes de Educación Secundaria: Variables moduladoras y redes sociales. *Electronic Journal of Research in Educational Psychology, 10*, 771–788.

Li, Q. (2008). A cross-cultural comparison of adolescents' experience related to cyberbullying. *Educational* cyberbullying. *Educational Research, 50*(3), 223–234. doi:10.1080/00131880802309333.

Livingstone, S. (2007). Los niños en Europa. Evaluación de los riesgos de Internet. *Telos. Cuadernos de comunicación e innovación, 73*, 52–69. http://sociedadinformacion.fundacion.telefonica.com/telos/articulocuaderno.asp@idarticulo%3D2&rev%3D73.htm.

Martínez Rojas, J. G. (2013). La Ley de convivencia: una deuda pendiente con la educación colombiana. *Ruta Maestra, 4*, 18–23.

Matilde, D. (2012). Nuevas formas de violencia entre pares: Del bullying al cyberbullying. *Revista Médica de Uruguay, 28*(1), 48–53.

Menesini, E., & Nocentini, A. (2009). Cyberbullying definition and measurement. Some critical considerations. *Journal of Psychology, 217*(4), 230–232. doi:10.1027/0044-3409.217.4.230.

Mesch, G. S. (2009). Parental mediation, online activities, and cyberbullying. *Cyberpsychology and Behavior, 12*(4), 387–393. doi:10.1089/cpb.2009.0068.

Nocentini, A., Calmaestra, J., Schultze-Krumbholz, A., Ortega-Ruiz, R., Menesini, E., & Scheithauer, H. (2010). Cyberbullying: Labels, behaviours and definition in three European countries. *Australian Journal of Guidance & Counselling, 20*(2), 129–142. doi:10.1375/ajgc.20.2.129.

Olweus, D. (2011). Bullying at school and later criminality: Findings from three Swedish community samples of males. *Criminal Behaviour and Mental Health, 21*(2), 151–156. doi:10.1002/cbm.806.

Ortega, R., Elipe, P., & Calmaestra, J. (2009). Emociones de agresores y víctimas de cyberbullying: un estudio preliminar en estudiantes de secundaria. *Ansiedad y Estrés, 15*(2–3), 151–165.

Pavez, M. I. (2013). *Los derechos de la infancia en la era de Internet. América Latina y las nuevas tecnologías*. Santiago de Chile: Naciones Unidas.

Pimienta, D. (2008). Brecha digital, brecha social, brecha paradigmática. In J. A. Gómez Hernández, A. Calderón Rehecho, & J. A. Magán Wals (Eds.), *Brecha digital y nuevas alfabetizaciones. El papel de las bibliotecas*. Madrid: Biblioteca Complutense.

Price, M., & Delgleish, J. (2010). Cyberbullying: Experiences, impacts and coping strategies as described by Australian young people. *Youth Studies Australia, 29*(2), 51–60.

Shariff, S. (2005). Cyber-dilemmas in the new millennium: Balancing free expression and student safety in cyber-space. Special issue: Schools and courts: Competing rights in the new millennium. *McGill Journal of Education, 40*(3), 467–487.

Shariff, S. (2009). *Confronting cyber-bullying: Issues and solutions for the school, the classroom, and the home*. Abington: Routledge (Taylor & Frances Group).

Shariff, S., & Churchill, A. (Eds.). (2010). *Truths and myths of cyberbullying. International perspectives on stakeholders, responsibility and children's safety*. New York: Peter Lang Publishing, Inc.

Third, A., Bellerose, D., Dawkins, U., Keltie, E., & Pihl, K. (2014). Children's rights in the digital age: A download from children around the world. Young and Well Cooperative Research Centre, Melbourne. http://www.youngandwellcrc.org.au/wp-content/uploads/2014/09/Childrens-rights-in-the-digital-age.pdf.

Twyman, K., Saylor, C., Taylor, L. A., & Comeaux, C. (2010). Comparing children and adolescents engaged in cyberbullying to matched peers. *Cyberpsychology and Behavior, 13*(2), 195–199. doi:10.1089/cpb.2009.0137.

Varela, J., Pérez, C., Schwaderer, H., Astudillo, J., & Lecannelier, F. (2014). Caracterización de cyberbullying en el gran Santiago de Chile, en el año 2010. *Revista Quadrimestral da Associação Brasileira de Psicologia Escolar e Educacional, 18*(2), 347–354.

Vega-López, M. G., González-Pérez, G. J., & Quintero-Vega, P. P. (2013). Ciberacoso: victimización de alumnos en escuelas secundarias públicas de Tlaquepaque, Jalisco, México. *Revista de Educación y Desarrollo, 25*, 13–20.

Zurita Rivera, U. (2012). Concepciones e implicaciones de tres leyes antibullying en México. *Diálogos sobre educación, 4*, 1–21.

Chapter 8
Cyberbullying in Eastern Countries: Focusing on South Korea and Other Eastern Cultures

Seung-Ha Lee

8.1 Introduction

Internet has been disseminated rapidly since the late 1990s in Asian countries. Currently, China has the greatest number of Internet users, and the majority of population in other eastern countries are Internet users: South Korea (92.4%), Japan (86.2%), Taiwan (80.0%), and Hong Kong (80.9%; Source: www.internetworldstats.com/stats3.htm). The great increase of Internet use and development of information and communication technology (ICT) had brought many benefits but also caused unexpected results. People have begun to be suffering from threatening, malicious images, or messages at anytime and anywhere. In South Korea, in the early 2000s, celebrities were targets for the malicious behaviors in cyberspace, and these were regarded as one of the main reasons of suicides of a couple of celebrities (i.e., *Jin-sil Choi, Yuni*). A public concern for cyberbullying was triggered by a middle school boy's suicide in 2011 in South Korea; a pupil committed suicide after serious school bullying including cyberbullying. The boy had been hit, insulted, extorted, and had been even subjected to waterboarding. This occurred repeatedly and continued anywhere through his mobile phone. This is not restricted to South Korea but is also noted, for example, in Japan. This chapter illuminates studies on cyberbullying in Far Eastern countries, focusing on studies in South Korea and other countries (i.e., China, Hong Kong, Japan, and Taiwan).

S.-H. Lee (✉)
Department of Early Childhood Education, Yeungnam University,
280 Daehakro, Gyeongsan-si, Gyeongsangbuk-do 712-749, South Korea
e-mail: seungha94@gmail.com

© Springer International Publishing Switzerland 2016
R. Navarro et al. (eds.), *Cyberbullying Across the Globe*,
DOI 10.1007/978-3-319-25552-1_8

8.2   Definition of Bullying and Cyberbullying

In some countries, there exist clear terms for cyberbullying. In South Korea, several terms are used to indicate bullying-like behaviors: *hakkyo-pokryuk* (school violence), *wang-ta, gipdan-ttadolim* (group isolation), and *gipdan-gorophim* (group harassment or group bullying). These terms are often used interchangeably, although there are some differences in the types of aggression each term includes (Lee et al. 2012). *Gipdan-ttadolim* and *gipdan-gorophim* imply group aggressive behaviors to one person used frequently in the late 1990s to the early 2000s. Recently, the term *hakkyo-pokryuk* has been mainly used as it indicates a wide range of aggressive behaviors, which happen among pupils such as physical attack, name-calling, *gipdan-ttadolim,* extortion of money, and sexual abuse. *Wang-ta* is a slang term emerged from pupils in the late 1990s, which means socially excluded person or excluding behavior. For terms for cyberbullying, cyber*gorophim* (cyber harassment), cyber*ttadolim* (cyber isolation), cyber*pokryuk* (cyber violence), and cyber *wang-ta* are used. Sometimes the English term *cyberbullying* is directly used. Many recent studies on cyberbullying in South Korea tend to use the term cyber*pokryuk* to indicate the corresponding phenomena to cyberbullying in Western cultures.

Although there is no consensus on the definition of cyberbullying in South Korea, researchers generally agreed that cyber*pokryuk* (cyber violence) is an individual's harmful behavior conducted by electronic communication equipment to (a) specified or unspecified individual(s). *Hakkyo-pokryuk Prevention and Counterplan Act* (2012.4.1) defines cyber*ttadolim* as "the behaviors affecting a pupil's distress; a pupil/pupils aggress(es) other pupil(s) repeatedly, consistently or spread(s) personal- or false information using information technology equipment such as Internet or mobile phone."

In Japan, the term *ijime* has been used to indicate a corresponding phenomenon to bullying in Western cultures. *Ijime* is strongly emphasized on group interaction process and victim's position in a group. It includes several types of aggressive behavior, such as name calling, teasing, mobbing, and excluding, and the victim is completely isolated in the group (Morita 1999). The term *netto ijime* can be a corresponding phenomenon to cyberbullying. This is used to indicate abusive use of mobile text messages and Internet sites or blogs (Toivonen and Imoto 2012).

In Taiwan, there was no clear term for indicating bullying behavior. The terms bullying and cyberbullying are not frequently used in Chinese culture, and even the direct translation of the world bullying *(ba-lin)* is not often used either (Huang and Chou 2010).

There are clear terms for indicating cyberbullying in South Korea and Japan. The meaning of the terms in both countries are common in respect of emphasizing the psychological effect on victims and victim's position, which are generally not considered in the definition of bullying in Western cultures. Apart from South Korea and Japan, in other Asian countries such as Taiwan and China few clear terms are known; however, the bullying phenomenon clearly exists in those countries as well.

8.3 Types of Cyberbullying

There were some differences in the types of cyberbullying investigated across studies. However, across cultures, studies are generally common in terms of some forms: including sending insulting contents (i.e., messages/text/images), sending sexual contents (sexting), misuse others' private information/profile, and spreading rumors or messages for defamation.

Among South Korean studies, cyberbullying was generally categorized by behavior rather than the media used for it. It was generally examined in terms of cyber*moyok/bibang* (insults); cyber*myungye-hweson* (defamation); cyberstalking; cyber*sungpokryuk* (sexting); *gaeinjungbo-youchul* (personal information drain); cyber*gangyo* (coercion); and cyber*ttadolim* (exclusion), cyber*gorophim* (harassment), or cyber *wang-ta*.

In Taiwan, Huang and Chou (2010) distinguished the types of cyberbullying by way of media used: e-mails, instant messengers, chat rooms, online polls, web forums, weblogs, and cell phone messages. They investigated whether—through those media—pupils have experienced threats, harassment, humiliation, insults, and any other emotional put-downs by means of words, taking pictures, "Peeping Tom" videos, or any combination of digital contents.

Some types of cyberbullying (i.e., cyber insults, cyberstalking, sexting, humiliation, harassment, etc.) are similar to or almost the same as with those of Western cultures. However, there is also a distinctive cyberbullying behavior. In South Korea, cyber*gangyo,* often called *"Wi-Fi-shuttle"* may be exclusive types. *Cyber-gangyo* indicates that a bully compels a victim to do/deliver whatever he/she wants. The victim buys what the bully demands and delivers to him/her. For example, the victim downloads charged data, game money, or game items on his mobile (the cost will be charged on his/her mobile fare) and sends the resources to the bully. Pupils usually called this *Wi-Fi shuttle* as this was executed by mobile or wireless service. If this is related to specific Internet game items, they call it *"game shuttle."* In fact, the boy introduced at the beginning of this chapter was a victim of this. Furthermore, this type of cyberbullying is likely to be deeply involved in bullying in school. A pupil/pupils target(s) the other pupil who is socially or physically weak in school (and the victim is often *wang-ta*) and use(s) him/her to obtain the materials he/she wants.

8.4 Incidence of Cyberbullying

Studies showed a wide range of percentages for prevalence of cyberbullying from 7 to 70% across countries. The variety of prevalence resulted from differences of types of cyberbullying or a reference period investigated across studies.

8.4.1 Doing Cyberbullying

A global study, which was conducted by Microsoft Corporation, provides useful information. Microsoft surveyed cyberbullying of youths aged 8–17 in 25 countries, including European, American, and some Asian countries (e.g., China, Japan, Malaysia, Singapore).

The Microsoft study (2012) showed that 9% of youth in Japan reported cyberbullying, followed by 5% of youths in UAE. The most frequent type of cyberbullying was "made fun of or teased" (10%), followed by "mean or unfriendly treatment" (7%), and "called mean names" (6%) in Japan (Microsoft 2012).

Although there is low prevalence of cyberbullying in Japan, it has been slowly increasing. Of the total bullying incidences in 2013, cyberbullying amounted to 4.7%—an increase of 4% compared with the previous year (*JapanTimes,* 19 January 2015). In contrast to Japan, China showed the highest rate (58%) of cyberbullying among 25 countries (Microsoft 2012). The most frequent type of cyberbullying was "called mean names" (48%) followed by "made fun of or teased" (38%) and "mean or unfriendly treatment" (28%) in China (Microsoft 2012).

In South Korea, the prevalence of cyberbullying varied across studies between 7 and 40%. Hwang et al. (2013) investigated the incidence of cyber*pokryuk* among 1500 elementary, middle, and high school pupils across national regions in South Korea. They offered the definition of each type of cyber*pokryuk* (cyber verbal violence, cyber defamation, cyber stalking, cyber sexual abuse, personal information drain, and cyber bullying (*ttodolim*)) and asked pupils' experiences for the last 1 year. The results indicated that 29.2% of the pupils had experiences of doing cyber*pokryuk*.

In addition, the National Information Society Agency (NIA 2013) in South Korea investigated cyberbullying at the national level. They surveyed 11,956 elementary (fifth and sixth graders, aged 11–12), middle, and high school pupils (aged 13–18). Figure 8.1 indicates the incidence of cyberbullying by its type; it shows that relational aggression (cyber*baejae* (exclusion)) was most common, and verbal aggression (cyber*bibang* (insults)) showed slightly less than that.

For the media for cyberbullying, in South Korea, cyberbullying was commonly conducted through messenger (*kakaotalk, mypeople, line,* etc.), cyber community (anti-café, social club), and social networking service (SNS; *Facebook, Twitter,* blogs, etc.; Hwang et al. 2013). In addition, for means of cyberbullying, mobile phone (58.5%) was the most common (Lee et al. 2013).

In Hong Kong, Wong et al. (2014) reported that less than one third of secondary adolescents showed cyberbullying experiences for the last 30 days. They reported that 31.5% of respondents had cyberbullying experiences; 13% had once, 11% of them had two to four times, and 7% had more than five times. Table 8.1 indicates the percentage by types of cyberbullying they investigated.

Interestingly, engaging social groups to insult another person was most common, which may reflect group aggressive behavior in collectivistic cultures. Another study in Hong Kong showed a similar result; among Hong Kong university

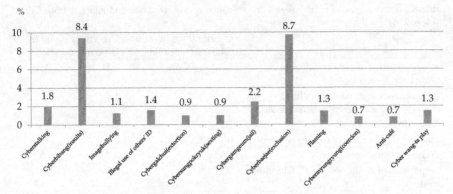

Fig. 8.1 Percentage of doing cyberbullying by its type. (Adapted from NIA 2013). Imagebullying means posting or spreading someone's photos or video clips to offend others. Cyber*gamgeum* indicates cyber jail, which confines someone in chat rooms of the Internet or a smartphone to swear at or insult him/her. Anti-café is an Internet community which is built up for excluding and slandering a particular person. Cyber *wang-ta* play is that several people make someone *wang-ta* (socially excluded person) using insulting, swearing, or denigrating him/her in cyberspace, and this is regarded as a play

students, the most frequent form of cyberbullying was "deliberately ignoring or excluding someone from an online activity" (47.9%), followed by "disseminating private information/messages or posting images/videos without permission" (24.7%; Xiao and Wong 2013).

A study in Taiwan showed that threatening or harassing (20.4%) was the most common type, followed by making jokes (18.2%) and spreading rumors (12.2%; Huang and Chou 2010).

Table 8.1 Percentages of doing cyberbullying among Hong Kong adolescents by its type (total 1917 respondents, multiple answers were possible). (Adapted from Wong et al. 2014, p. 137)

Types of cyberbullying	%
Involved in social groups whose purpose was to tease or insult another person on the Internet	14.3
Used online texts to insult, tease, socially isolate, or make jokes about another person	13.5
Use online communication tools to send annoying or vulgar message to another person	12.4
Maliciously spread fictitious rumors about another person on the Internet	10.7
Registered an online account using false information to make jokes about another person	10.7
Used multimedia forums such as photographs and videos to insults, tease, socially isolate, or make jokes about another person	10.1
Involved in an online social forum to hunt for another person's information and post it on the Internet for malicious purposes	9.7
Edited and posted another person's photographs on the Internet for humiliation purposes	7.6
Hacked into another person's online account to alter his or her personal information without permission	6.6

Table 8.2 Percentages of cyberbullying by reference period. (Exerted and adapted from Udris 2014, p. 256)

	Cyberbullying without time reference (%)	Cyberbullying for the last 6 months (%)
Upload/publish a picture or video online without permission	2.3	1.1
Spreading messages containing insults or bad rumors among classmates or acquaintances	2.7	1.1
Slander someone online	3.5	1.4
Send insulting or abusive messages/e-mails	0.7	0.2
Send sexual messages/e-mails	0.9	0.7
Tamper with or create someone's fake online profile	0.3	0.3
Abuse or slander someone on phone	0.7	0.5
Total	7.9	2.9

Udris (2014) surveyed cyberbullying of 877 adolescents aged 15–19 in Japan. The results showed that 7.9% of the pupils had experiences of cyberbullying, which is a slightly lower rate than that in the Microsoft study. The prevalence decreased to 2.9% when then they were asked about cyberbullying in the last 6 months. Table 8.2 indicates percentages of cyberbullying by its time and reference period. The most frequent type of cyberbullying was "slander someone online," which decreased to less than half when the reference period of cyberbullying was restricted into the recent 6 months.

Also, the middle or high school pupils were more likely than elementary school pupils to be involved in cyberbullying. In South Korea, elementary school pupils (7%) showed lowest rates, and middle school pupils (39%) and high school pupils (38.4%) showed much higher experiences of it (Hwang et al. 2013). Similarly, in Japan, high school pupils (19.7%) were more likely than elementary school pupils (1.4%) to cyberbully (*JapanTimes,* 2015.1.19). Similarly, Suzuki et al. (2012) reported that high school pupils showed higher means for cyberbullying than elementary or secondary school pupils in Japan.

Considering the results across the studies, verbal insults or threatening was one of the most common forms across countries. Furthermore, social exclusion or ignoring was the most frequent type in some studies both in South Korea and Hong Kong.

8.4.2 Receiving Cyberbullying

In South Korea, Hwang et al. (2013) reported that 30.3% of pupils received cyber*pokryuk;* about 40% of middle and high school pupils had cybervictim experiences during the recent 1 year, whereas only 7.4% of elementary school pupils had such experiences. Jung et al. (2011) reported that one third (34%) of elementary

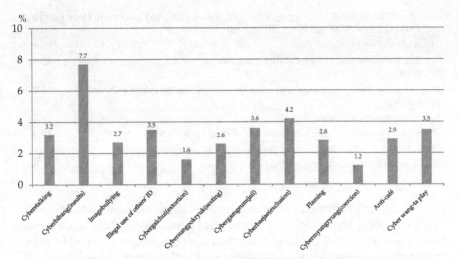

Fig. 8.2 Percentage of receiving cyber*poryuk* by its type. (Adapted from NIA 2013)

school pupils had experience of receiving cyber*pokryuk*; upper graders aged 10–12 (49.3%) had received cyber*pokryuk* three times more than lower graders aged 7–9 (13.0%).

Figure 8.2 indicates the percentages of receiving cyberbullying by its type (NIA 2013). The most common type of receiving cyberbullying was cyber*bibang* (insults), followed cyber*baejae* (exclusion).

Huang and Chou (2010) showed that junior high school pupils in Taiwan received threatening or harassing most commonly (34.9%), followed by making jokes (32.3%) and spreading rumors (25.2%).

In Hong Kong, 23% of the students replied that they had cybervictim experiences in the last 30 days (12.2% had one time and 10.8% had two to four times; Wong et al. 2014). The most common type of cyberbullying was using others' private photos or videos without permission ("had your own or a family member's photographs or videos uploaded to the Internet without your permission":12.5%). "Received annoying or vulgar messages through online communication tools such as email or online messaging" was the second highest (12.1%).

Among Hong Kong university students, 71.9% of respondents had experience of being cybervictims, and 51.7% of respondents had experience of being both cyberbullies and cybervictims (Xiao and Wong 2013). The most frequent form of cybervictimization was "disseminating private information/messages or posting images/videos without permission," which is consistent with the results of Wong et al. (2014). Table 8.3 indicates the percentages of receiving cyberbullying by its type among university students in Hong Kong.

Interestingly, in a Hong Kong sample, the most common type of cyberbullying was "deliberately ignoring or excluding someone from an online activity" whereas the most common type of cybervictimization was "disseminating private information/messages or posting images/videos without permission" (43.7%).

Table 8.3 Percentages of receiving cyberbullying among university students in Hong Kong by its type. (Adapted from Xiao and Wong 2013, p. 48)

Types of receiving cyberbullying	%
Sending threatening, harassing, humiliating, insulting, and teasing messages, images, or videos	42.4
Disseminating private information/messages or posting images/videos without permission	43.8
Spreading rumors or gossips	14.2
Deliberately ignoring or excluding someone from an online activity	29.9
Pretending to be someone to send or post messages in someone's name	11.8
Attacking online accounts or modifying others' profile	24.0

This may reflect that group cyberaggression such as excluding someone online might have been perpetrated on a few targeted pupils. While there might be relatively lower number of pupils who send threatening messages, images, or videos, they might have done these to a number of victims (less targeted than exclusion).

In the Microsoft study (2012), Japan showed the second lowest rate of receiving cyberbullying (17%), following UAE (7%), and China showed the highest cyber-victimization rate (70%).

The high prevalence of cyberbullying in the Microsoft study may be because there was no time reference, and the study included a wide range of ages (8–17 years). Studies which included the youth from upper elementary to high school or those older than 10 years showed lower prevalence than this.

For the type of cybervictimization, spreading, private information was most common in Hong Kong, and verbal threatening or insults were most frequent both in South Korea and Taiwan.

8.4.3 Sex Differences

Generally, boys were more likely than girls to be both cyberbullies and cybervictims across countries: South Korea (Hwang et al. 2013; NIA 2013), Taiwan (Huang and Chou 2010; Wong et al. 2014), and Japan (Microsoft 2012). However, in relational type of cyberbullying (i.e., cyberexclusion), there were more girls than boys involved in it.

For cyberbullying, in South Korea, boys were generally more likely than girls to do cyber*pokryuk* (Jung et al. 2011; Lee et al. 2013; Shin and Ahn 2013). More boys than girls were involved in cyber verbal violence, cyber defamation, cyber stalking, cyber sexual abuse, and personal information drain, whereas girls were more likely than boys to do cyber*ttadolim* (Hwang et al. 2013). NIA (2013) also showed that girls (61%) were generally more likely than boys (39%) to be cyberbullies only in cyberexclusion (called cyber*baejae*).

In Hong Kong, there were more boy perpetrators across all types of cyberbullying behavior, except for one case; there were more female than male students in the item "involved in social groups whose purpose was to tease or insult another person on the internet" (Wong et al. 2014). Inconsistently, another study in Hong Kong showed that male students were less likely than female students to engage in cyberbullying (Xiao and Wong 2013).

For cybervictimization, boys were more likely than girls to receive cyberbullying, but this varies by types of cyberbullying. In South Korea, boys were more likely than girls to be cybervictims in cyber verbal violence, cyber defamation, and personal information drain, but in cyber sexual abuse, girls were more likely than boys to be victims at middle and high school levels (Hwang et al. 2013).

Also, in some types of cyberbullying, girls were more likely than boys to be cybervictims (i.e., sexting, cyberexclusion, anti-café, cyber *wang-ta* play; NIA 2013). Particularly, cyberexclusion showed the biggest sex differences: The victims in cyberexclusion were more girls (60.8%) than boys (39.2%).

Similar to South Korea, a study in Hong Kong showed that there were more boys than girls in cybervictimization (Wong et al. 2014). However, in Japan, girls (21%) tended to be more cyberbullied than boys (12%; Microsoft 2012). In China, girls and boys showed similar rates of receiving cyberbullying, although girls (71%) showed slightly higher rates than boys (69%; Microsoft 2012).

Sex differences of cyberbullying or cybervictimization are not consistent across studies; boys are more likely than girls to be both cyberbullies and cybervictims in South Korea or Hong Kong, but this is not noted in studies from China or Japan. Also, girls are more likely than boys to be involved in relational cyber aggression such as cyberexclusion even if boys were more likely to be cybervictimized in South Korea.

8.5 Awareness of Cyberbullies

Many pupils were aware of the names of cyberbullies. In South Korea, nearly or more than half of the respondents perceived who cyberbullies were. Forty-three percent of victims were aware of cyberbullies; they were cyberbullied by their peer(s) in the same school (Lee et al. 2013). Also, more than half of the cyberbullies reported that they did cyber*pokryuk* to a pupil/pupils whom they knew in their schools (Hwang et al. 2013); 54.3% of elementary school pupils, 52.3% of middle school pupils, and 64.6% of high school pupils. Similarly, Lee et al. (2013) reported that 55.4% of cyberbullies chose the target from the same school in South Korea. This is more so in the Taiwanese sample, many adolescents perceived who the cyberbullies are; 74.9% of victims and 57.9% of bystanders were aware of bullies' identity (Huang and Chou 2010).

Reflecting the findings, cyberbullies tend not to try to hide or disguise themselves in cyberspace. Authors suggested that it might be because the account names were exposed when users logged in (Huang and Chou 2010). Alternatively, it may reflect that face-to-face bullying may be continued in cyberspace to the same pupils.

8.6   Motivations for Cyberbullying

In South Korea, "for fun" and "upset with the victim" were most frequent answers
for the reason for doing cyber*pokryuk* (Hwang et al. 2013; NIA 2013). The most
common reasons were somewhat different by school levels. Among elementary
school pupils, "for fun" was the highest (elementary: 45.7%, middle: 29.7%, high:
33.3%), but in older ages such as middle and high school pupils, "upset with the
victim" was most common (elementary: 34.3%, middle: 68.2%, high: 64.1%;
Hwang et al. 2013). Additionally, "no reason" (elementary: 22.9%, middle: 11.8%,
high: 11.5%) and "getting along with friends" (elementary: 20.0%, middle: 5.6%,
high: 12.5%) were also frequent responses (Hwang et al. 2013).

8.7   Responses After Being a Cybervictim or Witnessing
Cybervictimization

Passive reactions such as "no response" or "ignoring the cyberbullying" were very
common across cultures. In South Korea, "get back in the same way"(39.4%) was
the most common answer as a response after being cyberbullied, followed by "demand deletion or correction of the message to the cyberbully (ies)" (17.6%) and
"claiming apologies" (17.1%). There was also a high frequency who replied "no
response" (36.5%; Jung et al. 2011).

By school levels, mid or late adolescents chose a more direct solution by confronting the cyberbullies; in South Korea, middle school pupils (50.3%) and high
school pupils (40.9%) were more likely than elementary school pupils (29.7%)
to demand the cyberbully (ies) to delete or correct the harmful writing or message
(Hwang et al. 2013). Younger pupils tended to report and ask help from others;
"Telling friends" (elementary: 35.1%, middle: 27.4%, high: 22.2%) and "telling
parents/families" (elementary: 24.3%, middle: 16.8%, high: 6.4%; Hwang et al.
2013). However, among the responses of asking help from someone, "telling school
teacher" (elementary: 8.1%, middle: 9.1%, high: 4.9%) showed low percentages
in relation to telling friends or parents/families (Hwang et al. 2013). Reporting to a
legal or formal institution was less common than other ways of reporting. "Reporting police, *Wee*centre (bullying intervention centre in South Korea), calling 117, or
cyber bureau of national police" showed the least frequent responses (elementary:
5.4%, middle: 7.1%, high: 4.4%; Hwang et al. 2013).

Forty-two percent of pupils who received cyber*pokryuk* reported that they did
not do anything because "it may be not helpful" (64.4%); particularly, elementary
school pupils were afraid of being isolated more seriously after reporting the incident (28.6%; Hwang et al. 2013).

In Taiwan, a lot of cybervictims (78.4%) reported their cybervictimization to
someone: 33.4% of them reported to classmates, 16.1% to siblings, 11.6% to
parents, and only 5.9% of them told teachers (Huang and Chou 2010). Similar to

South Korea, Taiwanese adolescents' common reasons for not reporting were "being afraid of getting into trouble" and "feeling a sense of uselessness in looking to adults for assistant" (Huang and Chou 2010).

In Hong Kong, "withdrawal or avoidance" (i.e., "I can tolerate although I am not happy") was the most common response, followed by "passive responses" (i.e., "delete the webpages or messages") and "take revenge" (i.e., "take revenge on the person who is responsible for the bully"). Active responses (i.e., "inform family, teachers, or social worker") were the lowest (Wong et al. 2014).

Taking no action against cyberbullying is a common response among bystanders. In South Korea, about 37% of middle and high school pupils and 12.6% of elementary school pupils had experience of witnessing cyber*pokryuk* (Hwang et al. 2013). Almost half of them (48.6%) did not do anything because they thought that "it is nothing" (45.6%). Among younger pupils (i.e., elementary school pupils), "don't know what to do" is a common reason, whereas among older pupils (i.e., middle and high school pupils), "it is nothing" was the most common reason (Hwang et al. 2013).

In Taiwan, more than half of the pupils witnessed cyberbullying: making jokes (64.4%) and threatening or harassing (63.5%) were commonly witnessed, followed by spreading rumors (60.9%; Huang and Chou 2010). However, 58.7% of the bystanders did not report bullying to anyone; they tended to think it as neither their business nor their responsibility. Some of them even suggested that reporting bullying which did not happen to themselves means involvement in others' privacies (Huang and Chou 2010). This may indicate serious moral disengagement about bullying behavior.

Many pupils who are victimized or witnessed cyberbullying in Taiwan and South Korea seem to be afraid of the bully's revenge or threat and unsure of adults' help for their cyberbullying experiences. This may explain why passive responses were common after cybervictimization.

8.8   Effective Coping Strategies

In South Korea, across school levels, "telling friends" was most helpful for stopping cyberbullying (elementary: 69.2%, middle: 75.9%, high: 60.0%), followed by "telling parents, siblings, families." Around half of the pupils who asked cyberbullies to "delete or correct the messages" found this strategy helpful (elementary: 45.5%, middle: 55.6%, and high: 48.2%). "Telling teachers" was fully useful (100%) among elementary school pupils, but it was not among older pupils (38.9% in middle and 30.0% in high school pupils thought it as useful; Hwang et al. 2013).

Half of the elementary school pupils who reported the incidents to the police, *Wee*centre, 117, or cyber bureau of national police thought it as helpful, and 42.9% of middle school pupils and 44.4% of high school pupils reported this as effective (Hwang et al. 2013).

8.9 Related Variables

8.9.1 Psychological Variables

Studies reported that psychological variables such as aggression, impulsiveness, self-control, self-esteem, or guilty feeling were involved in cyberbullying, and both cyberbullies and cybervictims suffered from a lower level of psychological well-being.

Aggressive traits of pupils positively predicted cyberbullying behavior. In South Korea, boys' aggressiveness predicted cyberbullying but not girls' (Kim and Yoon 2012a). Also, aggression of both boys and girls showed positive correlation with cyberbullying behavior (Nam and Kwon 2013; NIA 2013; Sung et al. 2016). Impulsiveness (Nam and Kwon 2013) and low self-control ability (NIA 2013) influenced cyberbullying behavior. Upper elementary pupils (aged 11–12) who had experiences of cyber*gorophim* showed lower self-esteem than pupils who did not (Oh 2011). Also, awareness of the guilt of cyberbullying negatively predicted cyberbullying behavior (Nam and Kwon 2013).

Xiao and Wong (2013) studied personal and environmental factors affecting cyberbullying among 288 university students in Hong Kong. They found that Internet self-efficacy and motivation were all significantly related to cyberbullying behavior (Xiao and Wong 2013). High level of Internet self-efficacy is related to cyberbullying behavior. Also, motivation for cyberbullying such as wanting to obtain power, attention, or peer approval predicted cyberbullying behavior. Similarly, cyberbullying behavior was negatively correlated to self-efficacy, empathy, and psychosocial well-being in Hong Kong (i.e., overall happiness and relationships with family, peers, and teachers; Wong et al. 2014).

South Korean studies showed that cybervictim experiences predicted internalizing (i.e., depressive symptom) and externalizing problems (i.e., aggressive traits; Oh 2013; Kim 2013). Low level of self-control was related to cybervictim experiences (NIA 2013). Also, cybervictim experiences increased the tendency of suicidal thinking (Seo and Cho 2013).

8.9.2 Social Variables (Parents/Schools)

Parents and school variables were related to cyberbullying across studies. Relationships between adolescents and parents were involved in adolescents' cyberbullying behaviors. Adolescents' attachment to their parents predicted cyberbullying behavior. In South Korea, adolescents who are less attached to their parents are more likely to do cyberbullying (Sung et al. 2006). Also, witnessing parental violence and receiving abusive experiences from parents are positively related to cyberbullying behavior (Kim and Yoon 2012a).

An individual's adaptation to schools was related to cyberbullying. In South Korea, low level of school satisfaction was associated with cyberbullying (NIA 2013). In the same line with this, the sense of belonging to school and harmonious school was negatively correlated to cyberbullying in Hong Kong (Wong et al. 2014).

Parental support is useful for preventing cyberbullying. Yang et al. (2014) investigated the role of parental support to high school pupils' flow to Internet in China. They surveyed 1203 high school pupils and found that parental support decreased the pupils' Internet addiction and increased exploratory behavior. This supportive parental attention leads children's Internet usage to a healthy way.

Cybervictim experiences were related to parental attention and degree of parental control to their children's Internet usage; these were negatively related to children's low level of cybervictim experiences (Cho 2013). Parent–child communication skills negatively predicted adolescents' cyber delinquency, and authoritarian or controlling parental attitude were related to it in South Korea (Kim 2014).

Having delinquent peers and positive attitudes toward cyberbullying were associated with cyberbullying. In South Korea, having or contacting delinquent peers was a significant factor for cyberbullying behaviors (Kim 2013; Nam and Jang 2011). Lee and Jeong (2014) investigated factors which may predict willingness for cyberbullying behavior among 514 middle and high school pupils in South Korea. They found that having delinquent peers and positive subjective norms of cyberbullying (e.g., how other people perceive my cyberbullying) predicted willingness to cyberbullying behavior. Consistently, an individual's social norm related to cyberbullying was a significant predictor, which increased the likelihood of cyberbullying behavior in Hong Kong. University students in Hong Kong who had positive normative beliefs about cyberbullying behavior (i.e., they believed that people who were important to them approved the behavior) were more likely to adopt it (Xiao and Wong 2013).

Psychological and social factors such as parent/peer influence are related to cyberbullying in South Korea or Hong Kong; however, this should be carefully interpreted as many of them generally do not mean causal relationships, except for a few studies. Longitudinal studies are needed for examining variables influencing cyberbullying.

8.10 Relationships Between Traditional Bullying and Cyberbullying

Bully or victim experiences in traditional bullying are related to cyberbullying. Many studies (e.g., Cho 2013; Ryu 2013; Sung et al. 2006; Wong et al. 2014) indicated strong relationships between a bully in cyberspace and a victim in traditional bullying.

In South Korea, Ryu (2013) examined 1088 middle and high school pupils' cyberbullying experiences in relation to their traditional school bullying experiences. The author indicated that cyberbullying experiences are positively correlated both to victim's and bully's experience of traditional bullying. Also, in Hong Kong cyberbullying behavior was positively related to traditional bullying, traditional victim, and cybervictim experiences. (Wong et al. 2014).

In South Korea cybervictim experiences were predicted by bully or victim experiences in traditional bullying among adolescents (Cho 2013). There were significant relationships between *gipdan-ttadolim* (group isolation) and cyberbullying. Both bullies and victims of *gipdan-ttdolim* were more likely than non-victims to cyberbully or be a cybervictim (Lee et al. 2013).

In addition, being a cybervictim was predicted by being a cyberbully or traditional victim in the Hong Kong sample. (Xiao and Wong 2013). However, traditional bullying behavior did not predict cyberbullying behavior in Hong Kong (Wong et al. 2014).

The relationship between traditional bullying and cyberbullying may reflect that victimization in school could continue in cyberspace, and cyberbullying can influence the cybervictim. However, the findings are dependent on correlation; only a few studies showed cause and effect relationships. Further longitudinal studies are needed to explain the relationships.

8.11   Perspectives to Cyberbullying

Studies about perception of cyberbullying are very lacking. Only a few studies investigated pupils' sense of ethics in cyberspace or guilty consciousness of cyberbullying. In South Korea, pupils who are more tolerant to violence tend to cyberbully (Kim and Yoon 2012a). Also, victim and cybervictim experiences increase tolerance of violence, which positively influenced cyberbullying behavior (Kim and Yoon 2012b). Some pupils justify their cyberbullying behavior. Lee et al. (2013) indicated that middle school pupils justified their bad reply on the Internet: They perceived that bad replies written by themselves were less problematic than those written to themselves.

Many pupils did not show guilt for the cyberbullying behavior. In South Korea, elementary school pupils showed a high percentage of "I don't feel it as fault because I have done it for fun" (25.7%). "Sorry for the person" and "regret" were also common feelings after cyber*pokryuk* among pupils, ranging from 22.9 to 29.7% (Hwang et al. 2013).

Moral insensitivity or indifference to cyberbullying tends to increase as pupils grow older. In South Korea, "don't feel anything" was also a common answer for cyber*pokryuk*, which was higher in older pupils: middle school pupils (28.7%), high school pupils (24.0%), and elementary school pupils (20.0%; Hwang et al. 2013). In South Korea, many pupils (92.8%) were aware of the legal punishment for cyberbullying (Lee et al. 2013). Likewise, most middle and high school pupils (92%) perceived legal punishment for cyber*pokryuk*, and 67.8% of elementary school pupils knew about this. Girls were more likely than boys to be aware of this (Hwang et al. 2013).

Pupils' moral or ethical sensitivity was related to cyberbullying. In South Korea, Sung et al. (2006) reported that cyberbullying experiences were negatively predicted by the sense of ethics of information communication and experiences of punishment.

Teachers' perception of cyberbullying plays an important role in cyberbullying. In Japan, Kumazaki et al. (2012) investigated the impact of teachers' instructions on cyberbullying and school bullying. Teachers were asked about their instructions of cyberbullying, and students were requested to share their experience of cyberbullying for the past month. The results showed that "teachers' immediate reaction to a bully was effective to decrease cyberbullying." Also, classrooms in which teachers tell the entire class that bullying is not acceptable did not reduce cyberbullying.

In contrast, those cases in which teachers tell the entire class that the teacher is in charge of bullying other students showed a decrease in cyberbullying. This reflects that confirming that the teacher is responsible and emphasizing supportive attitude toward cyberbullying was more powerful for intervening cyberbullying than simply telling about prohibition of cyberbullying. At the elementary school level, there were more significant differences in cyberbullying and bullying incidence than at middle school levels, depending on teachers' active strategies. This implies that if intervention should be started at early stages, it may be more influential to prevent cyberbullying.

8.12   Prevention and Intervention

Studies or programs for prevention or intervention of cyberbullying have started since around 2010. Across cultures, these were less likely to be studied in comparison with the prevalence of cyberbullying. In Japan, only 9 % of schools had formal written policies for cyberbullying, and 28 % of schools performed education for it (Microsoft 2012). Also, a specialized legal system of cyberbullying was very lacking.

In Taiwan, the Ministry of Education provides definition, guidelines, and information about the procedure to prevent and stop bullying through "Regulations on the prevention of school bullying." Although there is no anti-cyberbullying legislation in Taiwan, this provides a variety of online resources for students, parents, and teachers (The Taiwan Ministry of Education cited in Bhat et al. 2013).

In South Korea, the *hakkyo-pokryuk Prevention and Intervention Act* from 2012 indicates that schools must form a *hakkyo-pokryuk* committee if an incidence of *hakkyo-pokryuk* is reported: The committee consists of experts from several areas (i.e., teachers, judges, lawyers, or medical doctors) and parents. The committee decides on actions for stopping bullying: protection for victim, punishment to bully, conciliation between victim and bully, and forcing intervention program for the bully and bully's parents, etc.

Websites managed by governmental institutions were created to take immediate action on cyberbullying incidences. In South Korea, the Ministry of Education established an anti-bullying website called *stopbullying* in 2012 (http://www.stopbullying.or.kr). This guarantees users' anonymity; thus, an individual can report their victimization without worrying about revealing their status or position. They can call 117 or ask for help by accessing the website or sending a mobile text message. The person then would be helped and provided with counselling service and coping strategies.

Educating netiquettes and forming ethical or moral culture in the use of Internet or SNS have been emphasized. In South Korea, Korea Internet Security Agency (KISA) established a website (https://www.iculture.or.kr) to foster sensitivity of information ethics and create a healthy and beneficial Internet culture. This provides information on the usage of Internet and SNS and varied educational guidelines for elementary, middle, and high school levels. In Japan, Kumazaki et al. (2011) showed the moderating effects of netiquettes on cyberbullying: Pupils who had a high level of netiquettes did not increase the frequencies of cyberbullying even if the use of technology was increased.

Repeated warning can be effective to prevent cyberbullying. In Japan, Yasuda (2010) conducted a prevention program for cyberbullying using a leaflet. The researcher pointed out that students do not perceive that mobile phone and Internet can be strong weapons. Students can learn to understand the information society and many social factors consisting of it; their behavior can be affected by other social factors (other person) which urge them to behave with responsibility in cyberspace. The author developed a leaflet program: Homeroom teachers distributed leaflets every morning, and it took only 1 min to read them. The leaflet cautions students not to cyberbully and indicates the safe usage of technology or technology information. After students have read the leaflet, they pass it to their parents at home. In Yasuda's (2010) study, the school practiced this for 3 years, and the results showed that it was highly effective to decrease problems related to mobile phone or Internet in school. Also, 73 % of guardians thought that school guidance using leaflets was useful (Yasuda 2010).

A program using peer support system was developed in South Korea. NIA in South Korea operated programs for information ethics education. Volunteer teachers are trained and equipped with knowledge on cyberbullying and the need of prevention. They then organize a club consisting of pupils called *areumnuri-jikimi*. This consists of 30–40 pupil volunteers; they learn about cyberbullying and their responsibility for preventing it by the trained teachers. After training, they begin to work in various ways in order to create a healthy culture in cyberspace. They pass on their knowledge on cyberbullying and conduct a campaign for right Internet use.

Some web sites for prevention of cyberbullying or prevention programs in South Korea provide very useful information, but the effectiveness of those programs has not been evaluated yet.

8.13 Conclusion

This chapter has reviewed studies on cyberbullying in Asian cultures. Across cultures, there were common aspects such as the tendency of sex differences in prevalence and type of cyberbullying that were investigated. Interestingly, group cyber aggression such as engaging in social groups to tease someone or excluding one person in cyberspace was the most common type: Cyberexclusion was one of the most common forms in Hong Kong and South Korea. Sex differences in cyberbullying and cybervictimization were inconsistent across countries. It would be interesting to examine the main types of cyberbullying between Western and Eastern cultures in terms of individualism–collectivism dimension.

In comparison with studies about prevalence, there is a serious lack of studies on pupils' or teachers' attitudes toward cyberbullying. The findings of pupils' indifference to cyberbullying occurring to others give important points for prevention strategies. That is, responsibility for and attention to others' well-being could be important factors to prevent cyberbullying, which is related to morality. Therefore, a critical issue to decrease cyberbullying is to increase sensitivity to morality of doing cyberbullying.

The ethical concept of technology had not been required when pupils started to use ICT. Pupils had learned only those skills of ICT which were required for their needs and may not have even perceived why ethical attitudes are needed when they use their own media (mobile, computer, etc). Emphasizing ethics in cyberspace and increasing moral sensitivity and responsibility in cyber behavior are necessary for preventing cyberbullying. Some web sites in South Korea and a prevention program using leaflets in Japan provide good examples for this.

Research on cyberbullying among Far Eastern Asian countries is encouraging; however, there remain many further steps to go. Many studies focused on the frequency or prevalence of cyberbullying; a qualitative approach could be useful to illuminate pupils' motivation of cyberbullying. Also, studies for developing prevention/intervention programs and examining the effects of them are needed. In addition, communal efforts in family, school, and governmental levels should be consistently provided for preventing and intervening with cyberbullying.

References

Bhat, C. S., Chang, S. H., & Ragan, M. A. (2013). Cyberbullying in Asia. *Education About Asia, 18*, 36–39.

Cho, Y-O. (2013). 청소년의 사이버불링 피해실태 및 피해유발 요인연구 [A study on the factors associated with cybervictimization]. 한국공안행정학회보 *[Korean Association of Public Safety and Criminal Justice Review], 53*, 303–328.

Huang, Y. Y., & Chou, C. (2010). An analysis of multiple factors of cyberbullying among junior high school students in Taiwan. *Computers in Human Behavior, 26*(6), 1581–1590. doi:10.1016/j.chb.2010.06.005.

Hwang, S.-W., Cho, J-S., Oh, Y-H., Lee, J-H., Lim, D-K., & Kim, S. (2013). *2013 사이버폭력 실태조사 [2013 Survey of cyberpokryuk].* Seoul: KISA: Korea Internet & Security Agency.

Jung, G-H., Ryu, J-H., Kim, B-Y., Lee, E-J., Shim, D-W., Lee, Y-H., Kim, K-E., & Ryu, J-S. (2011). 인터넷 윤리문화 실태조사 *[Survey of ethical cultures in internet].* Seoul: KISA: Korea Internet & Security Agency.

Kim, K-E. (2013). 청소년의 사이버폭력에 영향을 미치는 위험요인: 비행친구의 매개효과를 중심으로 [Influential risk factors for youth cyber violence: With priority given to the mediating effects of delinquent friends]. 미래청소년학회지 *[Journal of Future Oriented Youth Society], 10*(4), 133–159.

Kim, K-H. (2014). 초기 청소년의 부모-자녀 의사소통과 부모의 양육태도가 학업스트레스 및 사이버비행에 미치는 영향 [Effects of early adolescents' parent-child communication and parents' rearing attitudes on academic stress and cyber delinquency]. 미래청소년학회지 *[Journal of Future Oriented Youth Society], 11*(2), 1–22.

Kim, K-E., & Yoon, H-M. (2012a). 청소년의 사이버폭력에 관련된 생태체계변인의 영향 [Influences of eco-systemic factors related to adolescents' cyber violence]. 청소년복지연구 *[Journal of Adolescent Welfare], 14*(1), 213–238.

Kim, K-E., & Yoon, H-M. (2012b). 청소년의 폭력피해경험, 폭력용인태도와 사이버폭력가해행동의 관련성 [Associations between adolescents' victimization of violence, tolerance toward violence, and cyber violence offending behavior]. 한국아동복지학 *[Journal of Korean Society of Child Welfare], 39,* 213–244.

Kumazaki, A., Suzuki, K., Katsura, R., Sakamoto, A., & Kashibuchi, M. (2011). The effects of netiquette and ICT skills on school-bullying and cyber-bullying: The two-wave panel study of Japanese elementary, secondary, and high school students. *Procedia-Social and Behavioral Sciences, 29,* 735–741. doi:10.1016/j.sbspro.2011.11.299.

Lee, K-E., & Jeong, S-H. (2014). 청소년의 사이버폭력행위에 영향을 미치는 요인에 관한 연구 [Predictors of cyberbullying behaviors among adolescents: Application of theory of planned behavior and social learning theory]. 사이버커뮤니케이션학보 *[Journal of Cybercommunication], 31*(2), 129–162.

Lee, S-H., Smith, P. K., & Monks, C. P. (2012). Meaning and usage of a term for bullying-like phenomena in South Korea: A lifespan perspective. *Journal of Language and Social Psychology, 31*(3), 342–349. doi:10.1177/0261927X12446602.

Lee S-D., Hwang, S-K., & Yeum, D-M. (2013). The exploratory research on recognition and actual condition of cyberbullying: Focused on middle school students in *Uiryeonggun.* 청소년문화포럼 *[Youth Culture Publishes Forum], 33,* 120–145.

Microsoft Corporation. (2012). *WW online bullying survey.* http://goo.gl/gGrRSW. Accessed 3 April 2015.

Morita, Y., Soeda, H., Soeda, K., & Taki, M. (1999). Japan. In P. K. Smith, Y. Morita, J. Junger-Tas, D. Olweus, R. Catalano, & P. Slee (Eds.), *The nature of school bullying: A cross national perspective* (pp. 309–323). London: Routledge.

Nam, J-S., & Jang, J-H. (2011). 청소년 사이버불링 피해에 관한 연구: 청소년 비행요인과 지역사회요인을 중심으로 [A study on the cyber-violence victimization of juveniles—focusing on the juvenile delinquency factor and local community factor]. 한국범죄심리연구 *[Korean Studies of Criminal Psychology], 7*(3), 101–119.

Nam, S-I., & Kwon, N-H. (2013). 청소년 사이버불링 가해에 영향을 미치는 변인 연구 [A study on the factors that influence adolescents' cyberbullying behavior]. 미래청소년학회지 *[Journal of Future Oriented Youth Society], 10*(3), 22–43.

NIA. (2013). 사이버불링 실태와 해법 세미나발표 자료 *[Prevalence and prevention of cyberbullying seminar. 2013. 12. 18.].* Seoul: NIA.

Oh, I-S. (2011). 초등학생 온라인 괴롭힘의 실태 및 오프라인 괴롭힘과의 비교분석 [Comparative analysis on characteristics of on-line bullying and off-line bullying in elementary schools]. 아시아교육연구 *Asian Journal of Education], 12*(3), 75–98.

Oh, T-K. (2013). 중학생의 사이버불링 피해경험과 정서행동과의 관계 [The relationship between cyberbullying victimized experience and emotional behavior of middle school students].

한국컴퓨터정보학회논문집 *[Journal of the Korea Society of Computer and Information], 18*(12), 207–215.

Ryu, S-J. (2013). 청소년들의 사이버 폭력과 오프라인 폭력 경험에 관한 연구 [A study of adolescents' experiences of cyberviolence and offline violence]. 한국언론학보 *[Korean Journal of Journalism & Communication Studies], 57*(5), 297–324.

Seo, H-W., & Cho, Y-O. (2013). 사이버불링 피해가청소년의 자살생각에 미치는 영향 [The impact of cyber victimization on suicidal thinking]. 미래청소년학회 *[Journal of Future Oriented Youth Society], 10*(4), 111–131.

Shin, N-M., & Ahn, H-S. (2013). 청소년 사이버폭력 현황 및 피해·가해관련변인에 관한 연구 [Cyberbullying among Korean adolescents: Facts and factors related to victimization and offending experiences]. 교육문제연구 *[The Journal of Research in Education], 26*(4), 1–21.

Sung, D-K., Kim, D-H., Lee, Y-S., Lim, S-W. (2006). 청소년의 사이버폭력 유발요인에 관한 연구: 개인성향, 사이버폭력 피해경험, 윤리의식을 중심으로 [A study on the cyber-violence induction factors of teenagers: Focused on individual inclination, cyber violence damage experience, and moral consciousness]. 사이버커뮤니케이션학보 *[Journal of Cybercommunication Academic Society], 19*, 79–129.

Suzuki, K., Kumazaki, A., Katsura, R., Sakamoto, A., & Kashibuchi, M. (2012). *Effects of mobile Internet usage on cyber- and school-bullying experiences: A two-wave panel study of Japanese elementary, secondary, and high school students 2011.* Paper presented at the 3rd Global Conference Bullying and the Abuse of Power. (Prague, Czech Republic).

Toivonen, T., & Imoto, Y. (2012). Making sense of youth problems. In R. Goodman, T. Toivonen, & Y. Imoto (Eds.), *A sociology of Japanese youth* (pp. 1–29). New York: Routledge.

Udris, R. (2014). Cyberbullying among high school students in Japan: Development and validation of the Online Disinhibition Scale. *Computers in Human Behavior, 41*, 253–261. doi:10.1016/j.chb.2014.09.036.

Wong, D. S., Chan, H. C. O., & Cheng, C. H. (2014). Cyberbullying perpetration and victimization among adolescents in Hong Kong. *Children and Youth Services Review, 36*, 133–140. doi:10.1016/j.childyouth.2013.11.006.

Xiao, B. S., & Wong, Y. M. (2013). Cyber-bullying among university students: An empirical investigation from the social cognitive perspective. *International Journal of Business and Information, 8*(1), 34–69.

Yang, S., Lu, Y., Wang, B., & Zhao, L. (2014). The benefits and dangers of flow experience in high school students' internet usage: The role of parental support. *Computers in Human Behavior, 41*, 504–513. doi:10.1016/j.chb.2014.09.039.

Yasuda, H. (2010). A risk management system to oppose cyber bullying in high school: Warning system with leaflets and emergency staffs. *Informatica: An International Journal of Computing and Informatics, 34*(2), 255–259.

Chapter 9
Cyberbullying Research in Belgium: An Overview of Generated Insights and a Critical Assessment of the Mediation of Technology in a Web 2.0 World

Wannes Heirman, Michel Walrave, Heidi Vandebosch, Denis Wegge, Steven Eggermont and Sara Pabian

In Belgium, scholars have put their efforts together to gain a better understanding of cyberbullying. In this context, the research group Media, ICT/Interpersonal relations in Organisations and Society (MIOS) has adopted the role of a Belgian pioneer in studying this form of negative online conduct among youngsters on the Internet and via mobile devices. The first aim of the chapter is to provide an overview of the outcomes of these research efforts. Both the prevalence rates, observed across five large-scale studies conducted by MIOS on cyberbullying, and the predictors of victimization and perpetration identified in these studies will be discussed. As a second aim, we critically assess the argument that cyberbullying has, due to the mediation of technology, an amplified impact as compared with the harm caused by traditional bullying.

9.1 Introduction

The technologies that young people employ constructively to consolidate friendships with peers are, as extensive research evidence has shown, also used for the purpose of inflicting pain and harm to others (mostly peers). Cyberbullying, as this phenomenon is being referred to, is a universal problem of which the prevalence has been evidenced in most developed countries (Mesch 2009). It started manifesting itself as soon as information and communication technologies (ICTs) started to permeate the family households (Ybarra and Mitchell 2004; Davies and Eynon 2013). Notwithstanding the fact that ICTs have been embraced by the youngest household

W. Heirman (✉) · M. Walrave · H. Vandebosch · D. Wegge · S. Pabian
Department of Communication Studies, University of Antwerp, Sint Jacobsstraat 2, 2000 Antwerp, Belgium
e-mail: wannes.heirman@uantwerpen.be

S. Eggermont
School for Mass Communication Research, Parkstraat 45,
University of Leuven, 3000 Leuven, Belgium

© Springer International Publishing Switzerland 2016
R. Navarro et al. (eds.), *Cyberbullying Across the Globe,*
DOI 10.1007/978-3-319-25552-1_9

169

members, their use has not remained limited to beneficial purposes, with alarming coverage of young people abusing these technologies for hurtful purposes including bullying. According to Smith et al. (2008, p. 376) a person is being cyberbullied when "an aggressive, *intentional* act [is] carried out by a group or individual, using *electronic* forms of contact, *repeatedly* and over time against a *victim who cannot easily defend him or herself*". In recent years, much scholarly attention has been devoted to this emerging form of negative online conduct as a host of harmful outcomes have been associated with it: What we know so far is that it tends to parallel the negative effects of traditional bullying (Bryce and Fraser 2013; Kowalski et al. 2012). Some observed consequences are decreased self-esteem, reduced concentration in classroom, feelings of embarrassment, social anxiety, depressive symptomatology and even suicide (Hinduja and Patchin 2007; Kowalski et al. 2014; Mason 2008; Mishna et al. 2009; Ybarra and Mitchell 2004).

Given its potentially severe impact on young people's mental and physical well-being, cyberbullying has attracted a great deal of policy-driven and government-funded academic research. Within the Belgian context, the research unit Media, ICT/Interpersonal relations in Organisations and Society (MIOS)[1] has become the leading pioneer in conducting research into this highly problematic phenomenon. So far, five large-scale studies have been conducted by MIOS on the topic of cyberbullying.

- The first project "Cyberbullying Among Flemish Youth"[2] was launched in 2005. It involved the administration of a paper-and-pencil questionnaire among 636 Flemish primary school children and 1416 secondary education pupils.
- In 2007 followed the study "Teens & ICT: Risks & Opportunities"[3] (TIRO), encompassing a self-administered survey among a total of 1318 Belgian adolescents.
- In 2010, the "Developmental Issues in Cyberbullying Amongst Adolescents"[4] (DICA) project was launched: The project epitomized a four-wave longitudinal paper-and-pencil survey with 6-month time intervals among 2312 respondents in the first wave and 2038 respondents in the final fourth wave.
- In the same year as DICA, another project was conducted, entitled "A Contextual Study of Cyberbullying in Early Adolescence: A Longitudinal and Social Network Approach"[5] (the "SNA project"). For the purpose of this study, 1458 respondents completed peer-nomination questionnaires allowing the full recon-

---

[1] The project was ordered by the Commission for Culture, Youth, Media and Sports of the Flemish Parliament. For more information, see https://www.uantwerpen.be/en/rg/mios/.

[2] This project was funded by Institute of Society and Technology. For more information, see http://ist.vito.be/nl/publicaties/rapporten/rapport_cyberpesten.html.

[3] This project was funded by the Belgian Federal Science Policy's programme on Society & Future. For more information, see http://www.ua.ac.be/tiro.

[4] This project was funded by the Bijzonder Onderzoeksfonds (BOF). For more information see, https://www.uantwerp.be/en/research-and-innovation/research-at-uantwerp/funding/internal-funding/university-research-bof/.

[5] This project was funded by the Research Foundation Flanders (FWO). For more information, see http://www.fwo.be.

struction of their online and offline friendship networks with pupils residing in the same grade.

- The most recent study, taking off in 2012, conducted by MIOS on the topic of cyberbullying is named Adaptive Technological Tools Against Cyberbullying (*Friendly ATTAC*)[6]. Although the main aim of this project is the development of a digital anti-bullying game, an online survey has also been conducted among 453 Flemish youngsters in the course of the project.

We will start this chapter by exploring the victimization and perpetration rates yielded by these studies. Subsequently, we will also discuss the most important predictors of online perpetration and victimization, as these have been identified in the course of these studies. Next, we will discuss at a more conceptual level some of the issues related with mediation of technology in the occurrence of cyberbullying and how these issues have evolved during the past few years, marked by a transformation to Web 2.0 filled with social media.

9.2   Prevalence of Cyberbullying in Belgium

Most studies exploring cyberbullying prevalence across the globe yield the rather consistent conclusion that a non-negligible percentage (ranging between 10 and 40 %) of contemporary youth is seriously affected by it (Tokunaga 2010). Nonetheless, we see that prevalence rates between studies vary strongly (Kowalski et al. 2012; Tokunaga 2010). These divergences appear not to be random but seem to depend on the specific study's *wideness of scope*, its deployed *age span*, the installed *time frame* and whether cyberbullying is *measured directly or indirectly*. We will discuss this in more detail in the following paragraphs:

The Wideness of Scope The operational definitions that are used for measuring young people's involvement in cyberbullying (in either *role*: as a *bully, victim, bully–victim*[7] or *bystander*) tend to vary from study to study in terms of specificity versus generality (Kowalski et al. 2014). Some studies are interested in examining adolescents' involvement in cyberbullying in general (Strohmeier et al. 2011; for Belgium, see Walrave and Heirman 2011), whereas other studies have a more narrow focus on specific types of cyberbullying (e.g. Moore et al. 2012: cyberbullying by means of *aggressive forum posts*; for Belgium, see Bastiaensens et al. 2014: cyberbullying *via social network sites*). The wider the scope of the study, the more negative online conduct falls under its focus of attention and, logically, the higher generally the yielded prevalence rates tend to be (Kowalski et al. 2014).

Age Span Also, the age difference among respondents across studies tends to vary from very narrow to very large. Some studies focus on respondents belonging to one specific study year (Fredstrom et al. 2011: only *ninth grade students*; for

---

[6] This project was funded by the Agentschap voor Innovatie door Wetenschap en Technologie (IWT) (2012). For more information, see http://www.friendlyattac.be.

[7] These are youngsters who are both victim and perpetrator of (cyber)bullying. According to various studies, this group of young people is most affected by the maladaptive conduct.

Belgium, see Wegge et al. 2014: only *eighth grade students*), whereas others have examined the behaviour among a more age-differentiated sample of adolescents (Brighi et al. 2012:*11–21-year-old* respondents; for Belgium, see Vandebosch and Van Cleemput 2009:*10–18-year-old* respondents). It is not entirely surprising that the choice of a specific age bracket also has repercussions for the prevalence rates observed across studies. Most cases of cyberbullying are typically found among 12–14-year-old respondents. As Table 9.1 shows, studies focussing on this narrow age group (e.g. Wegge et al. 2014) tend to find higher prevalence rates compared with studies with a wider age span (e.g. Vandebosch and Van Cleemput 2009).

The Time Frame Some studies are interested in finding out whether respondents have *ever* performed cyberbullying (e.g. Aricak et al. 2008; for Belgium, see Walrave and Heirman 2011), whereas other studies want to know more about young people's involvement within a given period (e.g. Bauman 2010: involvement in the *current school year*; for Belgium, see Vandebosch and Van Cleemput 2009: involvement during the *past 3 months*). Generally speaking, the wider the reference period for cyberbullying, the higher the prevalence rates tend to be (Kowalski et al. 2014).

Direct Versus Indirect Measurement Also, the way in which cyberbullying is questioned—either as *direct* or *indirect*—has possible repercussions (Aalsma and Brown 2008). Explicit direct questioning of cyberbullying of a victim may lead to underreporting, given the insight that endorsing the label as "a bully victim" could be emotionally difficult. Therefore, direct measurement of cyberbullying has been questioned as an appropriate way to assess its true prevalence, and installing a measure whereby respondents are asked to report their involvement in specific situations is considered by some scholars as more appropriate (Aalsma and Brown 2008).

Studies that have done so show that discrepancies between direct and indirect measurement turn out to be very large. For instance, the TIRO study found, compared with the prevalence rates based on direct measurement (34.2% victims and 21.2% perpetrators), far higher prevalence rates when pupils' involvement in cyberbullying was assessed using indirect methods of measurement. More than six out of ten respondents (64.3%) reported having experienced the consequences of at least one of the discerned types of negative online conduct, whereas nearly four out of ten (39.9%) reported having perpetrated at least one action (e.g. breaking in into an e-mail account and changing its password).

The Platform of Cyberbullying Prevalence rates also differ depending on the online venue where the bullying takes place. The Developmental Issues in Cyberbullying Amongst Adolescents (DICA) study provides more information on what type of cyberbullying occurs most: In its first wave the most common venue of cyberbullying was mobile text messages (44.9%) or social network sites (SNS; 44.9%). Less common platforms were e-mail (14%), gaming platforms and YouTube (3.1%). In the fourth wave of DICA, SNS were the most common venue for cyberbullying (50.4%), followed by text messages (41), gaming platforms (24.7%) and YouTube (12.0%).

The question that contemporary scholars are starting to ask is whether cyberbullying is a phenomenon on the rise (e.g. Kowalski et al. 2014; Olweus 2012). Only longitudinal data can elucidate this. The outcomes of the Belgian DICA study in Table 9.1 seem to suggest that prevalence rates are dropping, although we can-

Table 9.1 Cyberbullying prevalence in studies conducted by Media, ICT/Interpersonal relations in Organisations and Society (MIOS)

	Sample size	Age span (years)	Operational definition	Reporting time frame	Prevalence rate of victimization (%)	Prevalence rate of perpetration (%)
viWTA project (Vandebosch and Van Cleemput 2009)	2052	10–18	"Bullying someone through the Internet or mobile phone"	3 months before questionnaire	11.1	18.0
TIRO project (Walrave and Heirman 2011)	1318	12–18	"Bullying over the Internet or mobile phone"	Lifetime (not specified)	34.2	21.2
DICA project		9–18	"Bullying happens when people do or say mean things, when the bully has the intention to make others feel bad. The person being bullied has difficulties to defend him/herself. Bullying is not the same as arguing or teasing. […] Bullying can also happen on the Internet or mobile phone: How often did you bully someone over the Internet or mobile phone?"	6 months before questionnaire		
Wave 1	2312				11.1	10.5
Wave 2	2321				10.7	10.3
Wave 3	2101				6.8	7.4
Wave 4 (Pabian and Vandebosch 2014)	2038				6.7	5.7
SNA project (Wegge et al. 2014)	1458	13–14	Idem DICA: "Bullying happens […] Bullying is not the same as arguing or teasing." Bullying can also occur through electronic media, such as Internet or mobile phone Someone who bullies can, for example, send mean messages by SMS, post offensive reactions on Facebook, say things that are not funny on MSN or spread hurtful photos on a website. The following question *only* deals with bullying on the Internet or mobile phone *How often* were you bullied on the Internet or mobile phone during the past 6 months?	6 months before questionnaire	14.3	10.0

Table 9.1 (continued)

	Sample size	Age span (years)	Operational definition	Reporting time frame	Prevalence rate of victimization (%)	Prevalence rate of perpetration (%)
Friendly ATTAC (Bastiaensens et al. 2014)	453	13–14	The same as DICA: "Bullying happens [...] Bullying is not the same as arguing or teasing. Bullying can also occur through electronic media, such as Internet or mobile phone. Examples of SNS are MySpace, Flickr, Facebook, Hyves, YouTube, Twitter, Foursquare, Google+, Netlog, Pinterest, Wattpad. How often were you bullied on SNS during the last 6 months?"	6 months before questionnaire	15.9	13.4

VIWTA Vlaams Instituut voor Wetenschappelijk en Technologisch Aspectenonderzoek
ICT information and communication technology, *TIRO* Teens & ICT: Risks & Opportunities, *DICA* Developmental Issues in Cyberbullying Amongst Adolescents, *SNA* Social Network Approach, *ATTAC* Adaptive Technological Tools Against Cyberbullying, *SNS* social network sites

not exclude entirely that this is partially due to (1) an underrepresentation of self-reported victims and bullies in the last two waves of the study, that is, those students who self-reported as cyberbully dropped out of the study after completing wave 2 (because they refused further participation or changed schools). Another possible explanation would be the occurrence of an (2) *age effect*, that is, a fair deal of students who self-reported bullying in the first waves, stopped cyberbullying in the last waves. In such a scenario, it is likely that original cyberbullying pupils with their increasing age started realizing that bullying is a form of immature conduct and therefore stopped pursuing it.

What, however, is a conclusive and consistent finding observed both in the SNA and DICA projects is that traditional bullying remains the most dominant form of bullying in terms of prevalence compared with cyberbullying. Also other international studies came to a similar conclusion (e.g. Olweus 2012; Raskauskas and Stoltz 2007).

9.3 Why Do Some Youngsters Get Involved and Others Do Not?

A recurring finding in the five studies conducted by MIOS is that not all youngsters are equally likely to get involved (Friendly ATTAC 2012). Although we cannot 100 % accurately predict whether a particular child or teenager will get involved in cyberbullying, our research endeavours during the past decade have allowed us to identify some salient risk factors of be(com)ing a cyberbully or -victim. Providing an overview of these predictors allows us to draft a profile of cyberbullies and their victims. Such profiles may allow the identification of youngsters that are particularly vulnerable to victimization online and can fuel intervention and prevention strategies aiming to reduce cyberbullying.

9.3.1 Risk Factors for Online Victimization

9.3.1.1 Involvement in Traditional Bullying

The definitions of traditional bullying and cyberbullying share a lot in common: Both types are acknowledged as forms of aggression and encompass a power difference/imbalance between perpetrator and victim. Moreover, both are featured by repetition (Tokunaga 2010), thereby excluding singular acts of online negative conduct. Therefore, it is not surprising that a consistent finding in Belgian research has been that victimhood in cyberbullying is closely related with victimization offline. For instance, in the DICA study about two in three cybervictims (65.3 %) had also been bullied in the offline environment. Also in viWTA, strong correlations were found between both types of victimhood. Studies outside Belgium have confirmed this interrelation. Of those students who are cyberbullied, only a small minority did not experience bullying in traditional ways (Olweus 2012; Raskauskas and Stoltz 2007).

9.3.1.2 Involvement as Cyberbully

Although this may seem counterintuitive, a finding that emerged in TIRO, viWTA and the SNA projects was that an important predictor of victimization is one's *involvement as an online perpetrator*. For instance, in TIRO it was demonstrated that cyberbullies shared a sixfold increased likelihood of being victimized compared with non-cyberbullies. Also in other international research, a significant association has been observed (Espelage and Swearer 2003; Li 2007; Ybarra and Mitchell 2004).

9.3.1.3 Gender

Across Belgian studies, a consistent finding is that girls are more often victimized compared with male students. For instance, in the DICA study 14.1 % of female pupils reported being an online victim, whereas only 8.1 % of male pupils admitted being bullied online. This finding was corroborated by the TIRO study, the SNA project and in the online survey conducted in the context of the Friendly ATTAC project. Other international studies have produced mixed findings with respect to the influence of gender on young people's likelihood of victimization in the online realm. Some studies did not detect any significant gender differences at all (e.g. Patchin and Hinduja 2006; Raskauskas and Stoltz 2007; Slonje and Smith 2007).

9.3.1.4 Age

Research demonstrates that cyberbullying mostly occurs between elementary school and college. The majority of studies situate the peak in cyberbullying prevalence in the early years of secondary education, when pupils are between 12 and 14 years old. Studies, however, also tend to differ with respect to the direction of the association: Most studies find that cyberbullying declines with increasing age (e.g. Slonje and Smith 2007), whereas other research suggests an increased likelihood of cyberbullying with increasing age (Kowalski and Limber 2007).

9.3.1.5 Internet Experience

In both viWTA and TIRO, it was found that victims of cyberbullying tend to use the Internet more intensively. In addition, in TIRO it was found that victims of cyberbullying estimated their expertise in online activities as higher compared with other non-bullied students. Similar findings in viWTA and TIRO also show that involvement in other types of online risk behaviour (e.g. talking with online strangers, revealing passwords) helped in predicting teenagers' likelihood of victimization.

9.3.1.6 Person-Related Determinants of Cyberbullying Victimization

In Belgium, considerably less research has been devoted to the role of personality-related factors in predicting victimization. There are, however, some notable exceptions. For instance, in the course of the viWTA study it has been found that students featured by rather high degrees of Internet dependency were significantly more likely to become victimized in the online realm. Also, victims of cyberbullying tend to rate their self-esteem as lower as compared with non-victimized youth.

9.3.2 Risk Factors for Online Perpetration

9.3.2.1 Involvement as Cybervictim

In the previous section, we already referred to the strong interrelation between the role of bully and victim in cyberbullying. This goes in both directions: Not only are cyberbullies more likely to become online victims, cybervictims are also more inclined to become cyberbullies. An explanation is that they are possibly partially driven to do so for retaliation purposes (e.g. Bauman 2010; Vandebosch and Van Cleemput 2009). In the TIRO study, it was found that victims of cyberbullying have a nine times greater chance of perpetrating cyberbullying, a result which was echoed in viWTA.

9.3.2.2 Perpetrators in Traditional Bullying

What we know from extant Belgian research (viWTA and the SNA project) is that there is considerable overlap between being involved in traditional bullying as a perpetrator and adopting the perpetrator role in the online realm. These observations have been found in other studies outside Belgium (Olweus 2012; Perren and Gutzwiller-Helfenfinger 2012). As Olweus (2012) states, "to cyberbully others seems to a large extent to be part of a general pattern of bullying, where use of the electronic media is only one possible form". According to Sticca and Perren (2013) there are only few cyberbullies who have limited their actions to the online realm.

9.3.2.3   Person-Related Determinants of Cyberbullying Perpetration

Scrutinizing the *attitudes* expressed by cyberbullies in TIRO suggests that they tend
to minimize the impact of their acts. Perpetrators share a more positive attitude
towards cyberbullying. This finding was also observed in DICA, in which it was
shown that youngsters do a balancing exercise between the advantages and disadvantages of cyberbullying (Pabian and Vandebosch 2014). The most common
advantages are parallel with the main motivations to perform electronic bullying:
acquiring status, feeling powerful, combating boredom, etcetera. Possible disadvantages are peer rejection, being punished by adults or losing online access (Friendly
ATTAC 2012). The DICA study showed that significantly more cyberbullies than
non-cyberbullying youth tend to agree with statements, such as "cyberbullying
makes you more popular among peers". An additional DICA finding was that cyberbullies tended to estimate the disadvantages (e.g. getting punished) of cyberbullying
as relatively small: 16% of cyberbullies agreed with the statement that "perpetration in cyberbullying is unlikely to involve adult punishment", whereas only 11.4%
of non-cyberbullying youngsters agreed.

9.3.2.4   Gender

According to DICA, male pupils (12.4%) are more likely to adopt the cyberbully
role in comparison to females (9.9%), which is a replication of a similar finding
in the TIRO study (Walrave and Heirman 2011) and other international research
(Slonje and Smith 2007; Li 2006). Gender, however, was no significant predictor of
perpetration in the viWTA study (Vandebosch and Van Cleemput 2009).

9.3.2.5   Age

Extant research paints a mixed picture with regard to age differences. Some studies
find significant differences, and others suggest that age is not important (Patchin
and Hinduja 2006; Smith et al. 2008). Cyberbullying usually peaks somewhere in
lower secondary education (Slonje and Smith 2007; Vandebosch and Van Cleemput
2009). Cyberbullies tend to be slightly older than their victims (DICA and viWTA;
Ybarra and Mitchell 2004).

9.3.2.6   Educational Level

Belgium has an educational system that consists of three educational types in secondary education: *general secondary education* schools, which provide broad theoretical education preparing for further education at college or university; *technical
secondary education* schools, which focus more on technical skills and practical
matters; and *vocational secondary education*, which directly prepares pupils for

employment after secondary school. Both in viWTA as well as in TIRO, it was found that the highest-level pupils (general secondary education) were significantly less involved as perpetrators than pupils in other types of secondary education.

9.3.2.7   ICT Features

Cyberbullies usually are heavy Internet users as was found in viWTA. Also in the TIRO study it was observed that teenagers who spend more time on the Internet were more likely to become perpetrators of cyberbullying. Moreover, empirical evidence was provided that teens scoring high on self-rated ICT expertise were more likely to become a cyberbully. Also in TIRO, the possession of one's own computer and regular computer access in their bedroom were found to increase the likelihood of perpetrating cyberbullying. In the viWTA study, it was found that respondents whose parents are less involved with their Internet use have a higher perpetration chance.

9.3.2.8   Positive Normative Climate

A DICA finding suggests that when adolescents feel a positive subjective norm regarding cyberbullying among the significant others in their lives, they feel more inclined to perform it (Pabian and Vandebosch 2014). When they experience negative norms, they feel less motivated to engage in cyberbullying. This result was corroborated by other Belgian research (Heirman and Walrave 2012).

9.4   Issues and Concerns on the Mediation of Technology in Cyberbullying

In the previous section, we have reviewed extant Belgian cyberbullying research. At this moment, studies have succeeded in mapping its prevalence, but now other questions have started arising, such as "What are the middle-long and the long-term outcomes of cyberbullying?" In this regard, some argue that cyberbullying may amplify some of the harmful consequences that have been typically associated with victimization in traditional bullying (e.g. Willard 2007; Ybarra and Mitchell 2004). In reviewing literature on cyberbullying, we have detected five typical features of ICT that are said to enable this aggravation of harm. In this chapter, we critically appreciate their potentially amplifying impact. These characteristics include (1) the potential for bullies to stay anonymous (e.g. Kowalski and Limber 2007; Patchin and Hinduja 2006), (2) the furtive nature of online communication (e.g. Williams and Guerra 2007), (3) the absence of non-verbal cues in online communication (e.g. Kowalski and Limber 2007; Kowalski et al. 2012; Patchin and Hinduja 2006; Ybarra and Mitchell 2004), (4) the 24/7 attainability provided by online communication (e.g. Kowalski and Limber 2007; Patchin and Hinduja 2006) and (5) the quick distribution of electronic messages to infinite audiences (e.g. David-Ferdon and Hertz 2007; Kowalski and Limber 2007; Kowalski et al. 2012). The different issues raised will be scrutinized based on the following four interrogations:

a. Can these issues differentiate the impact of cyberbullying?
b. Can these issues also have a beneficial outcome?
c. Do these issues merely manifest themselves online or can they also be applied in traditional bullying forms?

A final aspect is related to the question of how cyberbullying has evolved in a Web 2.0 environment. Before the introduction of the static Web 1.0, cyberbullying was not really an issue: "[t]echnology had not advanced to the point where cyberbullying even was an issue" (Kowalski et al. 2012, p. 56). In the meantime much has changed. The online environment has transformed from a static platform to a dynamic and interactive Web 2.0 environment. Web 2.0 is also filled with animated effects and audiovisual content. Whereas online content in the dawn of the Internet was mainly produced by highly literate software engineers, in the Web 2.0 era nearly everyone with some computer literacy can create online content (Davies and Eynon 2013). Some known applications of this new participatory Web are blogs, SNS (e.g. Facebook), microblogs (e.g. Twitter, Instagram) and other picture and video-sharing platforms (e.g. YouTube). With these online applications the nature of cyberbullying may have altered. What is for sure is that new forms of cyberbullying have emerged that exploit some of the specific features of the Web 2.0 environment. For instance, *notify wars* are a type of cyberbullying in which adolescents abuse the report button that is typically present on most social media. They deliberately report the content written by their target/victim as problematic, which can lead the content provider to suspend the victim's account (Aftab 2014). Also other innovative 2.0 applications (e.g. Snapchat, Tinder, Ask.fm) have been abused for cyberbullying purposes. For instance, in case of Snapchat the print screen function has been used to distribute sensitive information. In 2013, there was a growing list of children and teenagers driven to commit suicide, at least in part, after being bullied online through a new collection of texting and photo-sharing cell phone applications. Therefore, we will ask ourselves:

d. Has the role of technological mediation in cyberbullying changed with the transformation towards Web 2.0?

9.4.1 Online Anonymity

In comparison to traditional bullying, cyberbullying is relatively easy to perform without the perpetrator revealing his/her identity. The easy possibilities of online anonymity in CMC communication are mentioned as one of the most worrying aspects in focus group conversations devoted to the topic (e.g. Agatston et al. 2007; Bryce and Fraser 2013). Anonymity is considered problematic for several reasons, the first being that it may lead to a *reduction of punitive fears* among young people who are thinking about victimizing others in the online realm. Indeed, one of the central findings of an early American focus group study into primary motivations for cyberbullying was that some participants admitted perpetrating it because they believed it was "safer" than traditional bullying due to the heightened possibility to cover true identity (Agatston et al. 2007; Li 2007). In addition, the DICA project demonstrates that this belief is indeed present among approximately one third of respondents, with 30.5 % (in the fourth wave) of respondents agreeing that cyberbullying is easier to perform because it can be accomplished anonymously. A second aspect that makes anonymity problematic is that it may enhance *feelings of disinhibition* among adolescents (Diener 1980; Bryce and Fraser 2013). In other words, it can reduce adolescents' restraint to perform maladaptive behaviour (Bryce and Fraser 2013). Essentially, the concept of disinhibition encompasses that people will say and do things anonymously that they would not say or do in face-to-face interactions. This may fuel youngsters' motivation to engage in cyberbullying perpetration, whereas they did not engage in traditional bullying, because it is more difficult to remain anonymous in offline bullying (Kowalski et al. 2014). Finally, the third and probably most problematic aspect related to anonymity in cyberbullying is that it may impede a solution for the victim as the source of maladaptive behaviour remains unknown (Moore et al. 2012). In this way, anonymity provides the cyberbully with an imbalance of power, as the victim's capacity to apply preventative techniques for avoiding aggressive behaviours is undermined (David-Ferdon and Hertz 2007).

Anonymity in technology-mediated communication can also turn out positive and beneficial for young people's well-being, to say the least, because it enables them to experiment with their identity. This may be especially important for shy and introverted youth. The ability to leave one's real persona behind and to adopt a new alter ego or an avatar in the online environment is designated by Suler (2004, p. 322) as *dissociative anonymity*: "When people have the opportunity to separate their actions online from their personal lifestyle and identity, they feel less vulnerable about self-disclosing and acting out." By offering people the opportunity to hide their identity, ICTs allow people to share the most intimate aspects of their lives with others in such a way that it cannot directly be linked to the rest of their lives, which may entice them to divulge extensive information to people they do not know in real life. This phenomenon is also called "the-stranger-on-the-train-effect", allowing people to express their emotions, which has proven to be beneficial under certain circumstances for one's personal and mental well-being (Bargh et al. 2002).

Although anonymity is fairly often mentioned as one of the features differentiating traditional bullying from cyberbullying (Smith et al. 2008; Kowalski et al. 2012), we think this is a debatable point of view. Many examples of anonymous offline bullying exist, for instance, when a victim's properties (e.g. a lunchbox) are stolen. The existence of anonymous instances in offline bullying can also be inferred from the formal distinction that is being made in traditional bullying literature between direct ("in the face") and indirect ("behind the back") bullying (Stassen Berger 2007; Vandebosch and Van Cleemput 2009). Moreover, most cyberbully studies suggest that the anonymity of the online perpetrator should be taken with a serious grain of salt. In the DICA study, only 24.26% of victimized adolescents (in wave 4) did not know the true identity of their online harassers. This implies that more than half of cybervictimized adolescents had a rather precise idea about who is targeting them in cyberspace. Also other studies outside the Belgian context confirm this: Juvonen and Gross (2008) have found that about three in four (73%) respondents in their study were pretty to totally sure about the identity of their online harasser. In addition, although many Internet users feel anonymous online, computer experts (e.g. Vishik and Finocchiaro 2010) argue that most online activities from non-professional ICT users can easily be traced back to a source. This is moreover evidenced in some of the most widely covered cyberbullying incidents in media, in which the real cyberbullies were tracked down and eventually identified.

With regard to the impact of anonymity on the perceived severity of cyberbullying, a Swiss study demonstrated that anonymous incidents of (cyber)bullying were considered as having a more severe impact compared with cases in which the identity of the online perpetrator was known (Sticca and Perren 2013).

Does anonymity remain a salient characteristic of cyberbullying in a *Web 2.0* environment? In the light of what we wrote above, it is somewhat remarkable that a fair deal of studies (e.g. DICA, Friendly ATTAC) found that SNS, typically *nomynous* environments (i.e. the user's identity is known and displayed), are the most commonly used venues for cyberbullies to perform their malicious acts. In its 1.0 version the World Wide Web was in the first instance an anonymous environment featured by high fragmentation. With the rise of 2.0 applications, the Web has become increasingly integrated and moreover a more personalized environment. Personalization implies less anonymity. So, if anonymity has decreased in Web 2.0, why are then the 2.0 applications among the most used venues for perpetrators to pursue their online acts? Several explanations are possible: First, although it is true that most young people are identifiable on SNS, this does not exclude the possibility for youngsters to impersonate as someone else online by creating a false SNS account. Second, although much of the content in Web 2.0 is available for a larger audience to consult, the most used applications have retained private chat functions (that have more or less the same functionality as text messaging and instant messaging). From early research, for instance viWTA, we know that these venues in which the name of the conversation partners is known were also the most commonly used platforms of cyberbullying.

9.4.2 Escaping Adult Supervision

In general, there are different aspects in the online environment that enable youngsters to relatively easily mask what is said and done from adult supervision (Davies and Eynon 2013). First, computer and cellular screens do not lend themselves efficiently to adult control. Second, many teenagers are savvy enough to think about ways to circumvent adult monitoring by means of several techniques (e.g. physically distancing themselves from adults when using mobile digital devices, using a smart button on a keyboard making communication screens disappear; Bovill and Livingstone 2001). Third, even if cyberbullying is detected by the adult eye, it is not so clear which group has the (legal) capacity to apply sanctions. Whereas teachers and school administrators are considered as obvious enforcers or agents to stop traditional bullying among pupils, this role is less self-evident in cyberbullying contexts (Tokunaga 2010). Fourth, cyberbullying is hard to supervise because a considerable share of victims decide not to tell anything about it. Some scholars suggest that a considerable share of cybervictims do not see how adult intervention can ameliorate the painful situation that victims have to endure (Juvonen and Gross 2008; Li 2007). On the contrary, many are convinced that involving adults in tackling cyberbullying will only aggravate the situation and increase humiliation.

Admittedly, some forms of cyberbullying can take place in a very sneaky way, and it is not easy for adults to detect them. The same, however, also applies to incidents of traditional bullying that share an increased likelihood of getting passed unnoticed in front of the adult supervising eye. Especially relational bullying (e.g. isolating a pupil from peers) and verbal bullying (e.g. making derogatory remarks) are in many cases likely to remain unnoticed (Griffin and Gross 2004). Conversely, physical bullying is the most obvious and visible type of bullying behaviour: A punch in the face is recognized not only by adults but also by children of the peer group (Smith et al. 2002). Research has found that teachers tend to intervene more quickly in this overt type of bullying since the physical integrity of victimized pupils is directly at stake (Bauman and Del Rio 2006) and that children are more likely to report these direct types of bullying (Griffin and Gross 2004). Intervention by adults is less likely for covert types of bullying. Williams and Guerra (2007) found that young people may be facilitated to engage in covert types of bullying because they believe that adults and bystanders are unlikely to intervene.

A beneficial aspect of the fact that online communication lends itself relatively difficult for adult supervision is that ICT provides youngsters with a *censorship-free* environment to initiate, maintain and reinforce friendships. Many adults would be disturbed by some of the things that young people send to each other online but the ability to do so is important for young people to achieve their developmental goals (identity construction and intimacy creation). Without the privacy and distance from the adult eye offered by CMC, teenagers' communication would be featured by far less spontaneity and honesty. From a developmental perspective it is not desirable to allow adults to constantly monitor youngsters' online communication.

In some literature, it is being hypothesized that with the emergence of *Web 2.0*, teenage content is exposed to an increasing influx of adults in teenagers SNS friend lists. It is possible that hereby possibilities for adult supervision are increased, although it seems that teens have enough means at their disposal to avoid such adult intervention. Options for customized privacy settings allow adolescents to precisely define what content is watchable for which specific person or group (Kowalski et al. 2012). Moreover, although many adults are active on Facebook, there remain plenty of platforms available that are *more teenage-oriented* (e.g. Snapchat).

9.4.3 Cockpit Effect

Many of the non- and para-verbal cues typically present in traditional modes of face-to-face communication get stripped away during young people's online communication. Indeed, most incidents of cyberbullying do not take place in a face-to-face setting, where both the perpetrator and the victim are jointly present. This entails that chances are small that the perpetrator has the occasion to witness how the victim emotionally reacts (Sticca and Perren 2013; Ybarra and Mitchell 2004). Given the lack of emotional feedback, the person perpetrating the negative online activities may feel less inclined to modulate his/her behaviours. In a paper dating back to 2008, we referred to a striking analogy between the absence of non-verbal communication cues and the lack of direct face-to-face contact among fighter pilots with their on-ground targets in World War II: the so-called *cockpit effect* (Heirman and Walrave 2008). This effect is said to work as a separating mechanism, decreasing empathy with others in the social environment (De Laender 1996). Konrad Lorenz (1974) studied the mental condition of soldiers after their participation in World War II. His study led to the remarkable result that infantrymen with high war-zone exposure in direct face-to-face confrontation with their individual enemies (infantrymen of the other side) reported higher levels of post-traumatic stress syndromes than fighter pilots. The latter, however, had caused far higher damage: Flying in the air and dropping bombs from the sky, they devastated entire villages and killed hundreds of people. Sitting in a cockpit, at large inobservable distances from their (suffering) targets, pilots did not have to "face" their actions, making it relatively easier for them to kill with less psychological damage (De Laender 1996). In a similar vein, a cyberbully may sit in front of his digital device and like a pilot in a cockpit may feel disinhibited. Like modern weapon technology, modern ICTs can, if used in an antisocial way, create distance between perpetrator and target and hereby eliminate the inhibiting effect that pity and empathy normally have in face-to-face interactions (De Laender 1996; Suler 2004). Indeed, previous studies have observed a significant association between young people's level of cognitive empathy and their self-reported engagement in cyberbullying (Ang and Goh 2010; Kowalski et al. 2012; Steffgen et al. 2011). Moreover, it is possible that the invisible suffering entails that the perpetrator thinks that what he/she is doing is not harmful. In psychology, the phenomenon that emerges when people are convinced that their virtual persona and online activities only exist online is being referred to as "dissociative imagination" (Suler 2004). This may explain why some cyberbullies indicate that they are performing their online harming activities "for fun" (Kowalksi and Limber 2007). They are genuinely convinced that they are not doing anything wrong and consider cyberbullying as merely an "imaginary act" of bullying. Studies such as DICA suggest that the lack of non-verbal feedback on behalf of the victim is a salient issue in explaining the prevalence of cyberbullying: About 25 % agreed that it is easier to perform cyberbullying because it prevents you from seeing the victim. The study by Bryce and Fraser (2013) was one of the first to provide empirical evidence for the fact that young people's perceived lack of face-to-face interaction and the inability to witness the impact had a direct effect on young people's cyberbullying intentions.

Disinhibition does not always lead to decreased empathy but can also drive opposite effects. It can motivate people to share their innermost feelings in a very sincere and honest way (Kowalski and Limber 2007). In this way, the lack of non-verbal cues may diminish restraint to tell stories that in a face-to-face setting would have remained untold, for instance, due to misinterpreted non-verbal or para-verbal signals (Ybarra et al. 2007).

In some instances of traditional bullying, the bully is also not present in the direct neighbourhood of the victim. Especially in the area of behavioural bullying, it is not so difficult to conceive situations in which a perpetrator does not see the emotion on the victim's face—for example, when a pupil's lunch is stolen from his bag or other personal belongings of a pupil are deliberately damaged by a bully when the victim was not in his/her neighbourhood.

Technology develops very rapidly. Increasing technological capacities have enhanced online experience in the *Web 2.0* era. Broadband Internet now allows the streaming or exchange involving many non-verbal cues that had been stripped away in early forms of online communication. For instance, VoIP services enabling audio- and video-stream of chat are now integrated within most SNS. From this perspective, one could argue that the potential to transmit non- and para-verbal information online has increased during the past decade. Notwithstanding this, cyberbullies may be more appealed to pursue their negative online conduct using media or specific applications within media that do not entail their confrontation with the emotional feedback of the victim.

9.4.4   Infinite Audiences: Shareability and Reproducibility

An often voiced concern emerging in interviews conducted on the topic of cyberbullying is that a theoretically limitless audience can get involved (Kowalski et al. 2012; Sticca and Perren 2013): "With regard to reproducibility, the core issue is that a person can easily copy all friends on a message or forward gossip to his or her entire address book" (Kowalski et al. 2014, p. 2). The extent to which traditional bullying spreads is in most cases restricted to some members or—in the worst case—a considerable part of the local school community. In cyberbullying, hurtful messages, however, can spread to a very wide audience in a very short period of time and with very little effort (Kowalski et al. 2012; Patchin and Hinduja 2006). According to extant research, the degree of publicity is directly related with the perceived severity of online bullying (e.g. Slonje and Smith 2008). Public cyberbullying is perceived as most severe, which suggests that adolescents are more fearful of humiliation in front of a large online audience, whereas the deliberate transmission of viruses or private messages (e.g. by SMS) are perceived as having far less impact (Sticca and Perren 2013). Moreover, publicly spread cyberbullying may be perceived as more severe because it decreases the victim's ability to maintain control over the situation. The feeling that the victim has no control over his/her online victimization and which audience gets involved has been associated with feelings of helplessness in previous research (Kowalski et al. 2012).

Despite the embarrassment this causes for cybervictims, the quick distribution capacities of technology may also greatly benefit other youths' achievement of developmental tasks. These developmental tasks are oriented towards the achievement of psychosocial autonomy, which can be accomplished by developing identity, creating intimacy and emotional release/disclosure. The importance of having an audience to provide feedback on youngsters' identity especially manifests itself on SNS. These media have been developed to allow people to ventilate their feelings, show their interests and activities in daily life, and aspects of their identity to a broad audience. This may serve important developmental needs, especially during adolescence, when the formation of an own identity is one of the crucial tasks (Calvert 2002).

One of the key terms of *Web* is *2.0* "sharing". This encompasses the encouragement for users to spread content across an online audience. Users are explicitly encouraged to distribute their and other users' content by means of the share button that is typically integrated in Web 2.0 content (e.g. a status update on Facebook, a picture on Flickr). From this perspective, one could argue that the distributional process of forwarding or sharing online content with larger audiences has been facilitated, when compared with Web 1.0. The fact that online content is now so easily shareable has also inspired application developers to create online chat functions that aim to prevent unrestricted sharing. For instance, the application Snapchat automatically deletes a message shortly after it has been opened by the intended receiver. Snapchat's popularity among teenagers supports this age group's need for an application that fosters interpersonal online communication without the free distribution of what is being communicated to others. The snake in the grass is, however, that there remain plenty of ways for teenagers to record/register the content of Snapchat on their mobile devices. Hence, users could be stimulated to disclose more sensitive information in the belief that Snapchat protects their information from being spread, but tech-savvy adolescent Internet users with cyberbullying intentions can still manage to store this sensitive information.

9.4.5   24/7 Attainability

One of the most mentioned amplifying effects of cyberbullying versus traditional bullying is the victim's difficulty to escape from it because of its space- and time-independent nature. Cyberbullying, however, can happen 24 h a day, 7 days a week. There is nothing that prevents a cyberbully from causing online harm, even when the victim is at that moment not in his immediate physical proximity (Patchin and Hinduja 2006; Slonje and Smith 2007). In traditional school bullying, the home environment could be considered as a safe retreat, a "bully-free" zone. The walls of the home, however, do no longer function as an impenetrable bunker (Kowalski et al. 2012). Instead, victimized students are more likely to become perpetual targets for cyberbullies, as digital devices (smartphones) allow cyberbullying pupils to dispose over a precise and continuous target.

Notwithstanding the potentially aggravating impact of cyberbullying due the "always online" capacity of technology, there are also many beneficial outcomes for young people that are precisely enabled by this "always on" aspect of communication technologies. At the psychological level, the introduction of cellular phones has invoked the possibility to experience "privatized mobility": the possibility to feel at home without even being physically present at home (Moores 2000).

Although traditional bullying could also take place outside school hours, the 24/7 access to the victim is indeed a relatively new aspect in a bullying context. Never have victims of bullying been so easily reachable as now with ICT. Traditional types of bullying mostly take place at school, or on the way home to or from school. Of course, bullying can also occur elsewhere in community, for example, in youth or sport clubs, but even considering that, youth do not go to these places every day, whereas their mobile devices are always within their reach.

In the era of *Web 2.0*, adolescents' possession of smartphones—mobile phones with access to the Internet through Wi-Fi or 3G/4G—has seriously increased (Lenhart et al. 2010; World Internet Project 2012). This entails that, whereas in the past only the traditional mobile phone could be deployed to bully other pupils by means of text messages on a continuous basis, now—due to the increased mobility of Web-based applications—also online services can be used to harass others. In addition, many content providers have developed specific apps that can enhance the experience of their services for mobile users (e.g. the Facebook app for smartphone). These applications easily allow SNS users to readily access their profile even when they are away from their computer. Increased mobility entails consequences for involvement in cyberbullying as either a perpetrator or a victim. A fairly recent study by EU Kids Online shows that teenagers disposing of their own smartphone or a tablet show higher likelihood of reporting that they are involved in cyberbullying as either a perpetrator or a victim. This result suggests that with the introduction of mobile digital devices among young people, their opportunities to become involved in it have equally risen.

9.5 Conclusion

At its core, cyberbullying encompasses the performance of intentional harmful online conduct by means of technology-mediated communication (Kowalski et al. 2014). Research in Belgium shows that a fairly substantial deal of Belgian youth is confronted with it at a given moment in time. In this chapter, the authors have brought together the technology-related concerns in cyberbullying. Remarkable is that all of the features of technology that are worrisome in an online bullying context can also have beneficial outcomes in other areas of a youth's life, especially when prosocial purposes are intended. For people who experience difficulties in engaging in social relationships, online anonymity may lower the barriers to meet new friends. In addition, by using SNS, today's teens are able to reach large audiences to tell what is going on in their lives and how they are feeling. Furthermore, technology's potential to extend the period of time in which peers can communicate with each other may enhance collaborative learning efforts and consolidate offline peer relationships. In a similar way, the private nature provided by ICT attributes largely to the success of mobile phones and the Internet to communicate with peers beyond the borders of adult supervision. Finally, the absence of non-verbal communication may take away inhibitive elements to tell about fears, emotions and desires and thus fosters genuine communication among peers.

Another remarkable assessment is that most technology issues in cyberbullying are not as "new" in a bullying context as sometimes presumed. Only with respect to the 24/7 intrusion of peers' lives, it seems that cyberbullying is indeed something "new". Despite the fact that traditional bullying can occur elsewhere in the community than in school, cyberbullies as opposed to traditional bullies appear able to pursue their victim, even behind the walls of their home environment. If the victimized teen prefers not to switch off the cellular phone at night, he or she is indeed a perpetual target for cyberbullies, whereas the victim of traditional bullying can find a safe retreat at home.

References

Aalsma, M. C., & Brown, J. R. (2008). What is bullying? *Journal of Adolescent Health, 43*(2), 101–102. doi:10.1016/j.jaohealth.2008.06.001.

Aftab, P. (2014). How does cyberbullying work, in detail? http://www.aftab.com/index. php?page=how-does-cyberbullying-work.

Agatston, P. W., Kowalski, R. M., & Limber, S. P. (2007). Students' perspectives on cyber bullying. *Journal of Adolescent Health, 41*(6), 59–60. doi:10.1016/j.jadohealth.2007.09.003.

Ang, R. P., & Goh, D. H. (2010). Cyberbullying among adolescents: The role of affective and cognitive empathy, and gender. *Child Psychiatry and Human Development, 41*, 387–397. doi:10.1007/s10578-010-0176-3.

Aricak, T., Siyahhan, S., Uzunhasanoglu, A., Saribeyoglu, S., Ciplak, S., Yilmaz, N., & Memmedov, C. (2008). Cyberbullying among Turkish adolescents. *CyberPsychology & Behavior, 11*(3), 253–261. doi:10.1089/cpb.2007.0016.

Bargh, J. A., McKenna, K. Y. A., & Fitzsimons, G. M. (2002). Can you see the real me? Activation an expression of the "true self" on the internet. *Journal of Social Issues, 58*, 33–48. doi:10.1111/1540-4560.00247.

Bastiaensens, S., Vandebosch, H., Poels, K., Van Cleemput, K., DeSmet, A., & De Bourdeaudhuij, I. (2014). Cyberbullying on social network sites. An experimental study into bystanders' behavioural intentions to help the victim or reinforce the bully. *Computers in Human Behavior, 31*, 259–271. doi:10.1016/j.chb.2013.10.036.

Bauman, S. (2010). Cyberbullying in a rural intermediate school: An exploratory study. *Journal of Early Adolescence, 30*, 803–833.

Bauman, S., & Del Rio, A. (2006). Preservice teachers' responses to bullying scenarios: Comparing physical, verbal, and relational bullying. *Journal of Educational Psychology, 98*(1), 219–231. doi:10.1037/0022-0663.98.1.219.

Bovill, M., & Livingstone, S. (2001). Bedroom culture and the privatization of media use (online). http://eprints.lse.ac.uk/archive/00000672.

Brighi, A., Guarini, A., Melotti, G., Galli, S., & Genta, M. L. (2012). Predictors of victimisation across direct bullying, indirect bullying and cyberbullying. *Emotional and Behavioural Difficulties, 17*, 375–388. doi:10.1080/13632752.2012.704684.

Bryce, J., & Fraser, J. (2013). "It's common sense that it's wrong"; Young people's perceptions and experiences of cyberbullying. *CyberPsychology, Behavior & Social Networking, 16*(11), 783–787. doi:10.1089/cyber.2012.0275.

Calvert, S. L. (2002). Identity construction on the internet. In S. L. Calvert, A. B. Jordan, & R. R. Cocking (Eds.), *Children in the digital age: Influences of electronic media on development.* Westport: Praeger.

David-Ferdon, C., & Hertz, M. F. (2007). Electronic media, violence, and adolescents: An emerging public health problem. *Journal of Adolescent Health, 41*(6), S1–S5. doi:10.1016/j.jadohealth.2007.08.020.

Davies, C., & Eynon, R. (2013). *Teenagers and technology.* London: Routledge.

De Laender, J. (1996). *Het hart van de duisternis: psychologie van de menselijke wreedheid.* Leuven: Davidsfonds.

Diener, E. (1980). Deindividuation: The absence of self-awareness and self-regulation in group members. In B. P. Paulus (Ed.), *The psychology of group influence* (pp. 209–242). Hillsdale: Erlbaum.

Espelage, D. L., & Swearer, S. M. (2003). Research on school bullying and victimization: What have we learned and where do we go from here? *School Psychology Review, 32*(3), 365–383.

Fredstrom, B. K., Adams, R. E., & Gilman, R. (2011). Electronic and school-based victimization: Unique contexts for adjustment difficulties during adolescence. *Journal of Youth and Adolescence, 40*, 405–415. doi:10.1007/110964-010-9569-7.

Friendly ATTAC. (2012). *Zes jaar onderzoek naar cyberpesten in Vlaanderen, België en daarbuiten: een overzicht van de bevindingen* (p. 17). Antwerp: Friendly Attac.

Griffin, R. S., & Gross, A. M. (2004). Childhood bullying: Current empirical findings and future directions for research. *Aggression and Violent Behaviour, 9*, 379–400. doi:10.1016/S1359-1789(03)00033-8.

Heirman, W., & Walrave, M. (2008). Assessing concerns and issues about the mediation of technology in cyberbullying. *Cyberpsychology: Journal of Psychosocial Research on Cyberspace, 2*(1), 1–12.

Heirman, W., & Walrave, M. (2012). Predicting adolescent perpetration in cyberbullying: An application of the theory of planned behavior. *Psicothema, 24*(4), 614–620.

Hinduja, S., & Patchin, J. W. (2007). Offline consequences of online victimization. *Journal of School Violence, 6*(3), 89–112. doi:10.1300/J202v06n03_06.

Juvonen, J., & Gross, E. G. (2008). Extending the school ground? Bullying experiences in cyberspace? *Journal of School Health, 78*(9), 496–505. doi:10.1111/j.1746-1561.2008.00335.x.

Kowalski, R. M., & Limber, S. P. (2007). Electronic bullying among middle school students. *Journal of Adolescent Health, 41*(6), 22–30. doi:10.1016/j.jadohealth.2007.08.017.

Kowalski, R. M., Limber, S. P., & Agatston, P. W. (2012). *Cyberbullying: Bullying in the digital age.* Singapore: Wiley-Blackwell.

Kowalski, R. M., Giumetti, G. W., Schroeder, A. N., & Lattanner, M. R. (2014). Bullying in the digital age: A critical review and meta-analysis of cyberbullying research among youth. *Psychological Bulletin, 140*(4), 1073–1137. doi:10.1037/a0035618.

Lenhart, A., Ling, R., Campbell, S., & Purcell, K. (2010). *Teens and mobile phones* (p. 114). Washington, DC: Pew Internet.

Li, Q. (2006). Cyberbullying in schools: A research of gender differences. *School Psychology International, 27*, 157–170.

Li, Q. (2007). Bullying in the new playground. *Australasian Journal of Educational Technology, 23*(4), 435–455.

Lorenz, K. (1974). *Das sogenannte Bose. Zur Naturgeschichte der Aggression.* Amsterdam: Ploegsma.

Mason, K. L. (2008). Cyberbullying: A preliminary assessment for school personnel. *Psychology in the Schools, 45*, 323–348. doi:10.1002/pits.20301.

Mesch, G. S. (2009). Parental mediation, online activities, and cyberbullying. *Cyberpsychology & Behavior, 12*(4), 387–393. doi:10.1089/cpb.2009.0068.

Mishna, F., Saini, M., & Solomon, S. (2009). Ongoing and online: Children and youth's perceptions of cyber bullying. *Children and Youth Services Review, 31*, 1222–1228. doi:10.1016/j.childyouth.2009.05.004.

Moore, M. J., Nakano, T., Enomoto, A., & Suda, T. (2012). Anonymity and roles associated with aggressive posts in an online forum. *Computers in Human Behavior, 28*, 861–867. doi:10.1016/j.chb.2011.12.005

Moores, S. (2000). *Media and everyday life in modern society.* Edinburgh: Edinburgh University Press.

Olweus, D. (2012). Cyberbullying: An overrated phenomenon? *European Journal of Developmental Psychology, 9*, 520–538. doi:10.1080/17405629.2012.682358.

Pabian, S., & Vandebosch, H. (2014). Using the theory of planned behavior to understand cyberbullying: The importance of beliefs for developing interventions. *European Journal of Developmental Psychology, 11*(4), 463–477. doi:10.1080/17405629.2013.858626.

Patchin, J., & Hinduja, S. (2006). Bullies move beyond the schoolyard: A preliminary look at cyberbullying. *Youth Violence and Juvenile Justice, 4*(2), 148–169. doi:10.1177/1541204006286288.

Perren, S., & Gutzwiller-Helfenfinger, E. (2012). Cyberbullying and traditional bullying in adolescence: Differential roles of moral disengagement, moral emotions, and moral values. *European Journal of Developmental Psychology, 9*(12), 195–209. doi:10.1080/17405629.2011.643168.

Raskauskas, J., & Stoltz, A. D. (2007). Involvement in traditional and electronic bullying among adolescents. *Developmental Psychology, 43*, 564–575. doi:10.1037/0012-1649.43.3.564.

Slonje, R., & Smith, P. K. (2007). Cyberbullying: Another main type of bullying? *Scandinavian Journal of Psychology, 49*(2), 147–154. doi:10.1111/j.1467-9450.2007.00611.x.

Smith, P. K., Cowen, H., Olafsson, R. F., & Liefooghe, A. P. D. (2002). Definitions of bullying: A comparison of terms used, and age and gender differences, in a fourteen-country international comparison. *Child Development, 73*(4), 1119–1133. doi:10.111/1467-8624.00461.

Smith, P. K., Mahdavi, J., Carvalho, M., Fisher, S., Russell, S., & Tippett, N. (2008). Cyberbullying: Its nature and impact in secondary school pupils. *Journal of Child Psychology and Psychiatry, 49*(4), 376–385. doi:10.1111/j.1469-7610.2007.01846.x.

Stassen Berger, K. (2007). Update on bullying at school: A science forgotten? *Developmental Review, 27*, 90–126. doi:10.1016/j.dr.2006.08.002.

Steffgen, G., König, A., Pfetsch, J., & Melzer, A. (2011). Are cyberbullies less empathic? Adolescents' cyberbullying behavior and empathic responsiveness. *Cyberpsychology, Behavior, and Social Networking, 14*, 643–648. doi:10.1089/cyber.2010.0445.

Sticca, F., & Perren, S. (2013). Is cyberbullying worse than traditional bullying? Examining the differential roles of medium, publicity, and anonymity for the perceived severity of bullying. *Journal of Youth and Adolescence, 42*(5), 739–750. doi:10.1007/s10964-012-9867-3.

Strohmeier, D., Kärnä, A., & Salmivalli, C. (2011). Intrapersonal and interpersonal risk factors for peer victimization in immigrant youth in Finland. *Developmental Psychology, 47*, 248–258. doi:10.1037/a0020785.

Suler, J. (2004). The online disinhibition effect. *Cyberpsychology and Behaviour, 7*(3), 321–326. doi:10.1089/1094931041291295.

Tokunaga, R. S. (2010). Following you home from school: A critical review and synthesis of research on cyberbullying victimization. *Computers in Human Behavior, 26*(3), 277–287. doi:10.1016/j.chb.2009.11.014.

Vandebosch, H., & Van Cleemput, K. (2009). Cyberbullying among youngsters: Profiles of bullies and victims. *New Media and Society, 11*(8), 1349–1371. doi:10.11.

Vishik, C., & Finocchiaro, G. (2010). Relative anonymity: Measuring degrees of anonymity in diverse computing environment. In N. Pohlmann, H. Reimer, & W. Schneider (Eds.), *Securing electronic business processes* (pp. 197–205). Wiesbaden: Vieweg. doi:10.1007/978-3-8348-9363-519.

Walrave, M., & Heirman, W. (2011). Cyberbullying: Predicting victimization and perpetration. *Children & Society, 25*(1), 59–72. doi:10.1111/j.1099-0860.2009-00260.x.

Wegge, D., Vandebosch, H., & Eggermont, S. (2014). Who bullies who online: A social network analysis of cyberbullying in a school context. *Communications, 30*(4), 415–433. doi:10.1515/commun-2014-0019.

Willard, N. (2007). The authority and responsibility of school officials in responding to cyberbullying. *Journal of Adolescent Health, 41*(6), s64–s65. doi:10.1016/j.jadohealth.2007.08.013.

Williams, K. R., & Guerra, N. G. (2007). Prevalence and predictors of Internet bullying. *Journal of Adolescent Health, 41*(6), S14–S21. doi:10.1016/j.jadohealth.2007.08.018.

WIP. (2012). *World internet project: International report.* Los Angeles: World Internet Project.

Ybarra, M. L., & Mitchell, K. J. (2004). Online aggressor/targets, aggressor and targets: A comparison of youth characteristics. *Journal of Child Psychology and Psychiatry, 45*(7), 1308–1316. doi:10.1111/j.1469-7610.2004.00328.x.

Ybarra, M. L., Diener-West, M., & Leaf, P. J. (2007). Examining the overlap in internet-harassment and school bullying: Implications for school intervention. *Journal of Adolescent Health, 41*(6), 42–50. doi:10.1016/j.jadohealth.2007.09.004.

Chapter 10
Spanish Youth Perceptions About Cyberbullying: Qualitative Research into Understanding Cyberbullying and the Role That Parents Play in Its Solution

Raúl Navarro and Cristina Serna

10.1 Introduction

Studies on cyberbullying have been a recurring theme in psychological research over the past 10 years. These studies, as previously occurred with school bullying, have attempted to know the nature of this phenomenon and lower its prevalence, considering the negative consequences for both victims and perpetrators. However, given the epidemiological approach of initial studies, cyberbullying research has predominantly used a quantitative approach where surveys have been the most widely used methodology to evaluate cyberbullying.

Research from this quantitative methodology has been devoted to analyze cyberbullying prevalence and risk and protective factors related to this phenomenon. Less attention has been paid to the meanings that youth confer to cyberbullying, considering the social nature of such interactions as well as the role that socialization agents (e.g., the family) play in cyberbullying. In this sense, qualitative research offers new ways to know youth's perspectives about cyberbullying, not only their own definitions about this type of aggression but also what role they believe that adults have to play in preventing and intervening in cyberbullying. Indeed, during the past few years, qualitative research has been increasingly fruitful. Several studies have analyzed the way children and adolescents from different countries perceive cyberbullying, the behaviors that they include as part of it, the impact of cyberbullying on those who suffer it, the reasons why youths engage in cyberbullying, and the coping strategies they use to stop cyberbullying (Ackers 2012; Agatston et al. 2007; Bryce and Fraser 2013; Cassidy et al. 2009; Compton et al. 2014; Frisén et al.

R. Navarro (✉)
Department of Psychology, Faculty of Education and Humanities,
University of Castilla-La Mancha, Avda de los Alfares, 42, 16071 Cuenca, Spain
e-mail: raul.navarro@uclm.es

C. Serna
Department of Psychology, University of Castilla-La Mancha, Faculty of Social Work,
Edificio Melchor Cano Camino del Pozuelo, s/n 16071 Cuenca, Spain

© Springer International Publishing Switzerland 2016   193
R. Navarro et al. (eds.), *Cyberbullying Across the Globe*,
DOI 10.1007/978-3-319-25552-1_10

2014; Kofoed and Ringrose 2012; Mishna et al. 2009; Naruskov et al. 2012; Wilton and Campbell 2011). As a whole, these studies have provided crucial information to know youths' perspective about these interactions and have been determinant for planning and implementing actions against cyberbullying by teachers, parents, and policy-makers.

Given the importance of qualitative research, this chapter presents an analysis of the meanings that Spanish youths aged 10–16 years confer to cyberbullying. We offer a study based on focus groups during which, and according to former research, we asked males and females about what they understand by cyberbullying, if there were any differences between cyber and school bullying, the reasons that motivate people to such action, and the role that adults play in prevention and intervention actions. We believe that the direct information obtained from those who suffer, observe, or participate in these interactions will help us learn more about a conduct whose translation into other languages like Spanish is not always clear. We consider that this chapter can be of much interest to learn about some barriers and difficulties that psychological research and education practice on cyberbullying must face to advance in its cross-cultural analysis and also in its prevention.

10.1.1   Cyberbullying Definition

Many people believe that they know well what cyberbullying is and think that they can easily recognize it when they come across it. However, reality shows that the cyberbullying definition is extremely varied, even in the scientific community (Sabella et al. 2013). Generally speaking, cyberbullying is described as a type of indirect traditional bullying because it occurs more than once, continues over time, is intentional, and is a form of psychological violence (Dehue et al. 2008). Cyberbullying comprises many aggressive strategies, which include sending threatening messages, posting false information on social networks or blogs, seizing digital identities, or deliberately excluding people from Internet groups. Cyberbullying has been defined as any conduct done via digital or electronic media by an individual or group that intends to harm or bother others (Tokunaga 2010). Yet cyberbullying has some specific characteristics that distinguish it from traditional bullying. These include the fact that cyberbullying goes beyond barriers in the school setting and takes place wherever victims connect to the Internet. Perpetrators can remain anonymous, and the digital means in which their conduct takes place makes it difficult for perpetrators to be aware of their victims' emotional reactions. Repetition occurs when perpetrators constantly send harmful or threatening messages but also when they resend the messages or pictures they use to other people to make them aware of the harassment the victim suffers (Smith 2012).

Despite the existence of these different characteristics, the cyberbullying definitions that researchers employ vary, as does the behavior they measure to know prevalence. Apart from this problem, there is no equivalent word to bullying in many languages other than English, which makes its study and comparing data among countries difficult. For instance, it has several translations in Spanish, which employs terms such as *acoso* (harassment), *victimización* (victimization), and *maltrato* (mistreatment). In order to find the terms that schoolchildren employ to describe victimization among peers, researchers have conducted cross-cultural studies to determine equivalent terms to the English term *"bullying."* The results obtained in Spain demonstrate that the most widespread term was *meterse con alguien* (teasing, for both direct and indirect physical and verbal aggressions), followed by *maltrato* (mistreatment) and *abuso* (abuse), where *maltrato* comes closer to the English term *bullying* (Smith et al. 2002). More recently, Spanish adolescents have reported that the Spanish term that they would use to indicate cyberbullying would be *acoso* (harassment; Nocentini et al. 2010). Therefore, in Spanish-speaking countries, it is still important to know what people understand by cyberbullying exactly, what characteristics they attribute it, and what type of behaviors these interactions comprise.

10.1.2   Cyberbullying and Traditional Bullying as an Overlapping or Divergent Phenomenon

Recent research has analyzed to what extent cyberbullying is a phenomenon that is independent of traditional bullying or if they are part of the same aggressive pattern (in this same volume, see Giumetti and Kowalski 2015). Some researchers have suggested that cyberbullying forms part of the same block of aggressive behaviors, but people use different methods to hurt their victims (Dooley et al. 2009). To support this hypothesis, some studies have found that perpetrators and victims of school bullying tend to also be cyberspace perpetrators and victims (Cassidy et al. 2009; Cross et al. 2015; Hinduja and Patchin 2008; Juvonen and Gross 2008). This would suggest that both bullying types overlap. Other studies that support that cyberbullying and traditional school bullying are converging phenomena are those that demonstrate that the psychological and social consequences that victims suffer, and the problems that perpetrators face, are similar in both forms of aggression (Juvonen and Gross 2008; Kowalski and Limber 2013; Låftman et al. 2013). There is further evidence to help sustain the overlapping hypothesis in those studies that found similarities among the reasons that lead males and females to engage in both forms of bullying, for example, wishing to obtain a better status and more power among peers, fun-seeking, and wanting release from boredom (Ackers 2012; Compton et al. 2014).

However, some studies indicate the need to distinguish between both forms of aggression. These include those which show that both forms of bullying barely overlap. For example, several studies have found that many victims and perpetrators of school bullying do not engage in cyberbullying (Kowalski and Limber 2013; Kubiszewski et al. 2015). Other studies that support the hypothesis of divergence are those which find that psychosocial adjustment of victims differs according to the type of bullying suffered. For example, some studies demonstrate that school bullying has a stronger impact on victims (Ortega et al. 2009), while others indicate that the impact is stronger on cyberbullying victims (Hay et al. 2010). Additionally, studies that have analyzed the reasons why perpetrators engage in both bullying types indicate certain differences. For example, while cyberbullying involves reasons like avoiding punishment/retaliation, revenge, and anonymity, school bullying is more motivated by perceived differences in various attributes such as race, weight, or academic abilities and also for anger/frustration at having been a victim of bullying (Compton et al. 2014; Wilton and Campbell 2011; Dooley et al. 2009).

Although several studies have already explored the overlap between school bullying and cyberbullying, the results are often divergent and require qualitative analyses to confirm these results. For this reason, the present study attempts to learn if youths perceive cyberbullying or bullying as clearly different phenomena, or if, conversely, they believe that cyberbullying is a type of bullying that employs some form of technology.

10.1.3 Prevention and Intervention Efforts

There is still little empirical evidence for the efficacy of the efforts made to intervene in cyberbullying (Sabella et al. 2013). Researchers have argued that we should draw upon experience from traditional bullying to prevent online bullying (Campbell 2005). Anti-bullying policies, peer helper programs, or social skills development strategies have proved successful in traditional bullying (Ttofi and Farrington 2011). To reduce possible risk factors and to prevent online bullying, these responses may be effective together with parental monitoring and education in cybersafety (Perren et al. 2012). Consequently, it is necessary to take a holistic approach in developing responses to deal with traditional and online bullying, which involves teachers, parents, and, of course, students.

Regarding students, previous research has shown that instead of encouraging youths to turn off or to avoid technology, students should be educated with adequate skills to respond effectively to cyberbullying. These skills include talking with a trusted adult, get additional assistance, block harassing messages, and remove hurtful content after archiving it (Bryce and Fraser 2013; Sabella et al. 2013). Other responses expressed by students are to report the website where the messages and images appear, report to the police, ignore messages, and confront the perpetrator in person or to do the same to him/her (Frisén et al. 2014; Giménez-Gualdo 2014). So, it is not just important to know what strategies youths think are more effective to stop cyberbullying but also their willingness to help those who suffer it; and if, for example, this willingness depends on the existence of some kind of friendly relationship with the victim.

Regarding parents and teachers, previous research has shown that trust and open communication among parents, teachers, and youths is a protective factor against cyberbullying (Elgar et al. 2014; Navarro et al. 2013). Therefore, parents need to be prepared to respond to technology issues. They should be aware of their children's activity online and work to understand the technology that they use. Sabella et al. (2013) stated that teachers and parents are obliged to help children become knowledgeable about technology use and teach them to police themselves. It is especially important to educate children about how to protect their personal data, and so, it is important to know to what extent youths perceive their parents or other adults as a source of suitable support and the role they play in solving problems like cyberbullying.

10.1.4 Aims of the Present Study

The general aim of this work is to learn how a group of Spanish youths understand and interpret problems like cyberbullying, especially when we consider that no equivalent term exists in Spanish. We are actually interested in knowing: (1) the differences they find between cyberbullying and traditional bullying, (2) what motivates perpetrators, (3) what concerns youths about a subject that entails considerable public alarm, (4) inquire into what a victim should do to stop cyberbullying, and (5) understand the role they think adults should play, especially parents, in intervening in these problems.

In short, the intention of this work is to go beyond merely describing this phenomenon by approaching the way we understand these relations from the perspective of those people who suffer this problem more. The youths' discourse allowed us to know about their attitudes to cyberbullying.

10.2 Method

10.2.1 Design

In accordance with the aims of the study, a qualitative methodological framework was followed that adopted a youth participation design. This approach allowed us to study cyberbullying from the perspective of children and adolescents who had experienced or observed it. The design took the form of a multiple case study (Yin 1984), which, apart from obtaining representative results, provided solid convincing results when combined with various analysis units (gender and age). We did not ask participants to disclose whether they themselves had ever been a victim or perpetrator of cyberbullying in order to protect their confidentiality in the discussion groups.

10.2.2 Participants

We conducted the current study in a city of central Spain, whose approximate population was 60,000. The participants were 108 children and adolescents aged 10–16 years from two primary schools and two secondary schools. We selected the schools from each level of education with the help of the local education bureau and in accordance with the criteria that govern the geographical location: two centers on the outskirts and two in the city center. We contacted principals by e-mail and phone. Once they gave consent to participate, students listened to a talk by the first author, and each student received a form for parental consent. We recruited those children whose parents agreed they could participate. Participants included 55 girls and 53 boys. All the participants were Caucasian and with a middle-high socioeconomic background.

10.2.3 Data Collection Procedure

We collected data from semi-structured focus groups through informal discussions held with a moderator to obtain perceptions on a defined area of interest (Berg 2004). There were 18 focus groups, and each comprised 6–8 participants. Since the focal point of the discussion was not youths' personal experiences, the groups were either mixed or of the same gender. Twelve groups included homogeneous single-sex groups and six mixed-gender groups. The saturation point of the information justified the number of groups. We created all the groups after the first four-month period of the academic year. The moderators were the two authors of this chapter.

10.2.4 Focus Group Questions

Based on previous studies (Compton et al. 2014; Mishna et al. 2009; Navarro et al. 2013), the researchers devised questions to guide the discussion in each focus group. As this study was interested in determining how participants understood cyberbullying and what role they believed parents play in intervention, the questions focused on these key areas. We did not ask the participants about their own cyberbullying experiences in order to protect their confidentiality. The questions used to guide the discussion were:

1. What is cyberbullying?
2. What are the differences between cyberbullying and traditional bullying?
3. Why do you think some people engage in cyberbullying?
4. Do you think that cyberbullying is a serious problem?
5. Does cyberbullying worry you?
6. What should cyberbullying victims do to stop it?
7. Would you help someone suffering from cyberbullying?
8. Would you look for help if it happened to you?
9. Do you think that cyberbullying victims should talk about it to someone?
10. Should victims tell their parents about it?
11. What can parents do to help victims?
12. Do your parents monitor what you do on the Internet? Do they teach you how to use social networks or other websites on the Internet?

Following the study by Compton et al. (2014), after participants had provided their insight into question 1, we handed out the cyberbullying definition by Tokunaga (2010) to them on a printed sheet. Providing this definition ensured that participants had a shared cyberbullying definition to guide their discussion for the other questions.

10.2.5 Analytical Process

Having finished the transcripts, we analyzed the content of the obtained information following a thematic approach. The codification process corresponded to what is called "field format" (Anguera 1994). We started by organizing work, which primarily consisted in the thematic blocks deriving from the main focus group questions, and we initiated an inductive process to create the categories and subcategories. We grouped the relevant conversational units together in accordance with those repeated aspects that we noted in the participants' conversational fragments. This process enabled us to modify the categorization of themes and subthemes according to the analysis done of the textual information. This afforded greater flexibility when it came to interpreting the information and the possibility of offering a description of the problems studied according to the opinions provided by the study participants. We used the ATLAS.ti program to assign the conversational fragments to each theme and subtheme according to its versatility to reorganize data throughout the analysis process.

10.2.6 Elements to Judge the Accuracy of the Research

We validated the scientific precision of this research by adopting the following criteria that also complemented the research (Guba and Lincoln 1989).

10.2.6.1 Credibility (Internal Validity)

We confirmed credibility by including various researchers in the study context, continuous assessments and exchange between the authors of this study, previous participation by researchers in qualitative research processes with similar samples, and the process of triangulation of results. We organized session groups to comment on and revise the results. The authors and other researchers who belonged to the psychology department participated in these sessions.

10.2.6.2 Transferability (External Validity)

We can define qualitative approaches by their flexibility and open character when it comes to tackling the unique character of the phenomenon under study. However, the description of the provided methodology, together with the review of the different studies done in different contexts, will allow readers to judge the design and the way we conducted this research.

10.2.6.3   Dependability and Confirmability (Replicability and External Reliability)

We were able to validate consistency, thanks to the clear, concise way of explaining the data analysis process and the process of obtaining the results. Together with this, we used a field diary to make the researchers' position clear about the phenomenon under study, unify criteria during the research process, obtain more focus groups to compare the information, and explore new aspects.

10.3   Results

We organized the results into sections and subsections after bearing in mind the thematic blocks, themes, and subthemes that we grouped the different conversational fragments into. Despite dividing the sample according to age and gender, which we did with the focus groups, to prepare this report, we opted to consider all the transcriptions together as a global discourse that drew together all the conversational fragments. However, within the comments, and more specifically in the section devoted to discussion, we indicated differences in discourses according to age and gender.

10.3.1   Definitions and Views of Cyberbullying

While forming groups with the 10–12-year-old participants, we found out that many were unaware of the term "cyberbullying." However, there was always at least one participant who said he/she knew what we meant and used names in Spanish to explain what cyberbullying was to the other group members. Some of these terms were *acoso en Internet* (Internet harassment), *acoso virtual* (Virtual harassment), or *maltrato en la red* (Internet abuse). Other participants said that it was a type of bullying, an Anglo-Saxon term that they knew, and they explained that cyberbullying was a form of bullying that took place on the Internet.

Among the definitions obtained in the group discussion, a 10-year-old boy stated that cyberbullying occurred when "a person teased someone else on the Internet and this person not only wanted to laugh at the other person, but wanted many people to laugh at them." A 14-year-old girl stated that cyberbullying takes place when "a person uses the Internet to insult someone else or to threaten them. They show them up. This person constantly teases others, blackmails them, or posts something on the Internet that can really hurt them." When we asked the participants to give examples of the conducts they would include in the cyberbullying category, many participants resorted to the cases they knew from the media which had far-reaching international repercussions as a result of those who had suffered it, having committed suicide. Similarly, many participants talked about a case that had taken place in their city a few days before holding the discussion groups. This case involved an adolescent who murdered a classmate and previously sent threatening messages over the Internet and by mobile.

For the 10–12-year-olds, the number of conducts included in the so-called cyberbullying was much larger than for the older participants. This age group indicated that cyberbullying do not only include conducts among peers, like insults, threats sent in messages on social networks, and posting humiliating pictures and videos but also computing offenses like hacking websites, robbing personal data (bank details), or conducts that involve adults like grooming. The impression we got from the responses of the younger participants was that they were not certain about what is cyberbullying. From 12 years of age, the cyberbullying concept came over more clearly, and the participants spoke more specifically about it but limited it to those behaviors which take place among peers. Examples of cyberbullying were uploading personal photos, or writing false claims about harassed victims, using webcam recordings without the victim realizing, posting compromising photos of victims or in the nude, and also blackmailing, and stealing passwords and replacing identities on social networks. The behaviors that this age group discussed about the most frequently included compromising pictures, and, in many cases, this group linked cyberbullying with breaking off an affective relationship between those involved. For example, a 12-year-old girl told us about a case she had heard in which "a girl was taking a shower in a gym at her high school, and someone took a photo of her. Then they posted the photo on Internet forums and in WhatsApp groups. This victim did not want to go to institute because people laughed at her." A 15-year-old female explained that she knew another female "who sent naked photos to her boyfriend. One day she discovered that her boyfriend was seeing other girls and she left him. Then he took revenge by posting the photos of her in the nude on Facebook and he laughed at her. She had to report the case at the local police station."

10.3.1.1 Characteristics of Cyberbullying and Differences with Traditional School Bullying

When describing what characterizes cyberbullying, people compare it with traditional bullying. However, it is important to consider that although the participants established some differences between cyberbullying and bullying (especially those characteristics linked to the context in which either one or the other took place), they mainly talked about both bullying types forming part of the same phenomenon. From the participants' view, bullying and cyberbullying are in the same continuum where people are sometimes victims of traditional bullying and victims of cyberbullying other times. When describing these two phenomena, they did not always bear in mind the characteristic criteria that research has indicated, for example, imbalance of power, repetition, or the desire to harm victims. Some participants even considered that these conducts are not intentional in all cases, but there are times when they form part of jokes for which imbalance of power is not at all clear. Likewise, some participants saw cyberbullying as the consequence of a previous conflict that had shifted from a real setting to a virtual one, where those involved suffer and harass differently. Table 10.1 shows the various themes we can classify as the participants' responses to the questions: What is cyberbullying? What are the differences between cyberbullying and traditional bullying?

The participants stressed the possibility of perpetrators remaining anonymous, which is much more difficult for traditional bullying. Yet many participants thought that victims are aware of who their perpetrators are, and if they are not sure who they are initially, they discover their identity if the cyberbullying continues with time. In any case, they pointed out that the anonymity perceived by perpetrators makes cyberbullying a potentially more dangerous conduct because the people who play this role believe it is very difficult to find them out. Therefore, they use a more much higher degree of aggressiveness because they think that this would have no consequences for them. In line with this, they thought that technology helps place a distance between perpetrators and victims because it is hard to know victims' emotional reactions. Although some participants believed that, emotionally, the separation between perpetrators and victims is wider, they did not consider it a relevant aspect because they stated that perpetrators know very well what victims could feel, but they do not care. Along these lines, a 14-year-old girl said that "it's true that perpetrators can't see how the people who read what they write about them on social networks, or who send them an email threatening them, can react, but they know very well that they'll not laugh about the situation, they'll feel bad. They simply don't care because they want them to suffer."

The older participants mentioned the repetition criterion more frequently. The younger participants included more sporadic conducts in cyberbullying, such as having received some insult or negative remark in a posting on social networks. It is necessary to point out that for these participants, repetition takes place when the same fact occurs many times, for example, some constantly received messages with insults or threats. They did not think that the repetition criterion arises when, for instance, someone posts a compromising photo on the Internet and resend it to many other people. They believed that repetition involves posting several photos. Despite this notion, they considered that cyberbullying entails much wider public exposure since the information exposed on the Internet reaches a much larger audience. This aspect was most important for the 12–16-year-old group of participants, and they pointed that if other people are not aware of this information, they would not consider it cyberbullying. In line with this, they believed that if someone insults somebody using text messages or WhatsApp, and only the people directly involved are aware of these facts, they would not consider it cyberbullying, rather it would form part of traditional bullying, not even when the means used is a mobile or the Internet.

Finally, they were of the opinion that cyberbullying not only causes psychological harm to victims but also hurts those with access to this information, like family members and friends. During much of their discourse, they did not link the harm

Table 10.1 Themes formed from participants' answers to the question "What is cyberbullying? What are the differences with bullying?"

Theme	Theme description	Illustrative quotation
Anonymity	Exposing victims to cyberbullying performed by known and unknown people	"Bullying takes place between people who know each other, while you might, or might not, know them on the Internet. It's dangerous if the people you don't know can insult or harass you." —13-year-old boy
	Perpetrators' feeling of anonymity can make the victimization suffered more dangerous since they think that no one can discover them, so they are more daring than when they physically face someone	"Not being known makes it easier for some people to be more daring than when faced with their victim. People feel more freedom to do what they want because they think they can hide their identity." —14-year-old girl
Repetition	In order to consider an aggressive behavior to bullying and cyberbullying, it must take place over a considerable period of time	"I don't think that cyberbullying involves someone insulting you once or twice, but it continues for a long time. It must be repetitive and last a long time. If you receive emails for many days and for a long time, then it's cyberbullying." —15-year-old girl
Public exposure	Unlike bullying, cyberbullying can involve greater public exposure as many people access the information published on the Internet	"Cyberbullying is more dangerous because it involves intimate aspects. It can reach many people, and they can make you feel a bigger fool." —13-year-old girl
Psychological harm	In school bullying, harm can be physical and psychological, while cyberbullying only involves psychological harm	"Cyberbullying can really hurt you inside; it can make you feel depressed, you don't want to leave home, etc." —12-year-old-girl
Social repercussion	The repercussions of cyberbullying go beyond the harm it causes victims because what people post on the Internet can also affect family members and friends	"Cyberbullying harm can affect your family and friends. For example, your friends can think that what they publish about you is true, and don't want to be with you anymore." —13-year-old-boy
Separation from victims	Cyberbullying places a greater distance between perpetrators and victims because technology makes knowing victims' emotional reactions difficult	"If I harm someone by cyberbullying, I can't see their expression. I mean her father could be sat next to her reading what I'm saying about her, but you keep doing it. You keep keying the words in. You don't care about her feelings." —15-year-old-girl
Continuity between bullying and cyberbullying	Although both types of bullying can take place in an isolated fashion, they often represent a continuous phenomenon in which harassment occurs both online and offline	"Sometimes bullying turns to cyberbullying, or the other way round. I think that it's much more dangerous when cyberbullying later becomes physical aggression." —14-year-old-boy

caused with the fact that family relations and friends empathize with victims' suffering but with further harm because it is possible that those who saw the information posted on the Internet actually believe it, so they could negatively react to the victim. They also explained that when cyberbullying shifted to the real world and took the form of traditional bullying, it was much easier that the latter took the form of more severe physical aggression with worse consequences for victims. About this, one 15-year-old boy said that "cyberbullies begin by posting small insults on the Internet, which then become more and more intense, and then they get angrier. If they meet the victim in person, they cannot control themselves and cause more harm because they got angrier on the Internet."

10.3.1.2   Reasons for Cyberbullying

When listening to the discourse on what would motivate cyberbullies' conduct, we classified the reasons given into themes, which Table 10.2 provides. Specifically, youths considered that cyberbullies take it to be a form of fun and that it forms part of jokes in some cases. If it is a joke, the participants did not think it is very important, but considered it a trivial aspect, and not one that could harm the person who is the target of the joke. The participants also believed that cyberbullying could be a means to blackmail to obtain something from the victim or to somehow change their behavior. They understood cyberbullying to be a manifestation of a former conflict between victims and perpetrators, and cyberbullying would be the way to continue it on the Internet. Therefore, they did not examine cyberbullying to be a conduct that addresses people who cannot defend themselves, rather a strategy that both parties can adopt.

The other reasons referred to the characteristics attributed to perpetrators, for example, they have a bad personality and enjoy making their victims suffer. They also linked aspects with social status in peer groups and the desire to be in a higher position than victims are and to feel superior to them. In line with this, they also described jealousy as an emotion that leads perpetrators to behave as they did, although their behavior could also stem from a former episode of aggressive behavior or not feeling motivated by school, which could encourage them to engage in such conducts at school and virtually.

10.3.1.3   Concern About Cyberbullying

When we asked the participants to what extent they thought that cyberbullying is a serious problem, some pointed out that it is something to which everyone can be exposed to and should, therefore, be a matter of concern. A 12-year-old boy said, "it is something that was becoming more and more usual. People mention an increasing number of cases or you can see someone talking about it on TV, and you think it could be you someday." Other participants said that insults on the Internet are so normal that they do not consider them all that important and that people

Table 10.2 Themes formed from participants' answers to the question "What motivates cyberbullying?"

Theme	Theme description	Illustrative quotation
Fun	They see cyberbullying as a form of fun for perpetrators to laugh at others and to make them look fools	"The only thing cyberbullies want is to make fun of others." —13-year-old-boy
	Sometimes youths perceive cyberbullying as a joke where the perpetrator wants to entertain others and it should not be taken seriously	"It's not always a case of hurting someone. It might be part of a joke, something entertaining, and it's not dangerous." —14-year-old-boy
Revenge	The fact that a former conflict or confrontation existed between those involved can motivate cyberbullying. So, people view cyberbullying as a form of revenge for something the victim did to the bully in the past	"It can happen because of a fight or some bad vibe between these people. This happens a lot; you don't like someone because of what they did to you, and you criticize them, and things like that. Most people do this." —15-year-old-girl
Blackmail (obtaining something)	Cyberbullying can be a means for blackmailing, to obtain something in exchange for not telling secrets or private information. Cyberbullies want something that the victim has or the victim must do something that benefits them	"They threaten other people by saying things about them on the Internet so they do their homework for them." —12-year-old-boy "I know a boy who threatened his girlfriend to post some of her photos if she left him." —14-year-old-girl
Bad personality	People describe cyberbullies as evil people whose only motivation is to enjoy inflicting harm on others	"As they are bad people, you don't need a reason. They enjoy hurting the feelings of others, and don't care how they feel. I think they enjoy harming others." —15-year-old-girl
Feeling superior	Perpetrators wish to show feelings of superiority by overpowering classmates. Therefore, cyberbullying can be a means to manage social status in peer groups and to occupy leadership positions	"Many people try to become popular with these things, like sending a message so people clearly understand that they are superior to all the others." —13-year-old-girl
Feeling jealous	Youths perceive cyberbullying as a reaction to perpetrators feeling jealous about the way their victims behave and act	"I know a girl who they teased because she was very pretty and was a good student. They said things about her because they were jealous of her. They tried hurting those who they want to be like." —12-year-old-girl
School maladjustment	Youths describe bullies to be people who have school maladjustment problems, like not feeling motivated to study	"They are people who feel bored when they come to the Institute. They just want to spend some time there, and don't study or do anything." —14-year-old-boy
Psychosocial maladjustment	Youths describe bullies as people with psychosocial maladjustment problems who always get into trouble or have internal conflicts that lead them to harass other classmates	"They do all this because they feel frustrated. For some reason, they're not happy and don't want others to feel happy." —13-year-old-girl

were unaware of real cyberbullying cases because they tended to trivialize them. Likewise, others thought that it was not a problem to worry about because the cases that appeared on the media were isolated and extreme. One 13-year-old girl told us, "people make a big issue of it than it really is. People see cyberbullying everywhere, but it's not as bad as all that. Quite often it is part of jokes that don't last long." Other participants pointed out that considering such conducts to be cyberbullying or not depended on how the people receiving this aggression interpreted it. One 13-year-old girl said, "someone can be playing a joke, but the person on the other end of the joke can take it to be cyberbullying and what they do hurts them."

The participants stated that concern for these problems is more social than personal. The information broadcast on the media and the talks they received on the subject at their schools made them think that adults are more concerned. An 11-year-old boy said, "the police came and gave us some talks about us being careful what we do on the Internet. I think it's a matter of concern."

The participants seemed more concerned when they are the victims or people close to them are; otherwise, they considered it a distant problem. Yet when they personally knew a case, it makes them think on what they do on the Internet. A 14-year-old boy explained, "with the cases you know, you think more about what you do on the Internet. You start thinking about what others can do with the information you post on the Internet and you try to be more careful." It was interesting to verify that they worried more about traditional bullying than cyberbullying because the former can be immediately more dangerous because it can end up in physical aggression. An 11-year-old boy said, "they can hurt you over the Internet, but I'm more worried about coming across someone and them hitting me." The older the participants, the more importance they attached to cyberbullying because it could affect their social reputation more. They were particularly concerned about information uploaded on the Internet reaching a larger audience. Despite all this, they were also worried about cyberbullying shifting from a virtual setting to a real one and physical aggression taking place. They took cyberbullying to be a very serious worrying fact when someone had suffered it and committed suicide, or if someone became depressed, or had to change school or move to a different city/town.

10.3.2 Intervention Strategies

10.3.2.1 Coping Strategies

When we asked them what cyberbullying victims should do about stopping it, most participants assumed that it would be complicated to leave this situation behind them and were quite unaware how to solve it. They believed that victims should tell someone and seek help but also pointed out that a priori, they would try to solve it themselves before seeking help. Besides, most students believed that confronting cyberbullying implied the victim losing the right to access the network because they considered the best solution was to be less active on the Internet to avoid insults or threats. They also considered that suitable Internet account management is vital to raise the level of privacy in social networks, as is restricting information that others could view as much as possible by, for example, making Instagram accounts private. Another important form of action was, on the one hand, not responding to aggressions to make perpetrators' conduct less relevant and, on the other hand, not giving the perpetrator reasons to continue. However, they believed that the solution might not prove effective. In this case, they said that the victim should save everything the cyberbully had sent them or had posted on the Internet about them and must report it. A 15-year-old boy said, "the most important thing to do is to eliminate the perpetrator from all the social networks you participate in, you must block this person. If the problem is serious and continuous, you should report it because you will always be able to know who is behind it all."

Reporting to the police was an aspect that many participants said that they would do, and yet, they were unaware how this type of bullying could be reported and punished. They thought that remaining anonymous on the Internet provided perpetrators with protection. At this stage, they thought it important to seek help but pointed out that they would more likely tell a friend before telling an adult. A 13-year-old girl told us, "a friend can help you. If you tell your parents about it, they can't help because they don't feel the same way you do. But your friends feel the way you do and they see this situation as something normal." Therefore, as in school bullying, social support was extremely important because it buffered the effect of aggression. Friends could offer advice about directly confronting harassment and about improving computer skills by, for example, better managing social networks.

When we asked them if they would help someone suffering cyberbullying, most of the participants said they would help their friends and the people they know. An 11-year-old boy said, "I don't like them hurting other people, but I'm not that worried about people I barely know. Yet if victims are my friends, then of course I'd try to do something as they hurt me too because the victims are my friends." Yet when we asked them what they would do to help friends if they needed them, many of them acknowledged that they did not know how they would act. They said they would offer them advice about making accounts private, managing personal data, and restricting people who could view profiles on social networks (Table 10.3).

10.3.2.2   Telling Adults

As we previously mentioned, many of the participants explained that they would first attempt to solve problems with peers themselves, and if that failed, they would seek help. However, they also stated that they would do this because the problem they faced had become more serious. Yet they also stated that if they told someone about this situation, an adult would not be their first option. When we asked them why they thought that cyberbullying victims did not tell teachers, a 14-year-old girl explained that "telling a teacher something personal is embarrassing," and a 12-year-old boy told us, "if you tell a teacher, your parents are more likely to find out about it. Besides, if you tell a teacher, the whole school will find out, and the

Table 10.3 Themes formed from the participants' answers to the question "What should the victim do to stop cyberbullying?"

Theme	Theme description	Illustrative quotation
Managing personal data	Everyone must correctly manage their personal data on the Internet to avoid placing any personal or compromising data that someone could use to harass them with	*"First you must be careful with the personal data you place on the Internet. It is important to think what you post on the Internet or what photos you upload"*—15-year-old girl
Avoidance: less Internet activity	Avoiding technology or disconnecting for a lengthy period of time	*"You have to somehow do what you do when you are out of the Internet. If someone picked on you in a given place, you avoid going to that place. It's the same on the Internet; you have to avoid being present as much as possible so it's more difficult for them to pick on you than if you're updating information everyday."*—14-year-old boy
Internet account management	Emphasizing the need to learn how to manage different Internet profiles, to restrict access to strangers, and to make content private	*"They can still call you queer or whatever; but when you limit access to your social networks, it makes it more difficult for them to send you messages directly. For example, I don't understand why some of my friends have public Instagram accounts when having private ones makes it more difficult for these people to reach you."*—15-year-old boy
Not responding to any form of aggression/ Ignoring aggression	Youths do not consider confronting a bully online or offline to be a good solution since it can intensify cyberbullying. They perceive ignoring messages or threats from bullies to be a better solution	*"Just don't go on the attack. If you read a message that says "If I see you, you queer; I'll kill you", you mustn't answer. It might be unpleasant and worrying, but you have to learn to just ignore it, because if you answer, you're giving them more chances to carry on getting at you."*—13-year-old boy
Importance of social support	Youths perceive that support and help from those close to them is important to withstand cyberbullying consequences and to manage personal data to moderate cyberbullying or to prevent it	*"Being supported by the people you are with and appreciate you is very important, and they can help you to be more practical. Before my accounts weren't private and everyone could see my photos and comments. Now only my friends can see them. At least now they can't write anything on my wall like they did before."*—15-year-old boy

problem can get worse if the bully finds out." Other students stated that there are trained people to help you at the institute; people trained to deal with this matter confidentially. They said that if anyone is a victim, they should visit the counselor or a teacher they could trust and tell them what was happening to them to stop it.

When we asked them if they thought that victims should tell their parents, most said they should. However, many believed that victims did not usually tell their parents because they did not often know how they would react and because they thought their parents do not possess a competent level of technology and could not help them. A 13-year-old boy added, "victims can think that their parents won't take them seriously, or might not know what to do, or even punish them by taking away their mobile." A 15-year-old girl also said that "victims might feel embarrassed by their parents knowing what they face, and also because they don't know how to stop it." Other students explained that a bully could threaten some victims, so they would not tell anyone, while others pointed out that they would not wish to worry their parents. A 13-year-old boy explained that "my parents have enough problems anyway, and I wouldn't want to worry them with these things."

10.3.2.3   Parental Mediation and Family Communication

The participants perceived that creating a climate of trust and, therefore, good communication between parents and children is fundamental when communicating this type of problems. A 13-year-old girl told us that "it all depends on trust. The same happens to parents and to your friends: if there's not enough trust, you don't tell them anything." They generally expressed that the younger they are, the more they talk with their parents, and that they feel less open to talk with them the older they are. A 14-year-old boy explained, "the younger you are, the more you tell your parents, but as you grow older, some personal things form part of your privacy and you don't share them." When talking about cyberbullying, the older participants were more reluctant to talk about it because they did not think that their parents could do anything about certain problems. A 15-year-old girl said, "I wouldn't tell my parents because then they would say: why didn't you tell us about it all when it first began? Imagine if some compromising photos or videos have been sent. What would your parents do with them if other people already had them?" The participants were generally reluctant to talk with their parents about aspects that they thought were part of their intimacy, especially aspects relating with their interactions on the Internet. However, they acknowledged that there are some important things they would tell their parents before they find out elsewhere or before the problem become worse. A 14-year-old girl said, "although we don't talk to our parents about all this, we should. I always thought it best they find out from me and not from other people, but it's true that I tell them very few things." At this point, some participants said that it is much easier to tell siblings as they perceive them as more technologically competent than their parents and that siblings can be more direct speakers when they face problems on the Internet. A 12-year-old boy explained, "my brother is older than me, so if he has experienced some form of harassment, or something like that, he knows what to do. So he can tell me and help me."

Regarding family communication, we asked the participants if their parents monitored their Internet activity in some way and if they gave them advice about the pages they can visit or how to manage personal data on the Internet. Here the intention was to check what value the participants conferred to parental mediation on Internet use. As the themes that arose from these questions demonstrated (see Table 10.4), parental mediation was poor and with limitations in most cases to monitor the times spent using the Internet and certain contents or employing certain devices. Such monitoring was greater, the younger participants were, and very few participants mentioned doing joint Internet activities with their parents or receiving advice about managing personal data. They perceived that such aspects depended on their parents' knowledge of technology which, as the participants explained, is quite poor or they do not perceive it as sound knowledge. The participants generally judged parental mediation as poorly effective because, as they themselves indicated, they can deceive their parents or using mobile phones could make parental monitoring of such activities difficult.

When we asked what parents could do specifically to help them if they suffered cyberbullying, the participants answered that it would depend on their knowledge of technology. Thus, younger participants better trusted their parents' skills to solve some problem on the Internet. Some participants feared that their parents' reaction would be to limit their Internet use by confiscating their mobile. They were also afraid that parental intervention would make the problem worse when parents inform educational agents, like teachers, or attempted to talk with perpetrators. However, a considerable number thought that their parents could help deal with the problem by talking with their perpetrator's parents, helping them manage their Internet accounts (for example, taking measures with Internet providers), going to the police if necessary, or simply reassuring them. Many participants spoke about the need for parents offering them advice about how to manage their information on the Internet or what to do if someone teased them, but they did not always talk about such matters with their parents. One 13-year-old boy said, "I know I'm not old enough to use Facebook or Twitter, but I have accounts on them, and my parents know this. I'd like to sometimes ask them things about configurations and such, but I can't because my parents don't use these networks, and they don't know how they work."

10.4 Discussion and Implications for Practice

The discourse obtained during the discussion groups allowed us to conclude that Spanish youths' vocabulary includes the Anglo-Saxon term bullying. However, not all the participants were clear about its meaning, which we found when they had to tell us what cyberbullying was and what conducts they would relate with it. For both age groups that participated in the discussion groups (primary and secondary education students), it clearly came over as a form of harassment (*acoso* in Span-

Table 10.4 Themes formed from participants' answers to the questions "Do your parents monitor what you do on the Internet? Do they teach you how to use social networks and other Internet websites?"

Theme	Theme description	Illustrative quotation
No parental monitoring	Many parents do not monitor what their children do on the Internet. We can attribute lack of parental monitoring to reciprocal trust, and sometimes to carelessness	*"Parents trust us. I don't check their mobiles and they don't check mine."* —14-year-old girl
Limited technological competences	It is not infrequent to find that parents possess less technological knowledge than their children, who do not perceive them as competent enough to help them with their problems	*"My mother does not use a computer, and let alone Facebook. She doesn't know how it works nor what people place on it"* —13-year-old boy
Spying parents	Some parents watch their children's activities using their own accounts in social networks and check the list of the sites they browse or attempt to access their cildren's accounts	*"I know my mother opened a Twitter account with no photo to see what I placed there, but no matter how much I look for her, I can't find out who it is."* —14-year-old boy
Controlling times in relation to the time spent studying	Sometimes parental mediation is limited to control the time we use technological devices or the time spent on the Internet	*"In my case, I have to spend 4 hours studying one day, 3 hours another day … They take away my mobile during these hours and they give it me back when I finish studying and I can have it whenever I want."* —14-years-old girl
Making contents private	Some participants consider that their activity on the Internet is private and parents must not control it because it is their personal life	*"If they ask me, I don't mind telling them which social networks I use or why I use the Internet, but some things are private and you don't want your parents to ever see them, and there are other things I'm sure they wouldn't want to know."* —15-year-old girl
Resisting parental control	Many participants admit that their parents keep an eye on them, or can even feel worried, so they keep asking questions about their Internet activities. However, they admit that they can deceive them because they fear they will restrict their Internet use	*"They can keep an eye on you, ask you things, but you can deceive them. I've no idea how they might react if they find some things out."* —12-year-old boy

ish), which coincided with previous research on the terms employed in Spain to talk about cyberbullying (Nocentini et al. 2010). However, the cyberbullying concept for the 10- and 12-year-old participants was much broader and included conducts such as grooming, which would not form part of cyberbullying as research defined it. The term became more accurate among the older participants that described cyberbullying as aggressive interactions between peers but did not always appear to follow research definition criteria, such as intention, repetition, harm, and imbalance of power. For example, most participants included sporadic conducts in cyberbullying, which contradicts the repetition criterion indicated by research (Smith 2012). Similarly, they did not always mention that imbalance of power formed part of cyberbullying. They often said that cyberbullying could form part of a conflict between peers where both parties used the Internet to continue mutual confrontation by sending messages or threats.

As argued by Sabella et al. (2013), there is a wide variability in the way we define cyberbullying, which includes any form of conflict between peers, and even when the aforementioned defining criteria are unmet. For this reason, we believe that educational action is still necessary to help understand what cyberbullying is and to distinguish between the conducts included in this form of harassment and those that are not. The fact that the information offered by the media affects youths' opinions does not always help them to form a suitable idea of what conducts form part of cyberbullying. In any case, teachers and parents should employ the cases they know from TV and the facts they have witnessed to explain what cyberbullying is and is not.

Although the participants stated that someone can suffer cyberbullying without ever suffering school bullying before, and vice versa, most participants seemed to understand that both forms of aggression were interrelated phenomena rather than different conducts. In line with previous results reported in other countries (Cassidy et al. 2009), some works have often described cyberbullying as a reaction to an incident that took place offline at school and which later took an online form. The participants thought that the combination of both forms of harassment was potentially more dangerous because we can add physical damage to the psychological harm caused by cyberbullying. Cyberbullying, however, for the participants involved certain differences due to the means it occurred in, such as a greater possibility for the perpetrator remaining anonymous; more difficult to empathize with the victim as there is no physical contact between the parties involved; and a wider public repercussion since more people can view the insults, threats, or images about the victim on the Internet.

Academics and researchers have described these differences with school bullying to be specific characteristics of cyberbullying (Wingate et al. 2013). However, many participants pointed out that many victims knew who their bully was, given the continuity between both forms of bullying. They also mentioned that cyberbullying took place between classmates and even friends as a previous research work demonstrated (Fenaughty and Harré 2013; Jackson et al. 2013). The older participants even said that cyberbullying was a reaction to effective relationships ending. Although there is more work available on this matter with university students, some studies have indicated that they can often identify their "ex" as the bully and also as the cyberbullying victim (Crosslin and Crosslin 2014). These results must attract the attention of teachers, parents, and policy-makers about the need to intervene and that these interventions must simultaneously deal with both forms of bullying, given the relation between both forms. Then, there is also the matter of working on aspects linked to affective relationships since cyberbullying can act as a means by which to harass and control a partner (Burke et al. 2011). Preventing such conducts could mean having to do parallel preventive work into another type of mistreatment relations in adult relationships (Diaz-Aguado and Martinez 2014).

As for what motivates cyberbullying, it is interesting to note that youths understood it as a form of fun, and even a joke, where the idea was not to harm the person to whom these actions are targeted. If this were so, such conducts would not fulfill with the intention criterion that characterizes actions like cyberbullying, but in fact, these remarks could form part of the arguments that perpetrators could offer to justify their conduct. Yet previous studies have found this very result (Compton et al. 2014) and have related it with the fact that perpetrators do not witness victims' reactions and are not aware of the harm they cause. Many of our participants believed that perpetrators were well aware of the harm they caused but did not care. They even described them as evil people who enjoyed harming others. Yet we can link the fact that they viewed cyberbullying as part of a joke with lack of social keys in online contexts, which makes classifying them as a true threat, or not, more difficult (Bryce and Fraser 2013). In any case, these results suggest the need to implement measures that improve empathy to others and not only for perpetrators but also for all other peers who are aware about what goes on but do nothing because they consider it is not a serious matter (Ackers 2012).

In line with this, and despite some clashing views, many participants did not take cyberbullying seriously and even believed that existing public alarm does not match the real situation. Our participants often stated that cyberbullying involved isolated events or events that form part of reciprocal aggression among those involved. They generally viewed it as a problem that does not cause much concern, especially when it does not affect them. This view relates with their willingness to help someone suffering cyberbullying. They would help their friends but not their classmates or people they did not meet much. This outcome indicates just how important it is to work to change these attitudes to intervene in bullying episodes. While youths experience these problems as a distant aspect that does not directly affect them, they are not likely to engage in any form of intervention taken from institutes or other organizations that plan them (Price et al. 2014; Rigby and Bortolozzo 2013).

Other reasons that participants gave about why people are involved in cyberbullying coincided with former research, such as instilling fear, inflicting harm, feeling superior, or obtaining something from victims (Compton et al. 2014; Wilton and Campbell 2011). People have also viewed cyberbullying as a way to get revenge (Law et al. 2012). This may relate to those studies that have indicated how victims of school bullying can use cyberbullying to harm their perpetrators (Dooley et al. 2009). Our participants indicated that this aggression stemmed from a previous conflict between those involved. In such interactions, the perpetrator and victim roles are not clear, and both parties participate with reciprocal harassment. This fact once again indicates that what youths perceived about cyberbullying did not always respond to the criteria set by researchers and indicates the need to consider how they use the term as they do not always use the imbalance of power criterion in their definitions.

Regarding coping strategies, many participants admitted that they did not know what to do, nor what advice they could give to someone who was a victim of cyberbullying. As in former research studies, our participants said that it is important to manage the personal data they uploaded to the Internet; to make sure that social networks are private; to block perpetrators; and to quickly eliminate all the remarks, insults, or threats in order to minimize the public repercussion that cyberbullying could have (Giménez-Gualdo 2014). When harassment continued for long periods, they recommended reporting it to the police, although they were not very clear about how to report harassment as many believed that perpetrators' assumed anonymity protected them from legal actions. They were not always aware that it was necessary to save any evidence of harassment in order to report it. Hence, parents and teachers should know what legal consequences cyberbullying can have and should teach youths that the Internet does not protect perpetrators.

A fundamental element in the prevention of and intervention in cyberbullying is social support. However, our participants admitted not seeking help when they had a problem. They found it much easier to seek help from a friend than from an adult. Therefore, peer helper programs might prove most useful. Through these programs, cyberbullying victims, or any other young person, can find help from classmates who have received training about responsible technology use, and the risks faced, which include cyberbullying and strategies to cope with it (Sabella et al. 2013). Research also needs to analyze in more detail the role that siblings can play in coping with cyberbullying because the participants perceived them as more technologically competent than adults and think that youths can better cope with cyberbullying given their age and similar use of technology.

Adults were not their first option when seeking help. Indeed, they seemed reluctant to tell adults about their problems, especially adolescents, because they find it hard to admit that they are unable to solve the problem themselves. So, they could find telling them what happened quite embarrassing or they do not view adults having enough technological competence to suitably intervene in cyberbullying. Indeed the value they conferred to parental mediation of cyberbullying was low. Yet we found differences between younger and older participants. Both age groups considered that a climate of trust and good communication with parents are fundamental for them to talk to parents about what they experienced on the Internet, but such trust and communication are apparently lacking more among adolescents than the 10–12-year-old participants are. Recovering communication is fundamental if we wish parents to play a relevant role in solving cyberbullying (in this same volume, see Buelga et al. 2015). However, it is also important to train parents to be technologically competent, so youths can positively view them when they have to face problems like cyberbullying. Parents need to know what their children do online and how they can help them with the risks they face. Previous works have reported that parental mediation in cyberbullying is effective when establishing joint rules between parents and offspring (Navarro et al. 2013). We must make parents aware that they are obliged to teach about responsible technology use, so they themselves must learn to manage personal data and offer their children advice about how to make accounts on social networks private to protect against cyberbullying. Similarly, parents must show their children that they are willing to help them with any challenge they may face, and together, parents and children will seek the best solution to the problem without this entailing restricted technology use. Parents must understand that technology has become an essential element for young people to start and sustain relationships (Korchmaros et al. 2015), so it is no good making them not use it or ignoring what others say about them on the Internet. Parents need to be active in cyberbullying intervention and recover the trust that youths seem to have lost in the parental role to help solve online and offline problems.

10.5   Conclusions

The present work has attempted to present how Spanish youths perceive cyberbullying, when they do not have a similar term in their own language to define such aggressive online conducts. First, the results indicate that they have started to include the Anglo-Saxon term cyberbullying in their vocabulary, but their understanding of this phenomenon presents some differences with the definition used by researchers. Therefore, we need more research efforts to understand how youths approach a phenomenon like cyberbullying and to know to what extent research covers all the meanings that youths confer to this problem. Likewise, research has evidenced that not all youths know what cyberbullying is. Therefore, educational actions are still necessary to help them identify the conducts that make up cyberbullying and to improve their coping strategies. The youths' discourse in the present study reveals that it is necessary to reinforce parents' role in intervening in cyberbullying, improving their technological competences and their image as a source of social support for the risks that youths face on the Internet. This study evidences the necessity to train youths and adults in responsible technology use and in acquiring skills to manage personal data in order to prevent cyberbullying.

References

Ackers, M. J. (2012). Cyberbullying: Through the eyes of children and young people. *Educational Psychology in Practice, 28*(2), 141–157. doi:10.1080/02667363.2012.665356.

Agatston, P. W., Kowalski, R., & Limber, S. (2007). Students' perspectives on cyber bullying. *Journal of Adolescent Health, 41*(6), S59–S60. doi:10.1016/j.jadohealth.2007.09.003.

Anguera, M. T. (1994). *Metodología observacional en la investigación psicológica*. Barcelona: PPU.

Berg, B. L. (2004). *Qualitative research methods for the social sciences* (5th ed.). USA: Peason Education.

Bryce, J., & Fraser, J. (2013). "It's Common Sense That It's Wrong": Young people's perceptions and experiences of cyberbullying. *Cyberpsychology, Behavior, and Social Networking, 16*(11), 783–787. doi:10.1089/cyber.2012.0275.

Buelga, S., Martínez-Ferrer, B., & Musitu, G. (2015). Family relationships and cyberbullying. In R. Navarro, S. Yubero, & E. Larranaga (Eds.), *Cyberbullying across the globe: Gender, family, and mental health* (p. in press). New York: Springer.

Burke, S. C., Wallen, M., Vail-Smith, K., & Knox, D. (2011). Using technology to control intimate partners: An exploratory study of college undergraduates. *Computers in Human Behavior, 27*(3), 1162–1167. doi:10.1016/j.chb.2010.12.010.

Campbell, M. A. (2005). Cyber bullying: An old problem in a new guise? *Australian Journal of Guidance and Counselling, 15*(01), 68–76. doi:10.1375/ajgc.15.1.68.

Cassidy, W., Jackson, M., & Brown, K. N. (2009). Sticks and stones can break my bones, but how can pixels hurt me? Students' experiences with cyber-bullying. *School Psychology International, 30*(4), 383–402. doi:10.1177/0143034309106948.

Compton, L., Campbell, M. A., & Mergler, A. (2014). Teacher, parent and student perceptions of the motives of cyberbullies. *Social Psychology of Education, 17*(3), 383–400. doi:10.1007/s11218-014-9254-x.

Cross, D., Lester, L., & Barnes, A. (2015). A longitudinal study of the social and emotional predictors and consequences of cyber and traditional bullying victimization. *International Journal of Public Health, 60,* 207–217. doi:10.1007/s00038-015-0655-1.

Crosslin, K., & Golman, M. (2014). "Maybe you don't want to face it"—college students' perspectives on cyberbullying. *Computers in Human Behavior, 41,* 14–20. doi:10.1016/j.chb.2014.09.007.

Dehue, F., Bolman, C., & Völlink, T. (2008). Cyberbullying: Youngsters' experiences and parental percepcion. *Cyberpsychology & Behavior, 11,* 217–223. doi:10.1089/cpb.2007.0008.

Diaz-Aguado, M. J., & Martinez, R. (2014). Types of adolescent male dating violence against women, self-esteem, and justification of dominance and aggression. *Journal of Interpersonal Violence, 30*(15), 2636–2658. doi:10.1177/0886260514553631.

Dooley, J. J., Pyżalski, J., & Cross, D. (2009). Cyberbullying versus face-to-face bullying. *Zeitschrift für Psychologie/Journal of Psychology, 217*(4), 182–188. doi:10.1027/0044-3409.217.4.182.

Elgar, F. J., Napoletano, A., Saul, G., Dirks, M. A., Craig, W., Poteat, V. P., Holt, M., & Koenig, B. W. (2014). Cyberbullying victimization and mental health in adolescents and the moderating role of family dinners. *JAMA Pediatrics, 168*(11), 1015–1022. doi:10.1001/jamapediatrics.2014.1223.

Fenaughty, J., & Harré, N. (2013). Factors associated with distressing electronic harassment and cyberbullying. *Computers in Human Behavior, 29*(3), 803–811. doi:10.1016/j.chb.2012.11.008.

Frisén, A., Berne, S., & Marin, L. (2014). Swedish pupils' suggested coping strategies if cyberbullied: Differences related to age and gender. *Scandinavian Journal of Psychology, 55*(6), 578–584. doi:10.1111/sjop.12143.

Giménez-Gualdo, A. M. (2014). Estrategias de afrontamiento ante el cyberbullying. Un acercamiento cualitativo desde la perspectiva de los escolares. *Fronteiras: Journal of Social, Technological and Environmental Science, 3*(3), 15–32.

Giumetti, G. W., & Kowalski, R. M. (2015). Cyberbullying matters: Examining the incremental impact of cyberbullying on outcomes over and above traditional bullying in North America. In R. Navarro, S. Yubero, & E. Larranaga (Eds.), *Cyberbullying across the globe: Gender, family, and mental health* (p. in press). New York: Springer.

Guba, E. G., & Lincoln, Y. S. (1989). *Fourth generation evaluation.* Thousand Oaks: Sage.

Hay, C., Meldrum, R., & Mann, K. (2010). Traditional bullying, cyber bullying, and deviance: A general strain theory approach. *Journal of Contemporary Criminal Justice, 26*(2), 130–147. doi:10.1177/1043986209359557.

Hinduja, S., & Patchin, J. W. (2008). Cyberbullying: An exploratory analysis of factors related to offending and victimization. *Deviant Behavior, 29*(2), 129–156. doi:10.1080/01639620701457816.

Jackson, M., Cassidy, W., & Brown, K. N. (2013). "You were born ugly and you'll die ugly too": Cyber-bullying as relational aggression. *Education Journal: Special Issue on Technology and Social Media, 15*(2), 68–82. http://ineducation.ca/ineducation/article/view/57/538

Juvonen, J., & Gross, E. F. (2008). Extending the school grounds?-Bullying experiences in cyberspace. *Journal of School Health, 78*(9), 496–505. doi:10.1111/j.1746-1561.2008.00335.x.

Kofoed, J., & Ringrose, J. (2012). Travelling and sticky affects: Exploring teens and sexualized cyberbullying through a Butlerian-Deleuzian-Guattarian lens. *Discourse: Studies in the Cultural Politics of Education, 33*(1), 5–20. doi:10.1080/01596306.2012.632157.

Korchmaros, J. D., Ybarra, M. L., & Mitchell, K. J. (2015). Adolescent online romantic relationship initiation: Differences by sexual and gender identification. *Journal of Adolescence, 40,* 54–64. doi:10.1016/j.adolescence.2015.01.004.

Kowalski, R. M., & Limber, S. P. (2013). Psychological, physical, and academic correlates of cyberbullying and traditional bullying. *Journal of Adolescent Health, 53*(1), S13–S20. doi:10.1016/j.jadohealth.2012.09.018.

Kubiszewski, V., Fontaine, R., Potard, C., & Auzoult, L. (2015). Does cyberbullying overlap with school bullying when taking modality of involvement into account? *Computers in Human Behavior, 43,* 49–57. doi:10.1016/j.chb.2014.10.049.

Låftman, S. B., Modin, B., & Östberg, V. (2013). Cyberbullying and subjective health: A large-scale study of students in Stockholm, Sweden. *Children and Youth Services Review, 35*(1), 112–119.

Law, D. M., Shapka, J. D., Domene, J. F., & Gagné, M. H. (2012). Are cyberbullies really bullies? An investigation of reactive and proactive online aggression. *Computers in Human Behavior, 28*(2), 664–672. doi:10.1016/j.chb.2011.11.013.

Mishna, F., Saini, M., & Solomon, S. (2009). Ongoing and online: Children and youth's perceptions of cyber bullying. *Children and Youth Services Review, 31*(12), 1222–1228. doi:10.1016/j.childyouth.2009.05.004.

Naruskov, K., Luik, P., Nocentini, A., & Menesini, E. (2012). Estonian students' perception and definition of cyberbullying. *Trames, 16*(66/61), 323–343. doi:10.3176/tr.2012.4.02.

Navarro, R., Serna, C., Martínez, V., & Ruiz-Oliva, R. (2013). The role of Internet use and parental mediation on cyberbullying victimization among Spanish children from rural public schools. *European Journal of Psychology of Education, 28*(3), 725–745. doi:10.1007/s10212-012-0137-2.

Nocentini, A., Calmaestra, J., Schultze-Krumbholz, A., Scheithauer, H., Ortega, R., & Menesini, E. (2010). Cyberbullying: Labels, behaviours and definition in three European countries. *Journal of Guidance and Counselling, 20*(02), 129–142. doi:10.1375/ajgc.20.2.129.

Ortega, R., Elipe, P., Mora-Merchán, J. A., Calmaestra, J., & Vega, E. (2009). The emotional impact on victims of traditional bullying and cyberbullying: A study of Spanish adolescents. *Zeitschrift für Psychologie/Journal of Psychology, 217*(4), 197. doi:10.1027/0044-3409.217.4.197.

Perren, S., Corcoran, L., Cowie, H., Dehue, F., Garcia, D. J., Mc Guckin, C., Sevcikova, A., Tsatsou, P., & Völlink, T. (2012). Tackling cyberbullying: Review of empirical evidence regarding successful responses by students, parents, and schools. *International Journal of Conflict and Violence, 6*(2), 283–292.

Price, D., Green, D., Spears, B., Scrimgeour, M., Barnes, A., Geer, R., & Johnson, B. (2014). A qualitative exploration of cyber-bystanders and moral engagement. *Australian Journal of Guidance and Counselling, 24*(01), 1–17.

Rigby, K., & Bortolozzo, G. (2013). How schoolchildren's acceptance of self and others relate to their attitudes to victims of bullying. *Social Psychology of Education, 16*(2), 181–197. doi:10.1007/s11218-013-9213-y.

Sabella, R. A., Patchin, J. W., & Hinduja, S. (2013). Cyberbullying myths and realities. *Computers in Human Behavior, 29*(6), 2703–2711. doi:10.1016/j.chb.2013.06.040.

Smith, P. K., Cowie, H., Olafsson, R. F., & Liefooghe, A. P. (2002). Definitions of bullying: A comparison of terms used, and age and gender differences, in a fourteen-country international comparison. *Child Development, 73*(4), 1119–1133. doi:10.1111/1467-8624.00461.

Smith, P. K. (2012). Cyberbullying and cyber aggression. In S. R. Jimerson, A. B. Nickerson, M. J. Mayer, & M. J. Furlong (Eds.), *Handbook of school violence and school safety: International research and practice* (pp. 93–104). New York: Routledge.

Tokunaga, R. S. (2010). Following you home from school: A critical review and synthesis of research on cyberbullying victimization. *Computers in Human Behavior, 26,* 277–287. doi:10.1016/j.chb.2009.11.014.

Ttofi, M. M., & Farrington, D. P. (2011). Effectiveness of school-based programs to reduce bullying: A systematic and meta-analytic review. *Journal of Experimental Criminology, 7*(1), 27–56. doi:10.1007/s11292-010-9109-1.

Wilton, C., & Campbell, M. A. (2011). An exploration of the reasons why adolescents engage in traditional and cyber bullying. *Journal of Educational Sciences & Psychology, 1*(2), 101–109.

Wingate, V. S., Minney, J. A., & Guadagno, R. E. (2013). Sticks and stones may break your bones, but words will always hurt you: A review of cyberbullying. *Social Influence, 8*(2–3), 87–106. doi:10.1080/15534510.2012.730491.

Yin, R. K. (1984). *Case study research. Design and methods.* Beverly Hills: Sage.

Part III
Prevention and Intervention

Chapter 11
Intervention and Prevention Programmes on Cyberbullying: A Review

Conor Mc Guckin and Lucie Corcoran

11.1 Introduction

In this chapter, we explore prevention and intervention approaches to countering cyberbullying. For such an important, yet broad topic, the knowledge base regarding fundamental issues in the area is still in its infancy (e.g. operationally defining the area; Corcoran et al. 2015). With this, new approaches and considerations to prevention and intervention are emerging consistently in the academic and non-academic literature (e.g. digital citizenship and digital literacy skills for infants; Mooney et al. 2014).

For our work here, we are not seeking to provide an exhaustive list of available programmes or a historical review of how prevention and intervention programmes have developed. Nor do we set out to advocate any particular approach or programme. Rather, we seek to present some critical thought regarding the development, application, and evaluation of programmes in this important area. Through this approach, we are seeking to help the reader approach these various literatures and approaches in a more thoughtful and critical manner.

11.2 Thinking Back ... and Looking Forward

In thinking about our task for this chapter, we sat and thought, for a long time, about how we could construct a useful review of an issue that is as recent to society and our research endeavours as cyberbullying. One particular thought that kept arising for us was how to make this chapter useful for now, as well as an unknown future—

C. Mc Guckin (✉)
School of Education, Trinity College Dublin, Dublin 2, Ireland
e-mail: conor.mcguckin@tcd.ie

L. Corcoran
School of Arts, Dublin Business School, Dublin 2, Ireland

© Springer International Publishing Switzerland 2016
R. Navarro et al. (eds.), *Cyberbullying Across the Globe*,
DOI 10.1007/978-3-319-25552-1_11

not the far off future that we dream about in novels and films but the immediate future ahead of us. This appeared important for us because in our deliberations, we reflected upon how far our knowledge of bully/victim problems had come since the early studies of Olweus and from the initial gathering of colleagues in Stavanger in Norway. As psychologists and educators, we were also conscious of the fact that we are, in some instances, educating children and young people (CYP) for jobs that do not exist yet. So, it was almost like considering the enormous move from "analogue bullying" to "digital bullying" and like the early citizens of the industrial age before us, trying to figure out how the new technology could be used to make living conditions and society better (see Costabile and Spears 2012 for a useful overview of the impact of technology on relationships in educational settings).

Reflecting upon our own childhood development and our later research interests as adults, we were able to see the concurrent development of our own knowledge and that of society. There have been many remarkable developments in society and education since we first attended school (Conor in 1975 and Lucie in 1990). For example, we now view "inclusion" as "normal", with great focus on issues to do with early intervention (Carroll et al. 2013), a move from the medical model of disability and special educational needs to a more social model (Mc Guckin, Shevlin, Bell, and Devecchi 2013) and more inclusive research, practice, and student "voice" (Purdy and Mc Guckin 2015). With this, we can see the criticality of exploring previously unconsidered areas of bully/victim problems, such as disablist bullying (Purdy and Mc Guckin 2015) and alterophobic bullying (Minton 2012). With these developments, we can clearly see the importance of a "psychology of education" approach to theorising, researching, and helping with issues that affect CYP and hinder both educational and personal progress.

These developments and considerations are all important in their own way and provide a rich contextual backdrop to our focus in this chapter. As mentioned above, society is now much more pluralist and heterogeneous, with more discussion of "world issues" and "things" that are happening beyond the boundaries of our own little classrooms, schools, villages, towns, and cities—concepts like "globalisation", "time–space compression", and "global village". In other words, we need to remember the myriad of influences that affect CYP and that need to be considered by colleagues designing preventative and intervention approaches to cyberbullying. A useful and parsimonious theoretical model that has great applicability here is that of Bronfenbrenner's Ecological model (Bronfenbrenner 1977) or indeed a hybrid model drawing upon the Bildung model (Mc Guckin and Minton 2014). Such models allow for an understanding of the wider social, economic, political, philosophical, and "world order" factors that should be accounted for (e.g. Greene 1994; Greene and Moane 2000). As we discussed our own educational and personal development, we could see the influence of the meso- and macro-level factors mentioned in these models on our own development but also of the knowledge being generated in relation to the field.

When Conor was a schoolboy, whilst we knew what a bully was and what bullying behaviour was, the majority view in society and the research literature was that (a) this was not a particularly big problem at all, (b) it always happened somewhere else, and (c) it was a matter of "sticks and stones" (i.e. from the nursery rhyme—sticks and stones will break my bones but names will never harm me). In the intervening 10 or so years until Lucie began her schooling, perhaps the single biggest development in the research literature was the "new" view that perhaps girls could indeed be bullies. A very real and positive development was also evident across the educational sector—the acceptance that bully/victim problems happened in most (if not all) schools—even the best regulated.

From this starting point, we are fortunate that we have reached—in a small number of years—a stage whereby we have a sophisticated and nuanced understanding of the basic psychology regarding involvement in traditional bully/victim problems (see Smith 2014 for a pertinent and scholarly review). From this understanding, and largely underpinned by it, have been great advances in relation to the development of preventative and intervention approaches for what we now regularly refer to as face-to-face (f2f) bullying (Mc Guckin et al. 2010) or "traditional" bullying. This great work has been evident across society in terms of the marginalisation of erroneous views and "myths" about bully/victim problems—e.g. bullies as "thugs or thinkers" (Sutton 2001).

However, as with pioneering development in any area, many approaches to helping prevent or intervene in relation to the issues to do with traditional bully/victim problems were developed with good intentions. But good intentions alone do not evidence defensible findings. This chapter also reminds us that such a situation still exists today in relation to cyberbullying—perhaps, even more so because the Internet is available to anyone who wishes to publicise their own approach to countering such issues, with the attendant problem that content on the Internet is not peer-reviewed for accuracy and precision.

Negating the fact that the Internet is awash with helpful content, some more robust than others, seminal works in the area still act as beacons for those of us with an interest, whether professional or personal, in countering the insidious effects of involvement in bully/victim problems. For example, Smith et al. (2004) offered scholarly reviews of existing preventative and intervention approaches regarding traditional bully/victim problems. Farrington and Ttofi's (2009) Cochrane Review was a most welcome addition to the literature, in that it was formulated following the precise and scientific systematic literature review approach advocated by Cochrane collaborators. The ongoing development of robust programmes that are both theoretically and empirically informed continue to give us confidence that we are moving in the right direction—both in schools and society, more generally. Such work in the area of cyberbullying has demonstrated the value of including expertise from "sister disciplines" that did not traditionally contribute on a large scale to efforts to counter traditional bully/victim problems—e.g. law, business (see the review later of COST Action IS0801: https://sites.google.com/site/costis0801/).

11.3 Reviewing and Evaluating Programmes: What Should Be Considered?

Setting out to review preventative and intervention approaches to countering cyberbullying would appear, at first glance, to be a relatively straightforward endeavour. Surely, it is just a matter of exploring the academic databases for appropriate content, scouring the Internet for extra material not published in academic journals, and considering the grey literature (O'Brien and Mc Guckin in press). On one level, this could work. Indeed, it would work, if that was your usual approach to synopsising an area of scholarly work.

However, we are advocating a different approach here—one that we believe we should not have to emphasise, yet feel that this is indeed required. We advocate that developers of such programmes, whilst needing to be well-intentioned, also need to follow some basic theoretical and methodological rubrics so as to evidence programmes that are fit for purpose. Whilst not an exhaustive list, we detail some of these here in the hope that readers will reflect and consider their own approach to such issues as well as being able to critically analyse the programmes offered by others. On the whole, these are basic requirements and advanced programme developers would, we would expect, seek to further develop and supplement these.

In advancing our thesis, we would encourage colleagues to view our principles as yardsticks, and not templates, to approaching their good work regarding the development of preventative and intervention approaches. After all, our work in the social sciences with humans is akin to doing chemistry with dirty test tubes. Or, as Coolican (2007) argues, there is no one theory or approach that is absolutely correct or appropriate in all cases. Applying psychological interventions presents us with challenges different to those faced when applying medical or hard scientific interventions. "Working with and studying people is not like studying chemicals. People react; people know when they are under study; people have freewill and can change their mind or behaviour as a result of knowing what is expected of them, either to conform or to be contrary." (Coolican 2007, p. 3).

In the absence of such a standardised approach, we believe that some of what is currently available to end users has been developed on an ad hoc, but well-intentioned, reactionary basis. Some readers might assume that we are about to be severely critical of such approaches. We are not. Despite "our" well-intentioned rubrics, we accept that a purely "purist" approach to our endeavours in this area may not always result in the most relevant preventative or intervention programme for a particular population or "local" need.

As such, we are accepting of these "Desire Paths". The notion of desire paths comes from the literature regarding town and urban planning. The term desire path and it's associated names (e.g. desire line, social trail) refer to a pathway that has been created as a consequence of foot or bicycle traffic. The path usually represents the shortest or most easily navigated route between an origin and destination. Technical and measurable aspects of the path (e.g. width, depth, erosion) are indicators of the amount of use the path receives. In reality, desire paths are what we recognise in our built environment as shortcuts where the standard route seems to be too cumbersome or circuitous, or where a standard route does not even exist. For many of us, we would recognise a desire path as the route that we take to the bus stop or local shop—the route that cuts across the housing estate or rough land—nor the official route planned out on a map whereby the route relies on the road network, etc.

And so, what is it that we like about this borrowed concept from the world of town planning and other disciplines within the built environment?

As mentioned, we know that such an approach exists in relation to the development of preventative and intervention approaches to the amelioration of cyberbullying. Rather than being critical of the genetic background of these approaches in terms of their theoretical and methodological rigour, we can be more pragmatic and seek to understand their efficacy by means of measuring what data is available for them and treat them in a "quasi" manner.

Such research would explore the "deviation" between the de jure approach to preventative and intervention programmes (e.g. the programme, policy, etc.) as advocated by authority figures (e.g. the department of education, the researcher community) and the de facto approach that exists in reality (i.e. what is being implemented in schools). Schools and educators quite often develop and implement interventions and preventions that make "local sense" to their schools and pupils. Whilst some of these will mimic quite closely what is advocated by the authority figures, some will be so different that there is no convergence between what is being implemented on the ground and the approach envisaged by authority figures. Thus, in terms of desire paths, we could explore these non-standard (de facto) approaches by using methodology to explore the technical issues related to "width", "depth", and "erosion".

11.4 Reviewing and Evaluating Programmes: Useful Benchmarks

In the previous section, we discussed our views about whether we should always advocate a purist approach to programme development or whether a bespoke and "local" solution could also be considered as something useful. The commonality of both perspectives is that programmes are (a) developed with the very best intentions with regards to the safety and development of CYP and (b) can generate data that can be evaluated in a meaningful manner so as to determine efficacy.

Thus, whilst both approaches have the same starting and finishing points, it is to the points of divergence that we turn our attention to now. In developing robust programmes, we consider the following as important criteria. However, we also recognise that, depending upon the context, whilst some of the points below may be viewed as essential, others may simply be desirable:

a. That the programme is grounded in theory
b. That, where possible, the programme is evidence-informed
c. That the central tenets of the programme are operationally defined and clarified—e.g. traditional bullying, cyberbullying, cyber aggression, or all of these. That the target "audience" be clearly defined—e.g. all CYP in the target population or identified subsets of the population, such as disablist bullying (Purdy and Mc Guckin 2014) or alterophobic bullying (Minton 2012). That key variables and design parameters are considered as extensions to previous literature—i.e. that clear and precise comparisons can be made in terms of, for example, definitions, inclusion/exclusion criteria, time reference periods
d. That the incidence levels of involvement by the various actor groups can be assessed

e. That the programme be tested for effectiveness across different variables and contexts (e.g. social, personal, situational, cultural)—e.g. examining psychological and educational correlates, such as anxiety or academic performance, and ecological-level variables such as school policy, whole-school and whole-community approaches, school climate (e.g. Mc Guckin and Minton 2014)

f. That the programme be able to assess personal and situational factors, such as coping style (e.g. internal, external, resilience) and resources which mediate and moderate the relationship between the central concept and its correlates. The preponderance of research attention to date has been to the negative effects of involvement in traditional bullying and cyberbullying. There is a need to consider a positive psychology approach and associated constructs (e.g. empowerment, resilience, post-traumatic growth)

g. That the programme remains sensitive to the normative transitions made by CYP through, for example, chronological and interactional age development/stages, school systems, and their various transition points (e.g. from primary to post-primary). Programmes should also remain sensitive to the fact that transitions are not always linear and logical—e.g. for CYP with special educational needs and/or disabilities, whose transitions may resemble a more "scenic route" (Mc Guckin et al. 2013)

h. That the programme takes cognisance of the contemporary digital world that the CYP inhabit and seek to "future proof" the programme—e.g. incorporate attention to issues such as digital citizenship and digital literacy (Mooney et al. 2014), information and communications technology (ICT) engagement at personal, family, and school levels (e.g. European Union (EU) Kids Online, Net Children Go Mobile)

i. That consideration is given to the development of a longitudinal design or a quasi-longitudinal design

j. That advanced research methodology should be employed so as to explore effectiveness—e.g. a randomised control trial (RCT), psychometric evaluation of measurement instruments

k. That attempts are made to add to the database of knowledge regarding effective programmes—e.g. attempts are made to widely disseminate the technical information about the development and application of the programme and that results of applications be published

l. That analytical tools be used to ascertain user engagement of publically available resources for the programme (e.g. available via the Internet; Mc Guckin and Crowley 2012)

m. That materials and approaches be developed with consideration to use outside and beyond the confines of the programme. For example, in an era of high aspirations for life-long and life-wide learning, materials and delivery approaches should be developed with cognisance of the Bologna Process (Bologna Declaration, 1999) and be conversant with national frameworks of qualifications

n. That, before any of the criteria here are addressed (or not) and actioned, that two fundamental and non-negotiable points are agreed upon: (i) that "success" is defined (i.e. what would successful implementation look like? What objective assessment(s) would define success?) and (ii) that there is strict adherence to ethical issues regarding the potential effect that programme components could have on the CYP or other individuals, either involved or not involved in the programme—and where possible, external scrutiny of the programme be conducted by an ethics panel. For example, a programme may evidence a reduction in the incidence of cyberbullying by banning all use of technology in a school—is this fair to the students, not just in terms of personal technology but also pedagogical applications of ICT?

As noted above, we do not present these benchmarks as exhaustive or as a template for programme development. Rather, as yardsticks, these principles present an opportunity for programme developers to consider their work in a more holistic manner. They also allow for local issues that may necessitate bespoke planning of components or application (e.g. desire paths). They also present flexibility for the foreseeable future, where we can assume that the presentation and sequelae of cyberbullying will change—as society and consumer ICT will undoubtedly grow and change (e.g. Moore's law; Moore 1965).

In the next section, we move forward to an exploration of prevention and intervention approaches, with a focus on programmes, approaches, and materials that are contemporary, interesting, and show great promise.

11.5   Prevention and Intervention Approaches—What's Available?

With the benefit of distance and hindsight, the previous section explored a utopian view of criteria that programme developers should take heed of in their planning, development, implementation, and evaluation of programmes. In the current section, we move forward to an exploration of available prevention and intervention programmes, approaches, and information materials.

There have been many initiatives developed with a core intention of providing a managed response to cyberbullying incidents among CYP or intervening when such events occur. This section provides an overview of three of the early projects in the area of cyberbullying prevention and intervention. We believe that these seminal projects are worthy of attention here due to either their evidence-informed approach to programme development or have produced substantive knowledge that programme developers should take cognisance of. We believe that much of this early work has the potential to become the bedrock of future work in the area. Some examples of this newly emerging work are reported upon later.

11.6   CyberTraining

One early approach, specifically funded and designed to be evidence-informed, was the CyberTraining project (funded by the EU Lifelong Learning Programme: [Project No.142237-LLP-1-2008-1-DE-LEONARDO-LMP] http://cybertraining-project.org). The project provided a well-grounded, research-based training manual on cyberbullying for trainers. The manual includes background information on cyberbullying, its nature and extent in Europe, current projects, initiatives and approaches tackling the cyberbullying problem, best practice Europe-wide as well as practical guidance and resources for trainers working with the target groups of: (a) pupils; (b) parents; and (c) teachers, schools, and other professionals. The manual concludes with a comprehensive compilation of supporting references, Internet links, and other resources for trainers. Whilst the review material, manual, and resources are freely available on the Internet, the project was usefully also reported upon in Mora-Merchan and Jäger's (2011) edited collection.

Traditionally, much research concludes with a (hopefully) planned dissemination plan. Indeed, with funded projects like the CyberTraining project, it is generally a mandatory part of workflow and work package planning. However, for many researchers, the notion of dissemination is a one-way activity. That is, they view dissemination activities as "we published a paper", "we published a book", "we presented the findings at a conference", etc. Whilst laudable and part of the natural work of the researcher, this traditional view of dissemination does not take account of end-user activity. For example, is it not more important to know how many people attended the conference presentation, asked questions, made contact afterwards, etc.? This is not just a rhetorical question that we pose here. We have attended project update meetings with funders who have "suggested" that such an approach will be needed in future and that the old and traditional view of dissemination will not suffice.

As a pioneering approach to project evaluation and end-user engagement, Mc Guckin and Crowley (2012) reported on how they used Google Analytics tools to evaluate the effectiveness of the CyberTraining project. The interesting advance made by Mc Guckin and Crowley (2012) was that they were able to demonstrate how such analytical tools could help provide intelligence as to the access made by end users to project material available on the Internet. They demonstrated how these free and easy-to-use analytics tools can, for example, highlight the most accessed content, whether certain content should be positioned so as to be easier found, geographical spread of activity, etc. For example, do people from Ireland seek such material more often than their counterparts from Spain? Indeed, with enough website traffic, more fine-grained analysis would be possible—sudden spikes in access from particular intra-country regions could signify where extra resources may be needed in the school system.

11.7   CyberTraining for Parents (CT4P)

Following the success of their CyberTraining project, further funding was secured by the lead partners to develop a more focused and nuanced project specifically aimed at parents—CyberTraining-4-Parents (CT4P; http://cybertraining4parents.

org/ Project number: 510162-LLP-1-2010-1-DE-GRUNDTVIG-GMP). The CT4P project was specifically aimed at facilitating parent training in relation to cyberbullying, including self-directed online courses and moderated online courses for parents. Through its initial development and implementation, many of the principles that we outlined above can be seen in action in the CT4P project.

Partly building on the training material developed in the CyberTraining project, the CT4P project made provision for parents to gain a basic understanding of new ICT and Internet safety, as well as cyberbullying, its sources, prevalence and effects, legal issues at a national and transnational level, as well as strategies for preventing and tackling cyberbullying.

Interestingly, the materials and delivery approaches have been developed in such a manner that would allow easy translation into academic courses that would be conversant with national frameworks of qualifications. That is, we believe that it would not take too much effort to develop modules, courses, and programmes that take account of Bologna principles and the European Credit Transfer and Accumulation System (ECTS; Bologna Declaration 1999). This would add to the project's long-time sustainability.

Training courses were presented on two different levels: (a) on a national level the partner countries facilitated "face-to-face" training courses and (b) online courses targeting an international audience were facilitated online. Apart from theoretical introductions, the courses involved several practically oriented elements such as role plays, group work, and other interactive elements. The national courses were supported by an online forum that gave participants the opportunity to exchange with other participants of the courses, both on a national and transnational level.

Among other things, the courses contained clearly predefined learning goals; learning materials; recommended readings; and comprehensive lists of online resources, moderated online discussions between participants, online assessments of the learning outcome related to each of the modules, and individual feedback by the instructor. In terms of its learning environment, the courses combined three different platforms: (a) Moodle was used to host the main body of the courses, (b) asynchronous forums and assessments served as a document repository, and (c) weekly synchronous virtual meetings of all participants were held at a virtual campus in the virtual 3D online environment of Second Life—using the teaching facilities of the "virtual Anti-Violence-Campus" that were created in the EU funded Grundtvig project "Anti-Violence-Campus at Second Life" (AVC@SL).

11.8   COST Action IS0801

Whilst not developing a programme of intervention or prevention, the outputs from another EU supported project (COST Action IS0801: http://sites.google.com/site/costis0801) provide hugely beneficial inputs to any efforts to prevent cyberbullying or intervene when such issues arise.

COST Action IS0801 (Cyberbullying: coping with negative and enhancing positive uses of new technologies, in relationships in educational settings) brought together researchers, practitioners, and policy-minded colleagues from the field of traditional bullying, along with colleagues from disparate fields, such as law and telecommunications providers, so as to conceptualise and operationalise the field of cyberbullying.

Whilst one working group sought to determine the most appropriate manner in which to conceptualise the issue, another group worked on issues to do with national guidelines. Other groups worked on issues related to coping with cyberbullying, legal issues and input from mobile phone companies and internet service providers, and positive uses of new technologies, in relation to educational settings.

In terms of sustainability, the Action included short-term scientific missions to encourage the development of research capacity among younger researchers in the area. Large numbers of dissemination activities were carried out, with much of the content of these activities freely available on the Action website. Importantly, the key outcomes from the Action are also available freely, and we recommend that any programme developer in this area should consult these research-informed outcomes.

11.9 Prevention and Intervention: Newly Emerging Work

Reviewed above were three highly productive and influential early works in the area of preventing cyberbullying and educating those with a personal or professional interest in the area. Many highly useful programmes and approaches are available—each approaching the issue from different perspectives. For example, Ortega-Ruiz et al.'s (2012) ConRed Cyberbullying Prevention Program has three aims: (a) to improve perceived control over information on the Internet, (b) to reduce the time dedicated to digital device usage, and (c) to prevent and reduce cyberbullying. The influential KiVa Antibullying Program focuses on enhancing empathy, self-efficacy, and anti-bullying attitudes among those who are neither bullied nor victimised, namely bystanders (Williford et al. 2013). Toshack and Colmar (2012) have reported upon their psycho-educational programme for primary school children. The programme sets out with the aim that students would have a better understanding of cyberbullying, that they would have better knowledge of safety strategies, and that they would be encouraged to contribute to the management of such issues in their schools.

As noted at the beginning of the chapter, it is not our intention to either provide or review an exhaustive list of programmes. What we would like to do, however, is to provide overviews of four examples of the recently developed work in the area—programmes that have either demonstrated useful results already or have the potential to deliver useful results from their novel approach to programme design. These programmes incorporate guidance regarding the most appropriate ways of assessing effectiveness as well as highlighting the scope for both face-to-face and virtual delivery of material.

11.10   The FearNot! Programme

Sapouna et al. (2015) offered recommendations regarding efforts to counter cyber-bullying, which were based upon research which assessed the anti-bullying pro-gramme FearNot! The programme was designed to address traditional forms of bully/victim problems among primary school children and was tested cross-cul-turally in Germany and the UK. The central component of the programme was the education of children in relation to coping skills which would be effective for coun-tering traditional bullying. Interestingly, this education was achieved via role-play in a virtual environment, an approach based on experiential learning.

A strength of this programme was that it was informed by evidence that expe-riential learning can be an effective tool in allowing students to address social and emotional problems in school as they are given the opportunity to take the perspec-tive of another student with respect to thoughts, emotions, and behaviours, and in this way, there is an opportunity for empathy to develop. Because there are certain obstacles associated with implementing role play in a school environment, particu-larly in relation to a sensitive topic such as bullying, the virtual environment can provide a "safe space" to test out different coping strategies and responses to a bul-lying scenario. The components of the programme are directed by the literature on bully/victim problems, with emphasis on various forms of bullying, the bystander role, and effective/ineffective coping strategies. Children play the role of a friend of a character who is being bullied and in this way they have the chance to advise their friend in terms of how they can respond to victimisation. Children then receive immediate feedback in relation to how the strategy might work for the character.

Comparing a group who received the intervention with a control group, the FearNot! programme was assessed using pre- and post-measures of victim status, knowledge of effective coping strategies, and supportive bystander behaviour. Find-ings indicated that victims in the intervention group were significantly more likely to become escaped victims 1 week following the intervention. Some other differ-ences were culture-specific and may have been due to factors such as varying levels of anti-bullying intervention in both countries prior to beginning the study.

Based on the effectiveness of the FearNot! Programme, it would seem that it could be adapted to also counter cyberbullying in schools. According to the re-searchers, some important aspects of design that need to be considered for such as adaptation include the need to allow students and teachers to be involved in the development of the content and characters, the capacity for virtual characters to express themselves, the provision of sufficiently robust computers, the potential need for teachers to up skill in relation to computer use, and importantly, the incor-poration of this approach as just one component of whole-school system approach. However, another crucial component that we need to return to is the definition and delineation of cyberbullying/cyber aggression. If cyberbullying is merely an exten-sion or subtype of traditional bullying, then we can confidently apply the same prin-ciples and approaches to countering cyberbullying as we do to traditional bullying. However, we must be cognisant of the unique characteristics of cyberbullying/cyber aggression and design our intervention/prevention efforts accordingly (Corcoran et al. 2015).

11.11 A "Serious Game" Approach

Van Cleemput et al. (2015) provide a review of the initial stages of the design process for a digital game, which is to be used to counter cyberbullying in Belgian secondary schools. The target population was aged 12–14 years so as to reach young people who are most involved in cyberbullying. Highlighting the theoretical underpinning of the programme, Van Cleemput and colleagues describe "serious" games as appropriate for encouraging learning and behavioural change among young people because these games carry intrinsic motivation, they can facilitate learning and behaviour change through, for example, feedback, practice, reward, and they provide an appropriate fit for young people. In addition, the authors cite empirical support for the effectiveness of this approach in relation to learning and behaviour change.

There was focus on the initial phases of design, which followed an intervention mapping protocol so as to build a programme that could be effective in its aims. The game was primarily focused on the role of the bystander, considering that this is the most common role in cyberbullying scenarios, with research demonstrating that bystander-focused interventions can be particularly effective in terms of bullying reduction. Professional story writers were involved in the development of the story upon which the game would be based. With regard to narrative development, the researchers were guided by two key theories: transportation theory and the extended elaboration likelihood model. For instance, transportation theory suggests that when participants becomes more engaged with a story, their beliefs tend to reflect those of the story more closely and, moreover, they are less likely to develop counter opinions. Transportation can be affected by factors such as emotional empathy for the characters and lack of distraction from the real-world environment. The extended elaboration likelihood model also states that transportation can be affected by factors such as the appeal of the storyline and the quality of the production. The characters used in such a game can also be important as an attractive character can be a useful tool of persuasion. Furthermore, the authors have drawn on the social tearning theory by developing characters who can facilitate social modelling of desirable behaviour. The characters (if relatable for the children) can promote development of self-efficacy through changing their lives for the better.

Focus groups were conducted with Belgian secondary school children in order to retrieve feedback on an introductory clip for the game. It emerged that participants identified appealing aspects of the game whilst also offering critical feedback. The researchers examined factors, which could affect immersion in the story such as emotional response, participants' understanding of the story, and characteristics of the characters could make them more relatable for the target age group so as to identify aspects that needed further development. The researchers concluded that the background story should not be too predictable. In addition, they recognised the importance of craftsmanship when developing such an intervention as the professionally developed components of the programme were more popular with students than those that were generated by non-professionals.

Overall, in terms of our recommendations for programme developers, this programme provides a very useful template for setting out to develop an intervention in a rigorous manner with appropriate attention to relevant theory and empirical evidence.

11.12 A Web-based Approach

Jacobs et al. (2014) describe in detail the process of Intervention Mapping for developing a web-based intervention (Online Pestkoppenstoppen: http://www.pest-koppenstoppen.nl) to counter and prevent cyberbullying. The authors used a variety of sources for designing the intervention, including a review of the literature, a Delphi study with experts in the field, focus groups with the targeted group, as well as components of an effective anti-bullying programme. These researchers developed an online intervention which meets the specific needs of individual participants (victims of cyberbullying aged 12–15 years). There are three sessions in the intervention, which are delivered over a 3-month period.

The purpose of session 1 is to educate participants about how their behaviour is influenced by their thoughts and the way that they can identify and dispute irrational thoughts and form more rational thoughts. Session 2 teaches participants about the different ways that bullying can emerge and how their behaviour can affect bullying, whilst also recognising coping methods that can stop cyberbullying. Session 3 educates participants about the safe use of technology.

A strength of the design of the programme is the individualised approach, which fits to participants' own traits, such as personal coping style. The programme was pretested prior to implementation, and the researchers' plan for a RCT so as to assess effectiveness, primarily in terms of reducing cyberbullying and countering its negative correlates (specifically anxiety and depression).

Jacobs et al. (2014) set out to provide a programme which was theoretically sound and based on evidence. A web-based approach was chosen for this programme because the researchers felt it was most appropriate, considering findings such as, for example, that cybervictims are generally disinclined to report victimisation to an adult, they spend large amounts of time online, and can and conveniently access the programme.

- Step 1 in this design was to conduct a needs assessment, and Jacobs and colleagues report that there is a need for 12–15-year-olds beginning secondary school to improve their coping strategies in response to cyberbullying.
- Step 2 required the researchers to identify the change objectives of the programme. One objective was that, following the intervention, participants would cope in an effective manner when faced with cyberbullying experiences. Participants would be expected to perform specific behaviours, namely performance objectives. In order to facilitate participants meeting performance objectives, the 5G-schema was used to provide insight into the associations between an event, thoughts, feelings, behaviours, and consequences.

- Step 3 of the design stages was to assess the most important and changeable determinants of each performance objective, which literally required the researchers to decide which factors would determine whether a victim would, or is able to, perform each performance objective, such as, monitoring and evaluating thoughts following victimisation or recognising and regulating emotions. Jacobs and colleagues combined performance objectives and what they identified as their determinants and created 50 change objectives. An example of a practical application of modelling is the use of role models to enhance self-efficacy. The Online Pestkoppenstoppen programme utilised different methods including using a model to demonstrate behaviour and tailoring the programme delivery to the individual needs of participants.
- Step 4 of the design process required the researchers to produce programme components and materials. The intervention includes three advice sessions of approximately 45 min duration, as follows: (a) Think strong, feel better, (b) Stop the bully now!, and (c) You are doing great, can you do better?

Each session follows administration of questionnaires which measure tailoring and effect variables. The intervention was subject to pretesting as members of the target population completed the questionnaires and followed the advice. Focus groups were also conducted, and adaptations were made based upon the data collected from the pilot, pretest, and focus groups. The researchers will test the effectiveness of the intervention using a RCT with an experimental group, a general information group, and a waiting list control group.

11.13 "Let's Not Fall into the Trap" Programme

Menesini et al. (2015) provide a review of the effectiveness of an anti-bullying programme which has undergone assessment. They propose that, given the well-evidenced overlap between traditional and cyber forms of bullying, it is rational to extend existing anti-bullying programmes to also counter cyberbullying. However, they also highlight the argument that cyberspace has specific characteristics which do not pertain to the physical world, and for this reason, anti-cyberbullying initiatives should include some specific strategies. They discuss a programme called "Noncadiamointrappola!" (translation: "Let's not fall into the trap"), which has the objective of countering both traditional bullying and cyberbullying and promoting positive use of technology.

"Noncadiamointrappola!" has a prosocial perspective, facilitating provision of online support, encouraging positive online behaviours, and involving peers as educators in face-to-face and cyber settings. The researchers have been vigilant in creating a methodologically sound programme, modifying it over time in line with the latest findings from both their study and the recent research literature. Students were included in the design of aspects of the programme, such as the provision of materials and design of the logo. Whilst modest effects were found for the first edition of the programme (2009/2010), the researchers reported greater effects following the second edition, which included adaptations such as: giving equal consideration to both bullying and cyberbullying, greater emphasis on the bystander and victim roles, consideration of coping strategies, provision of peer-led face-to-face activities, increased focus on the ecological approach where teacher support of class activities is emphasised, and creation of a Facebook page which could complement the website's forum. Specifically, the second edition was related to a decline in bullying, victimisation, and cyber victimisation among those in the experimental group compared to the control participants. Furthermore, the experimental group was found to have a greater tendency towards adaptive/desirable coping whilst also displaying a decline in maladaptive coping.

Based on the results from earlier editions of the Noncadiamointrappola! programme, the researchers determined that when using a peer-led model, the role of the peer educators holds great importance with regard to overall effectiveness. They also discuss the group dynamics, which can contribute to the incidence of bullying and cyberbullying, suggesting approach coping styles making defending actions by bystanders more likely, whilst empathy and having attitudes against bullying are predictive of greater intervention by bystanders. Furthermore, they argue that in addition to developing individual attitudes and coping styles, it is also important to address the group as a whole.

For the third edition of the programme, the components remained largely the same, with some additional emphasis on, for example, peer-led activities and new components such as cooperative work. The newly added activities which were led by peer educators involved cooperative work focusing on empathy and problem-solving, with specific attention to the victim and bystander perspectives so as to indicate how change can be achieved.

The programme targeted bullying from an ecological perspective, focusing on a school-wide approach. A strength of this programme evaluation was that the researchers strove to achieve an evidence-informed programme. The evaluation was completed using two quasi-experimental trials with pre- and post-intervention testing. The control groups did not receive any intervention. Overall, results confirmed a significant decline in bullying, victimisation, cyberbullying, and cyber victimisation for the experimental group compared to the control group, although the effect size was not very strong. This research provides support for the peer-led model of intervention, which has received mixed effectiveness in the literature.

11.14 Moving Forward—Some Thoughts

We hope that you have found this chapter useful. At this point, we would like to offer a few words to reflect and consider as we move forward to a future that will continue to change and hold both wonder and fear for our young people.

As argued in the chapter, whilst there is no "best" programme or approach to combating either traditional bullying or cyberbullying, what we do have is the knowledge and professional skills to imagine and operationalise programmes that can keep CYP free from harm and harassment, allowing them to enjoy their education—in school, at home, and in society. After all, if we are to evidence a truly "inclusive" society, we need to consistently assert in a vigorous manner that the inhumane treatment of fellow citizens is a line in the sand that we should not cross. The minds of CYP are malleable enough for us to not lose faith in the good work that we do.

For the field of cyberbullying, we need to keep developing our understanding of fundamental issues related to definitional criteria and associated variables of concern (e.g. cyberbullying or cyber aggression?). For successful development of preventative and intervention programmes, we have highlighted key principles and benchmarks that we believe should be seen as yardsticks for future developments in the area. We trust that colleagues will heed such advice and strive for programme content and application (and evaluation) that evidences robust and appreciable findings. At all times, we strive to understand the phenomenon of cyberbullying whilst also attempting to be considerate of the national and international legal parameters within which cyberbullying operates and was not previously such a major issue of concern regarding traditional bullying (e.g. Purdy and Mc Guckin 2013).

To conclude, and as a cautionary note to us all regarding cyber-safety and CYP: if you don't understand it, you can't teach it! (Mc Guckin 2013).

References

Bronfenbrenner, U. (1977). Toward an experimental ecology of human development. *American Psychologist, 32,* 513–531. doi:10.1037//0003-066X.32.7.513.

Carroll, C., Murphy, G., & Sixsmith, J. (2013). The progression of early intervention disability services in Ireland. *Infants & Young Children, 26*(1), 17–27. doi:10.1097/IYC.0b013e3182736ce6.

Coolican, H. (2007). *Applied psychology*. London: Hodder. Arnold.

Corcoran, L., Mc Guckin, C., & Prentice, G. R. (2015). Cyberbullying or cyber aggression?: A review of existing definitions of cyber-based peer-to-peer aggression. *Societies, 5*(2), 245–255. doi:10.3390/soc5020245.

Costabile, A., & Spears, B. A. (2012). *The impact of technology on relationships in educational settings*. London: Routledge.

Farrington, D. P., & Ttofi, M. M. (2009). School-based programs to reduce bullying and victimization. *Campbell Systematic Reviews,* (6). doi:10.4073/csr.2009.4076.

Greene, S. M. (1994). Growing up Irish: Development in context. *The Irish Journal of Psychology, 15*(2–3), 354–371. doi:10.1080/03033910.1994.10558016.

Greene, S., & Moane, G. (2000). Growing up Irish: Changing children in a changing society. *The Irish Journal of Psychology, 21*(3–4), 122–137. doi:10.1080/03033910.2000.10558247.

Jacobs, N. C. L., Völlink, T., Dehue, F., & Lechner, L. (2014). Online Pestkoppenstoppen: Systematic and theory-based development of a web-based tailored intervention for adolescent cyberbully victims to combat and prevent cyberbullying. *BMC Public Health, 14*(1), 396. doi:10.1186/1471-2458-14-396.

Mc Guckin, C. (2013). School bullying amongst school pupils in Northern Ireland: How many are involved, what are the health effects, and what are the issues for school management? In A. M. O'Moore & P. Stevens (Eds.), *Bullying in Irish education* (pp. 40–64). Cork: Cork University Press. http://hdl.handle.net/2262/67694.

Mc Guckin, C., & Crowley, N. (2012). Using Google Analytics to evaluate the impact of the CyberTraining project. *Cyberpsychology, Behavior, and Social Networking, 15*(11), 625–629. doi:10.1089/cyber.2011.0460.

Mc Guckin, C., & Minton, S. (2014). From theory to practice: Two ecosystemic approaches and their applications to understanding school bullying. *Australian Journal of Guidance and Counselling, 24*(1), 36–48. doi:10.1017/jgc.2013.10.

Mc Guckin, C., Cummins, P. K., & Lewis, C. A. (2010). f2f and cyberbullying among children in Northern Ireland: Data from the Kids Life and Times Surveys. *Psychology, Society, & Education, 2*(2), 83–96.

Mc Guckin, C., Shevlin, M., Bell, S., & Devecchi, C. (2013). *Moving to further and higher education: An exploration of the experiences of students with special educational needs.* Research Report Number 14. A Study Commissioned by the National Council for Special Education (NCSE), Trim, County Meath, Ireland. http://www.ncse.ie/uploads/1/Report_HigherEd_22_10_13.pdf.

Menesini, E., Palladino, B. E., & Nocentini, A. (2015). Noncadiamointrappola! Online and School based program to prevent cyberbullying among adolescents. In T. Völlink, F. Dehue, & C. Mc Guckin (Eds.), *Cyberbullying and youth: From theory to interventions. Current issues in social psychology series.* London: Psychology Press/Taylor & Francis.

Minton, S. J. (2012). Alterophobic bullying and pro-conformist aggression in a survey of upper secondary school students in Ireland. *Journal of Aggression, Conflict and Peace Research, 4*(2), 86–95. doi:10.1108/17596591211208292.

Mooney, E., Mc Guckin, C., & Corcoran, L. (2014). Empowering young people through digital literacy skills in order to mitigate or cope with online risks (Symposium: Current Directions in Traditional and Cyberbullying). The Psychological Society of Ireland Annual Conference, Newpark Hotel, Kilkenny, Co. Kilkenny, Ireland, 12th–15th November, 2014. *The Irish Psychologist, 41*(1), S27–S28.

Moore, G. E. (1965). Cramming more components onto integrated circuits. *Electronics, 38*(8), 114–117.

Mora-Merchan, J., & Jäger, T. (2011). *Cyberbullying: A cross-national comparison.* Landau: Verlag Emprische Pädagogik.

O'Brien, A. M., & Mc Guckin, C. (in press). *The systematic literature review. SAGE cases in methodology: A unique collection of over 500 case studies for use in the teaching of research methods.* London: Sage.

Ortega-Ruiz, R., Del Rey, R., & Casas, J. A. (2012). Knowing, building and living together on internet and social networks: The ConRed cyberbullying prevention program. *International Journal of Conflict and Violence, 6*(2), 302–312.

Purdy, N., & Mc Guckin, C. (2013). *Cyberbullying and the law. A Report for the Standing Conference on Teacher Education North and South (SCoTENS).* Armagh: Centre for Cross Border Studies. http://hdl.handle.net/2262/67461.

Purdy, N., & Mc Guckin, C. (2014). Disablist bullying: What student teachers in Northern Ireland and the Republic of Ireland don't know and the implications for teacher education. *European Journal of Special Needs Education, 29*(4), 446–456. doi:10.1080/08856257.2014.952914.

Purdy, N., & Mc Guckin, C. (2015). Disablist bullying in schools: giving a voice to student teachers. *Journal of Research in Special Educational Needs, 15*(3), 202–210. doi: 10.1111/1471-3802.12110.

Sapouna, M., Enz, S., Samaras, M., & Wolke, D. (2015). Learning how to cope with cyberbullying in the virtual world: Lessons from FearNot! In T. Völlink, F. Dehue, & C. Mc Guckin (Eds.), *Cyberbullying and youth: From theory to interventions. Current issues in social psychology series.* London: Psychology Press/Taylor & Francis.

Smith, P. K. (2014). *Understanding school bullying: Its nature and prevention strategies.* London: Sage. doi:10.4135/9781473906853.

Smith, P. K., Pepler, D., & Rigby, K. (2004). *Bullying in schools: How successful can interventions be?* London: Cambridge University Press. doi:10.1017/CBO9780511584466.

Sutton, J. (2001). Bullies: Thugs or thinkers? *The Psychologist, 14*(10), 530–534.

Toshack, T., & Colmar, S. (2012). A cyberbullying intervention with primary-aged students. *Australian Journal of Guidance and Counselling, 22*(2), 268–278. doi:10.1017/jgc.2012.31.

Van Cleemput, K., Vandebosch, H., Poels, K., Bastiaensens, S., DeSmet, A., & De Bourdeaudhuij, I. (2015). The development a serious game on cyberbullying: A concept test. In T. Völlink, F. Dehue, & C. Mc Guckin (Eds.), *Cyberbullying and youth: From theory to interventions. Current issues in social psychology series*. London: Psychology Press/Taylor & Francis.

Williford, A., Elledge, L. C., Boulton, A. J., DePaolis, K. J., Little, T. D., & Salmivalli, C. (2013). Effects of the KiVa antibullying program on cyberbullying and cybervictimization frequency among Finnish youth. *Journal of Clinical Child & Adolescent Psychology, 42*(6), 820–833. do i:10.1080/15374416.2013.787623.

Chapter 12
Cyberbullying and Restorative Justice

Susan Hanley Duncan

12.1 Introduction

Hardly a day goes by without another cyberbullying incident and its devastating effects reported to the public. The following stories during the last year poignantly illustrate the magnitude of the problem.

- Parents file suit against the San Diego Unified School District after their high school-going son committed suicide following a video that went viral allegedly showing him masturbating in the bathroom (Snider 2014).
- A former Michigan high school student brought a Title IX claim against the school district for failing to investigate her claims of sexual assault and ignoring incidents of cyberbullying, forcing her to leave school (National Women's Law Center 2013).
- A Canadian teenager hung herself after explicit pictures of her were distributed by boys that allegedly raped her while she was intoxicated. The police did not press charges citing they did not have enough evidence of a crime (Bazelon 2014).

Parents, school officials, and policy-makers all seek to find solutions; however, nothing seems to adequately address the issue. Many states continue to revise their statutes criminalizing the behavior, while school districts implement policies prohibiting cyberbullying. Despite the good intentions behind these efforts, courts often strike down these laws or prohibit schools from disciplining students on constitutional grounds, leaving legislators and school administrators unsure how best to approach the problem. This chapter offers an alternative approach to use when addressing cyberbullying that focuses on restorative justice, principles, and practices.

S. H. Duncan (✉)
University of Louisville, Room 201 Wyatt Hall, Louisville, KY 40292, USA
e-mail: susan.duncan@louisville.edu

The original version of this chapter was revised. An erratum can be found at DOI 10.1007//978-3-319-25552-1_14

© Springer International Publishing Switzerland 2016
R. Navarro et al. (eds.), *Cyberbullying Across the Globe*,
DOI 10.1007/978-3-319-25552-1_12

Certainly not a silver bullet, restorative practices, however, offer hope to curb the cyberbullying epidemic currently existing in the lives of our young people. Restorative practices, unlike criminal justice sanctions or traditional school punishments, work better for this age group because it focuses on repairing harm and moving forward by teaching all involved powerful lessons of empathy and personal discovery.

This chapter will begin with a very brief overview of what cyberbullying is and how often it occurs since other chapters in this book will explore this in more detail. The chapter will then describe the current approaches to addressing the problem including laws and school discipline measures while also exploring the limitations inherent in these approaches. The third section will introduce the reader to the basic principles underlying restorative justice. Finally, the chapter will conclude by providing examples of restorative techniques being used in schools and other settings which appear to make a positive contribution to addressing cyberbullying despite their implementation challenges.

12.2   Part 1: What Is Cyberbullying?

Bullying typically involves a power imbalance with an intent to harass and intimidate over a repeated period of time (U.S. Department of Health & Human Services n.d., a). Cyberbullying is defined as bullying that utilizes technological devices (Cyberbullying n.d.). Because cyberbullying can be done 24 h a day, 7 days a week, and often times is anonymous, it differs significantly from traditional bullying (U.S. Department of Health & Human Services n.d., b). In addition, the permanency of cyberbullying distinguishes it from traditional bullying since posts may be difficult to delete (U.S. Department of Health & Human Services n.d., b). Despite these differences, cyberbullying produces some of the same harmful effects as traditional bullying. These effects manifest themselves in both physical symptoms such as stomachaches, headaches, and other health problems as well as more psychological issues including depression, anxiety, low self-esteem, and suicidal thoughts (Drake et al. 2003, p. 174). Victims of bullying often suffer academically in school or drop out of school, and some may even engage in violence themselves (Nakamoto and Schwartz 2010, p. 221, 234; Townsend et al. 2008, p. 29). Bullying also has detrimental effects on the bully and the bystanders (Copeland et al. 2013). Finally, cyberbullying many times negatively impacts school environments, disrupting the educational mission.

Grasping the true extent of the problem becomes difficult because bullying and cyberbullying remain underreported. In a recent study in Canada, researchers found that teens do not report cyberbullying to their parents for fear of losing their technological devices (MonoNews 2014). Research in other countries likewise shows an underreporting of cyberbullying by children (Kowalski and Limber 2007; Chadwick 2014). Even with underreporting, the cyberbullying statistics cause alarm. The National Crime Victimization Survey conducted in 2009 reported that 6% of the children surveyed or about 1,521,000 experienced cyberbullying (U.S. Department of Education 2011). In a survey 2 years later, 9% of the respondents answered positively to the question concerning cyberbullying, which translates to 2,198,000 children (U.S. Department of Education 2013). Other surveys report even higher numbers, with the Centers for Disease Control and Prevention reporting 14.8% children being cyberbullied in the last year (Centers for Disease Control and Prevention 2014).

These statistics should not be surprising as more and more children and teens use technological devices on a regular basis. Teens more than ever are technologically savvy and active users of technology. Recent surveys show:

- Ninety-five percent use the Internet (Pew Research Internet Project 2012)
- Ninety-three percent have a computer or access to a computer (Madden et al. 2013)
- Seventy-eight percent have a cell phone (Madden et al. 2013)
- Forty-seven percent have smartphones, up from 23% in 2011 (Madden et al. 2013)
- Seventy-five percent text (Pew Research Internet Project 2012)
- Eighty-one percent use some form of social media (Pew Research Internet Project 2012)

As fast as these statistics increase, so too do the types of platforms available for cyberbullying. Teens today often use more than traditional social media sites such as Facebook and gravitate to newer platforms including texting, Twitter, Snapchat, and Instagram. With the technological landscaping changing so quickly, no doubt new formats will be arriving soon providing additional platforms for cyberbullying.

12.3   Part 2: Responses to Cyberbullying

This explosion in types of technology and increased use of it by today's children and teens forces legislators, educators, and parents to play catch up. A review of state cyberbullying and sexting laws and policies show a wide range of approaches (Hinduja and Patchin 2013a, b). Bullying laws now exist in 49 states, with Montana being the sole state with a policy only. The laws vary greatly, with 20 of them specifically including cyberbullying. In addition to state laws, cities and counties impatient with the progress of their states now are passing ordinances aimed at criminalizing cyberbullying (Lueders 2012). Some of these laws require schools to develop anti-bullying policies, often with educational penalties (e.g., suspension), and impose a duty to report bullying incidents to governmental agencies (Hinduja and Patchin 2013a). The policies also may or may not include off-campus behaviors (Hinduja and Patchin 2013a).

The applicability of these laws and policies to off-campus behaviors makes dealing with cyberbullying particularly tricky under the law. Courts usually begin their analysis by discussing the famous Tinker–Fraser–Hazelwood trilogy of student speech cases, which all stand for the proposition that students' freedom of expression rights differ from those same rights for adults. The student First Amendment rights cases show the court's desire to more narrowly interpret what constitutes freedom of expression for students. In large part, whether a student's speech is protected depends on how it is classified. A brief background of three pivotal Supreme Court cases concerning student speech illustrates this point.

In 1969, in the midst of the Vietnam War protest era, the Supreme Court considered the case of *Tinker v. Des Moines Independent Community School District* (Tinker 1969). One junior high and two high school students filed a Section 1983 action after they were sent home and suspended from school until they removed black armbands they were wearing to protest the war (p. 504). No acts of violence or any other disruption in the school occurred because of the students' attire (pp. 509, 514).

In holding for the students, the court formulated a test to be used to determine the constitutionality of an attempt by a school to regulate student speech (p. 509). Restrictions on speech were constitutional only if the school administrators showed that the conduct somehow "materially and substantially interfere[d] with the requirements of appropriate discipline in the operation of the school" (Tinker quoting Burnside 1966, p. 749). The court specifically acknowledged that students had the same rights as other persons under the constitution and were entitled to free expression of their views in the absence of any disorder in the school (p. 511). From this case comes the oft-quoted language of Justice Fortas: "It can hardly be argued that either students or teachers shed their constitutional rights to freedom of speech or expression at the schoolhouse gate" (p. 506).

Less than two decades later, the court seemed to retreat from its earlier protection of student speech. In *Bethel School District v. Fraser*, the court expanded school administrators' authority to regulate student speech (Bethel 1986). A student was disciplined for giving a campaign speech for a fellow classmate that contained lewd language (pp. 677–678). There was no evidence that the speech, heard by 600 students, resulted in any substantial disruption (p. 677). Despite its holding in *Tinker*, the Supreme Court ruled that the First Amendment did not prevent the school administrators from disciplining the student for giving the speech (p. 685). The court carved out an exception to *Tinker* when the student's speech involves the use of vulgar or offensive language at a school-sponsored event (p. 685). Despite the fact that an adult's vulgar or offensive speech is more fully protected by the First Amendment, the court held that schools are not constitutionally required to give student speech the same latitude (p. 682).

In explaining its decision, the court noted that there must be a balance between students' right to advocate unpopular and controversial views and society's countervailing interest in teaching students the boundaries of socially appropriate behavior (p. 681). A school is not only obligated to teach its students academic subjects but also has a duty to teach "by example shared values of a civilized order" (p. 683). Thus, the court held that the school acted appropriately in disciplining the student for his lewd and indecent speech (p. 685).

The last case of the trilogy also conferred on school administrators more power to regulate student speech, even if similar speech could not be regulated outside of school. In *Hazelwood v. Kuhlmeier*, a high school principal prevented the printing of two articles from a student-run newspaper (Hazelwood 1988, p. 264). The first article described students' experiences with pregnancy, and the second article discussed the impact of divorce on students at the school (p. 263). The principal was worried that the articles might identify and embarrass students. He also felt the topic matter was inappropriate (p. 263). In ruling that a First Amendment violation had not occurred, the court held that a school need not tolerate speech that is inconsistent with its educational mission (p. 266). The test, therefore, for regulations that censor student-run newspapers or yearbooks was whether or not the rules "reasonably related to legitimate pedagogical concerns" (p. 273). The court distinguished Tinker, indicating that the Tinker test was not the appropriate test when school-sponsored speech, such as a newspaper, was involved (p. 273).

In summary, Tinker–Fraser–Hazelwood establish three examples in which student speech can be regulated without violating the First Amendment. A school can prohibit speech if it: (1) will cause a material and substantial disruption to the school, (2) is lewd or offensive, or (3) is related to a legitimate pedagogical concern.

In its most recent student speech case, the US Supreme Court continued to allow schools fairly expansive authority to regulate student speech (Morse 2007). In a 5–4 decision, the court upheld an Alaskan school's suspension of a student for holding up a sign with the words, "Bong Hits 4 Jesus" across the street from the school during a school-sanctioned event to watch the Olympic torch relay pass the school (p. 410). The court reasoned that the school's interest in protecting children from drugs justified their regulation of the student's speech and did not violate his First Amendment rights (p. 408). Because the sign could be viewed as promoting illegal drug usage, the school had a legitimate interest in regulating it (pp. 401–402).

In his dissent, Justice Stevens refuses to accept the majority's position that the student's speech promoted illegal drug use instead characterizing it as a "nonsense banner," a "ridiculous sign," and a "silly, nonsensical banner" (pp. 435, 438, and 446). He scolded the majority for engaging in viewpoint discrimination prohibited by the First Amendment for a message that did not advocate drug use (pp. 437–438). He also questioned how speech about drug use could be equated with other speech not protected by the First Amendment including fighting words, obscenity, and commercial speech (p. 446). Instead, he suggests that the better approach is to allow debate and dialogue about "the costs and benefits of the attempt to prohibit the use of marijuana" (p. 448).

Courts struggle when applying these cases to cyberbullying cases because often the speech is occurring off-campus and is not school-sponsored, distinguishing them from the trilogy and Morse. Courts remain unclear whether this speech in cyberbullying cases even meets the definition of school speech and, thus, whether the trilogy speech cases apply at all (Bendlin 2013). Most of the courts' analysis and discussion centers upon whether the geographical distinction of off-campus compared to on-campus speech makes the precedent case law completely inapplicable or does not matter and if a certain nexus must be established first before applying Tinker and the other cases (McDonald 2012, p. 736). The US Supreme Court has not weighed in on this issue yet and declined to hear these three cyberbullying cases: Kowalski v. Berkeley Cnty. Schs., 132 S. Ct. 1095 (2012) (mem.), denying cert. to

652 F.3d 565 (4th Cir. 2011); *Blue Mtn. Sch. Dist. v. J.S. ex rel. Snyder*, 132 S. Ct. 1097 (2012) (mem.), denying cert. to 650 F.3d 915 (3d Cir. 2011) (consolidated pursuant to Supreme Court Rule 12.4 with *Hermitage School District v. Layshock*); and *Doninger v. Niehoff*, 132 S. Ct. 499 (2011) (mem.), denying cert. to 642 F.3d 334 (2d Cir. 2011).

Until the Supreme Court accepts one of these cases, schools must try to decipher the lower court decisions, which appear to go both ways depending if the court finds that a substantial disruption occurred in the educational process or is likely to occur. For example, in *Kowalski V. Berkley County Schools* (2011), the Court upheld the school's 5-day suspension and 90-day "social suspension" of the student for creating a webpage called Students Against Sluts Herpes (S.A.S.H.; p. 3). Several classmates joined the page, and the group intimated that a fellow classmate had herpes (Id.). In finding for the school, the court noted that:

> Rather than respond constructively to the school's efforts to bring order and provide a lesson following the incident, Kowalski has rejected those efforts and sued school authorities for damages and other relief. Regretfully, she yet fails to see that such harassment and bullying is inappropriate and hurtful and that it must be taken seriously by school administrators in order to preserve an appropriate pedagogical environment. Indeed, school administrators are becoming increasingly alarmed by the phenomenon, and the events in this case are but one example of such bullying and school administrators' efforts to contain it. Suffice it to hold here that, where such speech has a sufficient nexus with the school, the Constitution is not written to hinder school administrators' good faith efforts to address the problem (p. 20).

The court also referenced several cases in which other courts found for the schools.

In contrast, other courts rule in favor of the student. For example, the court granted the student's motion for summary judgment on a First Amendment claim in a case involving the posting of a YouTube video that contained mean remarks about a classmate named C.C. (J.C. v. Bevery Hills Unified Sch. Dst. 2010). Comments in the video included such things as calling C.C. a "slut," "spoiled," talking about "boners," and using profanity (p. 1098). One of the participants called C.C. "the ugliest piece of shit I've ever seen in my whole life" (p. 1098). Although the court refused to impose a blanket rule that off campus speech could never be regulated, it still held for the plaintiff because it did not find a substantial disruption occurred at the school even though C. C. missed part of class because she was upset (p. 1117).

Not only do these split decisions cause confusion for school officials on their ability to discipline students, recent litigation also calls into question whether statutes criminalizing cyberbullying can survive a constitutional challenge. In a July 1, 2014 opinion, the New York Court of Appeals answered that question in the negative when reviewing a local law passed by the Albany County Legislature, criminalizing cyberbullying before the state of New York revised its bullying statute to include cyberbullying (People v. Marquan 2014, p. 15). The lawsuit arose from an incident involving a high school student who created a Facebook page, Cohoes Flame, commenting on alleged sexual activities of his classmates (p. 6). When charged under the statute, the student moved to dismiss, claiming the statute violated his First Amendment rights under the Constitution (p. 7). The city court denied his motion, and the county court affirmed, causing the student to appeal (pp. 6–7). On appeal, the student raised the doctrines of vagueness and overbreadth (p. 7). The Court of Appeals first found that cyberbullying could be regulated; however, the drafters made this particular statute too broad sweeping in protected speech and activities (pp. 8, 10). The County in its effort to uphold the law suggested the Court sever the objectionable parts, leaving a very narrow prohibition primarily to postings intending to inflict emotional harm on a child regarding posting of actual or false sexual activities (p. 12). Over a dissent, the majority refused to rewrite the statute for the County, which it classified as an encroachment on the legislative body, although it was sympathetic to the victims (p. 13).

12.4   Part 3: Restorative Justice

Much debate and commentary currently exists surrounding the desirability of criminalizing cyberbullying (Williams 2012). The new statutes and ordinances discussed above reflect a popular sentiment among many in favor of criminalizing this behavior. Frustrated with parental and school responses, advocates for criminalization contend that involving the criminal justice system will deter teens from cyberbullying (Patchin 2014). Not everyone, however, agrees citing concerns over the legality of these laws as well as their limited effectiveness in solving the underlying issues that cause the cyberbullying (Multiple Authors 2014).

Some of the same criticisms regarding the legality and limited effectiveness exist with traditional school disciplinary procedures (Williard 2011, p. 76). Popular during the last two decades as a result of school shootings, zero-tolerance policies have fallen from favor (Benefield 2014). Critics of zero-tolerance policies argue their implementation results in harsh consequences that make students less likely to remain in school. As a result of zero-tolerance policies, students may be expelled, suspended, or opt to drop out in frustration. Statistics illustrate that a link exists between suspensions and expulsions and the prison system (Curtis 2014; Brown 2013). Evidence also exists showing a disparate impact of these policies on minority populations (Hoffman 2014). Most educators agree that excluding students negatively impacts their academic achievement, rates of graduation, and future prospects.

Interestingly, in a footnote, the Court in the recent New York case offered "no opinion on whether cyberbullying should be a crime or whether there are more effective means of addressing this societal problem outside the criminal justice system" (People v. Marquan 2014, p. 9). Restorative justice very well may be a more effective means of addressing cyberbullying because it avoids the current legal uncertainties present with the criminal statutes and the disciplinary codes. In addition, restorative practices produce the added benefits of higher victim satisfaction, better education of the offender as well as involvement of bystanders and supporters.

Restorative practices offer an alternative approach to addressing conflict. The traditional punitive model focuses on punishing the person for the wrong they com-

mitted (Zehr 2002, p. 21). In contrast, the restorative approach centers upon relationships and not the wrong itself (Id.). Instead of punishing a wrongdoer, restorative practices involve exploring what harm occurred and how that harm can be
repaired (Id.). The emphasis is much more on individuals including the person who
caused the harm, the person who was harmed, and the supporters and community of
both of these individuals (pp. 14–18).

Restorative practices are nothing new. These practices originated in almost all
original societies. Aboriginal people in many countries around the world dealt with
conflict in their societies using restorative practices, although not to the exclusion of
retributive practices (Mulligan 2009, pp. 145–148; Johnstone 2002, pp. 47–48). Examples of these restorative practices can be found with Native Americans (Yazzie
and Zion 1996, p. 160, 171) in their peace circles, as well as the practices of native people in New Zealand (Pratt 1996, pp. 138–139) and Canada (Griffiths and
Hamilton 1996, pp. 175–192). These early inhabitants as well as religious traditions now inform the present day movement for restorative practices (Zehr 2005,
pp. 126–157). A belief that all people are valuable and necessary parts of the community underlies each of these traditions. Ancient communities could not afford to
remove one of its members for prolonged periods of time, so the conflict needed to
be resolved to reincorporate the member back into the fold.

Restorative practices can take on many shapes and forms, but family group conferencing would work the best for resolving cyberbullying incidents (National Institute of Justice 2007). Family group conferencing involves bringing together all the
parties to a conflict as well as their supporters to discuss the harm that has resulted
from the deed and then together develop a plan for repairing that harm. Trained facilitators conduct preconference meetings to prepare the participants for the actual
conference (Wachtel et al. 2010, pp. 190–197). Typically, the person causing the
harm along with his or her supporters as well as the person who was harmed and
his or her supporters attend. In addition, sometimes members of the community
may also attend (pp. 186–190). For example, in a school setting, teachers, coaches,
and administrators might be part of the circle since actions between two students
often cause ripple effects throughout a school. The facilitator takes the participants
through questions which seek to illicit what happened and how it impacts the people
at the conference (pp. 165–168). The person causing the harm usually starts by
describing what happened, what he or she was thinking about, and how it impacted
the people in the circle. Everyone has an opportunity to speak, and the facilitator
manages the discussion to avoid attacks on the person since the goal is to discuss
the harm and its impact (p. 207).

The second half of the conference focuses on the group brainstorming about
what the person causing the harm can do to make things right (pp. 216–218). All
participants can offer suggestions, and the group ultimately comes to a consensus.
While the facilitator drafts the agreement, the participants "break bread" together
(p. 219). This helps the healing process begin immediately for everyone involved
in the process.

A central value underlying restorative practices revolves around accountability
(McCold 1996, p. 87). A conference only occurs if the person causing the harm

admits fault and accepts responsibility for his or her actions. Facilitators will not conduct a conference unless all the participants willingly participate (Wachtel et al. 2010, p. 180). Mandatory conferences would not be effective and should never be held.

Current research identifies multiple benefits of restorative practices as compared to the traditional punitive model used by schools and the criminal justice system (Sherman and Strange 2007, p. 4). Studies show high outcome measures for victim satisfaction, offender satisfaction, restitution compliance, and recidivism (Bradshaw et al. 2006, p. 89). These benefits impact not only victims but offenders and bystanders and community members as well. Victims appreciate restorative practices because unlike traditional court proceedings, victims feel empowered with this process. Instead of the state taking over their cases, victims in restorative practices get to express their feelings directly to the person that caused them harm, as well as get their questions answered (Ministry of Justice, Module 1 2009, p. 6). People incorrectly assume that all victims want retribution and harsh punishments. Many victims also need restitution, validation of their feelings, and assurances that this will not occur again (Ministry of Justice, Module 2 2009, p. 5).

When victims hear the offender's side of the story, often it will change how they feel about the incident and the offender. Many conferences include moments of transformation between the parties (Vogel 2007, p. 576). Often, people arrive at the conference very angry but as it progresses, they begin to feel sympathy and even forgiveness. The healing process might be accelerated for victims because the discussions also lead to results that they prefer since they have input into what the offender will do to make things right.

Finally, victims want to feel safe going forward. Punishments meted out by the courts or school officials do little to ensure victims that the harm will not be repeated. The punishments may actually make an offender angrier and wanting to seek revenge, creating more apprehension for the victim (Ahmed and Braithwaite 2006, p. 353). Restorative practices allow victims the opportunity to get assurances that they will not be revictimized by the offender. Victim satisfaction numbers are high with restorative practices for all of these reasons.

Offenders also benefit from restorative practices. Specifically, conferences may build empathy in offenders. By forcing offenders to listen to the people they harmed including not only the victim but their supporters, often offenders gain new insights into the impact their behavior has on others. Traditional court proceedings offer little opportunity for offenders to reflect on the hurt they caused because no face-to-face discussion is happening with all the affected parties. The offenders often feel shame during the conferences. This shame is very different from the stigmatizing shame they experience in normal legal proceedings. John Braithwaite explains the difference between stigmatizing shame and reintegrative shame in his book *Crime Shame and Reintegration* (1989) and shows the value of shame in the entire process.

Opponents of restorative practices often mistakenly believe family group conferencing is too soft on crime (Mulligan 2009, p. 140). Anyone attending a conference can attest that these sessions are anything but that. Forcing the offender to sit across from the person he harmed and listen to their stories can be extremely difficult and uncomfortable for the child (Sanders 2008, f.n.61). Often, a free flow of emotions occurs during the conference, which rarely happens in a traditional court or school setting. Restorative practices also offer the offender a way to reintegrate back into society. Unlike typical punishments that ostracize the offenders and exclude them from the community, restorative practices look for ways to help offenders make amends and repair the harm they caused.

This opportunity to grow would seem particularly beneficial since cyberbullying involves mostly young people. We know now from research that human brains are not fully developed even at adolescence and in fact continue to develop throughout a person's twenties. Before a brain reaches full maturity, a person may not have mastered "complex cognitive tasks such as inhibition, high-level functioning and attention" (Human brain development does not stop at adolescence 2011). Often, adults wonder what a child is thinking, but the truth is that a child's brain does not allow for the advanced thought process of an older person. Instead of punishing children for impulsive, not well-thought-out behavior, perhaps, society should select a process that can educate the child and help the child develop social competencies. Restorative practices do not excuse the behavior but seek to help the child understand why the behavior is unacceptable.

This focus on teaching and developing a person aligns perfectly with goals of the educational system. Although not all people might agree, many educators and members of the public trust schools to educate students not only in academic subjects but also in character development (Lickona 1991, p. 22). Schools should teach and promote respect and responsibility as two critical values (p. 43). Respect and responsibility are the cornerstones of restorative practices. Engaging in family group conferencing develops these values in children much better than punishments do.

Supporters and community members also benefit because they play an integral role in the process, which rarely happens in other settings. Restorative practices can help ameliorate the very negative effects bystanders experience with bullying and cyberbullying. In addition, the supporters, in particular, play an important role with the offender because the shame offenders experience comes primarily from disappointing the people they are closest to and love the most, and they respond more readily to disapproval of their family and friends (Johnstone 2002, p. 101).

12.5   Part 4: Restorative Practices and Cyberbullying

Juvenile justice professionals engaged in restorative practices well before the schools started to use them. Now many schools utilize restorative practices as part of their tools in their toolboxes for dealing with behavior issues. Using restorative practices to combat bullying and cyberbullying makes perfect sense because "[b]ullying and restorative justice have a serendipitous fit; in that, bullying has been defined as the systemic abuse of power and restorative justice seeks to transform power imbalances that affect social relationships" (Morrison 2006, p. 372). Restorative principles fulfill schools' missions of educating students not just in subject matter areas but also for citizenship, which includes "shared values of a civilized social order" (Bethel 1986, pp. 675, 681, 683).

Recognizing the value of restorative practices, the US Department of Education and Department of Justice in a recent Dear Colleague Letter on the Nondiscriminatory Administration of School Discipline specifically recommend the use of restorative practices (Department of Justice 2014). The letter encourages schools to develop programs that "(1) reduce disruption and misconduct; (2) support and reinforce positive behavior and character development; and (3) help students succeed" (Department of Justice 2014). The Public Broadcasting Service (PBS) recently profiled a Colorado school district that uses restorative practices instead of more traditional discipline measures (Newshour 2013). Administrators found the number of incidents of defiance, disobedience, and use of profanity all declined after the integration of restorative practices in the school. During the 2007–2008 school year, 263 physical altercations occurred at the school, which dropped to 31 once restorative practices replaced suspensions and other disciplinary methods. Staff interviewed observed that practices help resolve conflict and displace anger unlike traditional discipline measures, which only add to a child's anger.

Many more examples exist throughout the USA and the world of schools using restorative practices specifically to address bullying and cyberbullying. Schools using restorative practices find they lead to an improved school climate. For example, the researchers conducting a recent study involving four schools in Brazil found restorative practices lead to "a healthier and peaceful school environment" (Grossi and dos Stantos 2012, p. 134).

In the Brazilian study, teachers and professionals from the selected schools underwent training on restorative practices before implementing them in the classroom. When conflicts arose, these teachers formed restorative circles attended by school administrators, teachers, the students involved and their family, as well as anyone else who chose to participate (p. 127). Most of these circles dealt with issues of bullying (p. 132). These circles addressed and solved conflicts using a democratic decision-making process. The study found that after these communal gatherings, the participant's rate of satisfaction was around 80 %, which the authors of the study attributed to the fact that everyone involved had something to gain from the agreement (p. 133). At the conclusion of the study, the schools involved experienced "reductions in behavior referrals to the principal's officers and in suspensions" (p. 133). Additionally, teachers reported positive feelings surrounding restorative circles. The implementation of restorative practices in these schools positively affected discipline at the schools and the overall well-being of the participants.

Research conducted by the International Institute of Restorative Practices likewise found a positive correlation between the use of restorative practices and school climate (International Institute of Restorative Practices 2009). Their report looks at experiences of six schools in the USA (West Philadelphia High School, Pottstown High School, Newtown Middle School, Palisades High School, Palisades Middle School, and Springfield Township High School) and two schools in both Canada (Kawartha Pine Ridge District School Board and Keewatin Patricia District Board School) and England (Bessels Leigh School (now Parklands Campus) and Hull).

Not all of the findings reported come from formal research studies but instead show a snapshot of various data collected by the schools. Quotes included from some of the community in the highlighted schools speak louder than any statistics or data could. Participants voiced the following opinions:

- "I used to get in a lot of trouble, but teachers talk to students and help you make the right decisions here. In homeroom we sit in a circle and talk about anything that needs to be brought up."
- Eighth-grade girl, Palisades Middle School, Kintnersville, PA, USA
- "When I first took over this school it was in 'Special Measures' and at risk of being shut down. Restorative practices helped it achieve 'Outstanding' status—the best it can possibly be."
- Estelle MacDonald, head teacher, Collingwood Primary School, Hull, England, UK

Qualitative data confirms and supports the views of the students, teachers, and administrators concerning the benefits of restorative practices.

Over and over, principals and teachers at the schools who participated in the International Institute of Restorative Practices research reported a before and after restorative practices culture at the school. The before culture is repeatedly characterized as a climate in which students felt disconnected from the school and the teachers, frequently with an "us verse them" feeling between the students and authority (pp. 9, 14, 27). Many of the school administrators reported that the climate was "discourteous and disrespectful and altercations were common" (p. 17). After the implementation of restorative practices, all the schools describe students and teachers feeling a greater sense of community (pp. 19, 27). Many of the schools commented that relationships between students and teachers improved. Most elucidative were the significant reductions in disciplinary actions in all the schools that participated in the study. School administrators frequently attributed this drop in misbehavior to students taking increased ownership in their behavior after seeing how their actions impacted others (p. 34).

School districts seeking to use restorative practices with cyberbullying might find the following school districts to be models or helpful resources.

12.5.1 Wright County, MN

A middle school in Minnesota utilized restorative practices after students distributed by cell phone sexually explicit photographs of a classmate found on her boyfriend's phone (Riestenberg 2014). Working collaboratively, school officials, court personnel, the county attorney, and the sheriff's office developed a protocol for handling sexting cases. This included holding a restorative group conference to resolve this incident. The conference included nearly 40 people including the students, parents, school administrators, and individuals representing law enforcement and the criminal justice system. This process has been repeated with over 200 students involved in sexting incidents.

Participants find the process extremely effective. Brian Stoll, a Wright County probation officer, supported using restorative practices for a number of reasons including that it made the child accountable but also provided a way to repair the harm without damaging his future. He also appreciated the opportunity for all people impacted by the incident to have a voice in the process.

12.5.2 Kawartha Pine Ridge District School Board, Peterborough, ON

This Canadian school district publishes a pamphlet providing cyberbullying information for parents (Kawartha Pine Ridge School District 2011). The pamphlet specifically informs parents that the school may use restorative practices when responding to cyberbullying incidents.

The principal also may recommend that the person causing harm, the individual harmed, witnesses, and families participate in a restorative circle. The person causing harm will be able to hear how the actions have affected others, will be encouraged to take responsibility for his or her actions, and will be supported to make things right. Restorative practice works only if all parties agree to and support the process. It should not proceed if the person causing harm has not accepted responsibility, the person harmed does not want to participate in it, or there is potential for further harm. It does not replace other consequences, such as suspension.

Cyberbullying requires a community approach because schools need the assistance of parents since schools do not have access to the various technological devices children use (Rockhill n.d.). Involving students, parents, and school officials in holding a child responsible for his or her actions and helping decide the consequences a student should face remains a superior option than other forms of discipline because it eliminates concerns over the legality of school officials' or law enforcements' actions (Siris 2013).

Although restorative practices hold much promise, some legitimate barriers do exist. First, restorative practices will not be appropriate for every situation. Conferences should not be held if the person who caused the harm refuses to be accountable for the actions or if danger exists of revictimizing the victim. Some may argue that the danger of revictimization would be high in a bullying situation since the very definition of bullying involves a power imbalance. They fear putting the bully and the target in the same room would be counterproductive and would only allow another venue for the bully to continue terrorizing the target (Christensen 2008). Family group conferencing with its multiple participants and trained facilitator lessens the risk as compared to a victim–offender mediation. In addition, if the supporters will not participate, it may be more difficult to conduct a conference, although surrogate representatives can sometimes fill the gaps. The preconference work with the participants becomes essential to vet out these issues in advance.

Restorative justice practices in domestic violence scenarios have faced similar criticisms concerning victim safety. Both domestic violence scenarios and bullying involve a relative power imbalance between the victim and the offender. Some studies have shown that restorative justice programs could put domestic violence victims at higher risk for reabuse (Kohn 2010, p. 573). However, victim–offender conferences in South Africa, youth justice care and protection family group conferences in New Zealand, and several programs in the USA offer restorative practices in domestic violence cases with measurable success (p. 576). In the South African victim–offender conferences, "[m]ost victims reported that they felt safe" (p. 574). Similarly, in the New Zealand youth justice and family group conference program, researchers studying the restorative interventions "reported that safety risks at conferences" were "negligible to nonexistent" (p. 575). Proponents of the use of restorative practices in domestic violence situations look to these positive examples as indicative of the possibility of more widespread use. Positive examples of restorative practices safe use in domestic violence scenarios indicate that in bullying cases, putting the bully and the target in the same restorative circle may be done safely.

Other concerns with restorative practices, whether it originates from the criminal justice system or the schools, include concerns about cost and time. Costs include someone to spearhead the program as well as the cost of training facilitators and possibly paying the facilitators. Several models of funding can be used including governmental funds as well as private donations from individuals as well as foundations. The Denver Foundation helped sponsor the project in the Aurora school district spotlighted by PBS. In Louisville, KY, funds come from anonymous donors, which match individual gifts as well as foundations such as the Kentucky Bar Foundation and the Gheens Foundation. In addition, Restorative Justice Louisville (RJL) hopes to secure a line item in the city's and state's budget.

Groups interested in starting restorative practices initiatives may want to calculate how much restorative practices cost compared to more traditional discipline methods. RJL crafted the chart below to illustrate how much money could be saved using a restorative justice approach. The court costs include data from various offices within the system including the sheriff, Department of Juvenile Justice (DJJ), the judge, court-designated workers, police, prosecutor, and public defender. These offices submitted a calculation of their average time spent on a case multiplied by their rate of pay. This chart does not even begin to quantify the savings of breaking the school to prison pipeline over the life of an individual.

12.5.2.1 Cost Analysis

Juvenile justice system costs per case

		h	Costs
Total	Court costs with probation	130	$3166.00
Total	Costs with placement in DJJ facility	180 days at $270 per day	$48,600

DJJ Department of Juvenile Justice

Restorative justice costs

		h	Costs
Total	RJL	23.75	$869.68
Total	RJL with court costs	28.7	$1014.00

RJL Restorative Justice Louisville

	ALS	Cost per day	Total
Secure detention	16	$250.00	$4,000.00

ALS average length of stay

Pretrial probation

	ALS	Cost per day	Total
HIP	32	$50.00	$1600.00
HSP	34	$40.00	$1360.00
APS	12	$182.00	$2184.00

HIP Home Incarceration Program
HSP Home Supervision Program
APS Alternative Placement Services
Based on 2012 average length of stay (ALS) in days

Lost instructional time

	Days lost	Instructional minutes per day	Total instructional minutes lost
Court process	6	370	2220
Referral to RJL	2	370	740

RJL Restorative Justice Louisville

Cost of lost instructional days

	Days lost	Cost	Total
Court process	6	$21.00	$126.00
Referral to RJL	2	$21.00	$42.00

RJL Restorative Justice Louisville

Allocation of time for restorative practices must also be compared with the savings it creates when schools or communities reduce the number of future harmful incidents. Although facilitating a conference may require a more substantial outlay of time compared to suspension or incarcerating a person, the benefits far outweigh the burdens. With restorative practices, the group addresses the underlying issues which hopefully can lead to a better result long term.

In addition, restorative justice practices take a fair amount of time when one considers not only the actual time devoted to a conference but also the time it takes to train facilitators and complete the preconference tasks. Other ways of addressing cyberbullying, however, also take time. Schools must spend time executing their disciplinary codes, and the courts spend time adjudicating disputes. The real question should be which time is better spent. In the long run, unpacking and addressing the core underlying issues will produce more permanent positive results, ultimately saving time.

12.6   Conclusion

Restorative practices may not be the cure-all for the cyberbullying issue, but it certainly holds great promise for many cases. Restorative practices avoid the legal pitfalls and uncertainties currently associated with cyberbullying statutes and school policies prohibiting cyberbullying. Even if those laws and policies could pass constitutional muster, restorative practices produce a better result because they involve the person who was harmed and educate and develop the person who caused the harm. Supporters and bystanders also contribute to the process and benefit from it. Policy-makers, school officials, and parents should focus on solving the underlying issues that spurred the cyberbullying through dialogue allowed by restorative practices instead of defaulting to a punishment only regime.

References

(23 September 2011). Human brain development does not stop at adolescence. *Medical News*. http://www.news-medical.net/news/20110923/Human-brain-development-does-not-stop-at-adolescence-Research.aspx.

Ahmed, E., & Braithwaite, V. (2006). Forgiveness, reconciliation, and shame: Three key variables in reducing school bullying. *Journal of Social Issues, 62*(2), 347–370. doi:10.1111/j.1540-4560.2006.00454.x.

Bazelon, E. (15 January 2014). The Online Avengers. *The New York Times*. http://www.nytimes.com/2014/01/19/magazine/the-online-avengers.html.

Bendlin, S. S. (2013). When is it "school speech" and when is it beyond the school's reach? *Northeastern University Law Journal, 5*, 47–76.

Bethel Sch. Dist. v. Fraser. (1986). 478 U.S. 675.

Benefield, K. (17 June 2014). Automatic suspensions falling out of favor in California. *Petaluma 360*. http://www.petaluma360.com/news/2000591-181/automatic-suspensions-falling-out-of.

Bradshaw, W., Roseborough, D., & Umbreit, M. S. (2006). The effect of victim offender mediation on juvenile offender recidivism: A meta-analysis. *Conflict Resolution Quarterly, 24*, 87–98. doi:10.1002/crq.159.

Braithwaite, J. (1989). *Crime, shame and reintegration*. Cambridge: Cambridge University Press. doi:10.1017/CBO9780511804618.

Brown, P. L. (3 April 2013). Opening up, students transform a vicious circle. *New York Times*. http://www.nytimes.com/2013/04/04/education/restorative-justice-programs-take-root-in-schools.html?pagewanted=all.

Burnside, v. Byars. (1966) 363 F.2d 744 (5th Cir. 1966).

Centers for Disease Control and Prevention. (2014). *Youth risk behavior surveillance—United States, 2013*. http://www.cdc.gov/mmwr/pdf/ss/ss6304.pdf.

Chadwick, S. (2014). *Impacts of in cyberbullying, building social and emotional resilience school.* New York: Springer. doi:10.1007/978-3-319-04031-8.

Christensen, L. (2008). Sticks, stones, and schoolyard bullies: Restorative justice, mediation and a new approach to conflict resolution in our schools. *Selected works of Leah Christensen.* http://works.bepress.com/leah_Christensen/7.

Copeland, W., Wolke, D., Angold, A., & Costello. E. J. (2013). Adult psychiatric outcomes of bullying and being bullied by peers in childhood and adolescence. *JAMA Psychiatry, 70,* 419–426. doi:10.1001/jamapsychiatry.2013.504.

Curtis, A. (2014). Tracing the school-to-prison pipeline from zero-tolerance policies to juvenile justice dispositions. *Georgetown Law Journal, 102,* n.p. http://www.lexisnexis.com/hottopics/lnacademic/?verb=sr&csi=7337&sr=TITLE(Tracing+the+School-to-Prison+Pipeline+from+Zero-Tolerance+Policies+to+Juvenile+Justice+Dispositions)%2B-AND%2BDATE%2BIS%2B2014.

Cyberbullying. (n.d.). http://www.merriam-webster.com/dictionary/cyberbullying.

Department of Justice & Department of Education. (8 January 2014). Joint dear colleague letter on the non-discriminatory administration of justice. http://www2.ed.gov/about/offices/list/ocr/letters/colleague-201401-title-vi.html.

Drake, J. A., Price, J. H., & Telljohann, S. K. (2003). The nature and extent of bullying at school. *Journal of School Health, 73,* 173–180. doi:10.1111/j.1746-1561.2003.tb03599.x.

Grossi, P. K., & dos Santos, A. M. (2012). Bullying in Brazilian schools and restorative practices. *Canadian Journal of Education, 35*(1), 120–136.

Griffiths, C. T., & Hamilton, R. (1996). Sanctioning and healing: restorative justice in Canadian aboriginal communities. In B. Galaway & J. Hudson (Eds.), *Restorative justice international perspectives* (pp. 175–192). Monsey: Criminal Justice Press. doi:10.1080/01924036.1996.9678572

Hazelwood, v. Kuhlmeier. (1988). 484 U.S. 260.

Hinduja, S., & Patchin, J. (2013a). State bullying and cyberbullying laws. *Cyberbullying Research Center.* http://cyberbullying.org/Bullying-and-Cyberbullying-Laws.pdf.

Hinduja, S., & Patchin, J. (2013b). State sexting laws. *Cyberbullying Research Center.* http://cyberbullying.org/state-sexting-laws.pdf.

Hoffman, S. (2014). Zero benefit: Estimating the effect of zero tolerance discipline policies on racial disparities in school discipline. *Educational Policy, 28,* 69–95. http://epx.sagepub.com/content/28/1/69.full.pdf+html.

International Institute of Restorative Practices. (2009). *Improving school climate. Findings from schools implementing restorative practices, IIRP.* http://www.iirp.edu/pdf/IIRP-Improving-School-Climate.pdf.

J.C. v. Beverly Hills Unified Sch. Dist. (2010). 711 F. Supp. 2d 1094 (C.D. Cal. 2010).

Johnstone, G. (2002). *Restorative justice: Ideas, values, debates.* Devon: Willan Publishing.

Kawartha Pine Ridge District School Board. (November 2011). *Cyberbullying information for parents.* http://eastnorthumberland.kprdsb.ca/cyberbullying.pdf.

Kohn, L. (2010). What's so funny about peace, love, and understanding? Restorative justice as a new paradigm for domestic violence intervention. *Seton Hall Law Review, 40,* 517–595.

Kowalski, R. M., & Limber, S. P. (2007). Electronic bullying among middle school students. *Journal of Adolescent Health, 41* (Suppl), S22–S30. doi:10.1016/j.jadohealth.2007.08.017.

Kowalski v. Berkeley County Schs. (2011). No. 10-1098, 2011 WL 3132523 (4th Cir. July 27, 2011). http://pacer.ca4.uscourts.gov/opinion.pdf/101098.P.pdf.

Lickona, T. (1991). *Educating for character: How our schools can teach respect and responsibility.* New York: Bantam Books.

Lueders, B. (11 November 2012). Vernon county ordinance targets cyber bullying. *Wisconsin State Journal.* http://host.madison.com/news/state_and_regional/vernon-county-ordinance-targets-cyber-bullying/article_58ef6248-2c0c-11e2-a1cd-001a4bcf887a.html.

Madden, M., Lenhart, A., Duggan, M., Cortesi, S., & Gossen, S. (2013). *Teens and technology 2013.* Pew research internet project. http://www.pewinternet.org/2013/03/13/teens-and-technology-2013/.

McCold, P. (1996). Restorative justice and the role of the community. In B. Galaway, & J. Hudson (Eds.), *Restorative justice: International perspectives* (pp. 85–102). Monsey: Criminal Justice Press.

McDonald, B. P. (2012). Regulating student cyberspeech. *Missouri Law Review, 77*, 727–759.

Ministry of Justice. (July 2009). Restorative justice facilitator induction training: Trainee module. http://www.justice.govt.nz/policy/criminal-justice/restorative-justice/restorative-justice-information-for-providers/documents/copy_of_MODULE-1-for-internet_1.pdf.

MonoNews. (9 July 2014). Survey reveals half of Canadian parents believe their kids could be cyberbullying others. http://www.mononews.ca/news/4292/survey-reveals-half-of-canadian-parents-believe-their-kids-could-be-cyberbullying-others.

Morrison, B. (2006). School bullying and restorative justice: Toward a theoretical understanding of the role of respect, pride, and shame. *Journal of Social Issues, 62*, 371–392. doi:10.1111/j.1540-4560.2006.00455.x.

Morse, v. Frederick. (2007). 551 U.S. 393.

Mulligan, S. (2009). From retribution to repair: Juvenile justice and the history of restorative justice. *University of La Verne Law Review, 31*, 139–148.

Multiple Authors. (2 April 2014). A gut check, please, on the Safe and Supportive School Act. *Minnesota StarTribune.* http://www.startribune.com/opinion/commentaries/253648041.html.

Nakamoto, J., & Schwartz, D. (2010). Is peer victimization associated with academic achievement? A meta-analytic review. *Social Development, 19*, 221–242. doi:10.1111/j.1467-9507.2009.00539.x.

National Institute of Justice. (2007). Family group conferencing. Resource document. *United States Department of Justice.* http://nij.gov/topics/courts/restorative-justice/promising-practices/Pages/family-group-conferencing.aspx.

National Women's Law Center. (2013). NWLC join title IX lawsuit against Michigan Public School for failing to address student's sexual assault. http://www.nwlc.org/press-release/nwlc-joins-title-ix-lawsuit-against-michigan-public-school-failing-address-students-se.

Newshour. (20 February 2014). To curb conflict a Colorado High School replaces punishment with conversation. *PBS.* http://www.pbs.org/newshour/bb/new-approach-discipline-school/.

Patchin, J. W. (2014). The criminalization of cyberbullying. http://cyberbullying.us/criminalization-of-cyberbullying/.

People v. Marquan M. (2014). _ N.E.3d _ N.Y. Slip Op. 04881 (N.Y. Ct. of Appeals. July, 1, 2014).

Pew Research Internet Project. (2012). Teens fact sheet. http://www.pewinternet.org/fact-sheets/teens-fact-sheet/.

Pratt, J. (1996). Colonization, power and silence: A history of indigenous justice in New England Society. In B. Galaway & J. Hudson (Eds.), *Restorative justice: International perspectives* (pp. 137–156). Monsey: Criminal Justice Press.

Riestenberg, N. (4 March 2014). Restorative group conferencing and sexting: Repairing harm in Wright County. *Cyberbullying Research Center.* http://cyberbullying.us/restorative-group-conferencing-and-sexting/.

Rockhill, J. (n.d.). Stopping cyber bullying requires a community effort. *Youth Service Bureau.* http://www.ysb.net/stopcyberbullying.aspx.

Sanders, L. C. (2008). Restorative justice: The attempt to rehabilitate criminal offenders and victims. *Charleston Law Review, 2*, 923–937.

Sherman, L., & Strange, H. (2007). Restorative justice: The evidence. *The Smith Institute.* http://www.restorativejustice.org/10fulltext/restorative-justice-the-evidence.

Siris, K. (2013). Out of school behaviors: A principal's responsibility. *Albany Law Journal of Science and Technology, 22*, 605–610.

Snider, B. (2014). Parents seek 1M from school after bullied boy's suicide. *FindLaw.* http://blogs.findlaw.com/injured/2014/07/parents-seek-1m-from-school-after-bullied-boys-suicide.html.

Tinker, v. Des Moines Independent Community School District. (1969). Des Moines Independent Community School District 393 U.S. 503.

Townsend, L., Flisher, A., Chikobvu, P., Lombard, C., & King, G. (2008). The relationship between bullying behaviours and high school dropout in Cape Town, South Africa. *South African Journal of Psychology, 38*, 21–32. doi:10.1177/008124630803800102.

U.S. Department of Education. (2011). Student reports of bullying and cyberbullying: Results from the 2009 School Crime Supplement to the National Crime Victimization Survey. http:// nces.ed.gov/pubs2011/2011336.pdf.

U.S. Department of Education. (2013). Student reports of bullying and cyberbullying: Results from the 2011 School Crime Supplement to the National Crime Victimization Survey. http:// nces.ed.gov/pubs2013/2013329.pdf.

U.S. Department of Health & Human Services. (n.d., a). What is bullying? http://stopbullying.gov/ topics/what_is_bullying/index.html.

U.S. Department of Health & Human Services. (n.d., b). What is cyberbullying? http://www.stop-bullying.gov/cyberbullying/what-is-it/.

Vogel, H. J. (2007). The restorative justice wager: The promise and hope of a value-based, dia-logue-driven approach to conflict resolution for social healing. *Cardoza Journal of Conflict Resolution, 8*, 565–609.

Wachtel, T., O'Connell, T., & Wachtel, B. (2010). *Restorative justice conferencing*. Pipersville: The Piper's Press.

Williams, J. L. (2012). Teens, sexts & cyberspace: The constitutional implications of current sex-ting & cyberbullying law. *William & Mary Bill of Rights Journal, 20*, 1017–1050.

Williard, N. (2011). School response to cyberbullying and sexting: The legal challenges. *Brigham Young University Education & Law Journal*, 75–125. http://heinonline.org/HOL/ Page?handle=hein.journals/byuelj2011&div=7&g_sent=1&collection=journals#77.

Yazzie, R., & Zion, J. (1996). Navajo restorative justice: The law of equality and justice. In B. Galaway, & J. Hudson (Eds.), *Restorative justice: International perspectives* (pp. 157–176). Monsey: Criminal Justice Press.

Zehr, H. (2002). *The little book of restorative justice*. Intercourse: Good Books.

Zehr, H. (2005). Covenant justice: The Biblical alternative. In H. Zehr (Ed.), *Changing lenses: A new focus for crime and justice* (pp. 126–157). Scottdale: Herald Press.

Chapter 13
Reading and Texts: Cyberbullying Prevention from Child and Youth Literature

Santiago Yubero, Elisa Larrañaga, Sandra Sánchez-García
and Cristina Cañamares

13.1 Literature As a Socio-educational Tool

Literature promotes an integrated approach to education and fits perfectly in the current concept of education in society. Books present scenarios, situations, contexts, and persons that are not very different from those of our own reality. Literary texts that present different social or cultural conflicts enable readers to understand that other people went through similar situations before them. Literature is not an aseptic thing; quite the contrary, it has intentionality and expresses feelings, concerns, circumstances, and ideologies. Literary texts have a series of elements through which authors show the world to us, intending to motivate our ability to reflect on and construe things. Books offer materials suitable for reflection and analysis, allowing readers to exercise decision-making and problem-solving (Yubero and Larrañaga 2011, 2014). Reading contributes to rebuild oneself against any loss affecting the meaning of life; it is a common experience that has been described by many authors (e.g., Petit 2008).

Readers can, no doubt, identify with situations described in the story and turn them into vicarious experiences, able to guide their attitudes and behaviors. We can immerse ourselves in the characters' lives and identify with them. This empathy process enables to understand the characters' problems and critically analyze their behaviors. Obviously, the power of literary texts to make readers experience emotions, to present different situations and behaviors to them, and even to get them to face their fears and concerns, makes reading a privileged instrument for

S. Yubero (✉)
Department of Psychology, Faculty of Education and Humanities, University of Castilla-La Mancha, 16071 Cuenca, Spain
e-mail: santiago.yubero@uclm.es

E. Larrañaga
Department of Psychology, Faculty of Social Work, University of Castilla-La Mancha, Camino del Pozuelo s/n., 16071 Cuenca, Spain

S. Sánchez-García · C. Cañamares
Department of Philology, University of Castilla-La Mancha, Cuenca, Spain

© Springer International Publishing Switzerland 2016
R. Navarro et al. (eds.), *Cyberbullying Across the Globe,*
DOI 10.1007/978-3-319-25552-1_13

259

intervention. For this reason, novels notably contribute to moral education of readers (Wollheim 1983). Telling and reading stories have been part of the learning ritual of social values very often. Therefore, the stories we were told in our childhood, those we were told subsequently, and those read by ourselves throughout our maturity process have contributed to construct ourselves as persons. It could be stated that most readings have played a key role in our development as persons, closely linked to the learning process of social values of our culture, helping us to integrate into society.

Books for children and young people can be a channel of socialization and cultural transmission, broadening dialog between children and society. When readers immerse themselves in texts, they create a mental picture of the story, get to identify with the characters and situations and can emotionally empathize with the text (Jauss 1982; Beach 1993). The events that take place throughout the story and the characters that come to life through words become vicarious experiences that may have an impact in the way our attitudes and behaviors are geared, besides influencing our own moral judgments (Borgia and Myers 2010). The role models represented by the characters of the texts become the focus of literary communicative interaction thanks to the processes of empathy or identification with the characters and their vicissitudes within the world of fiction (Jauss 1982). The different association relationships created between readers and characters[1] from complex psychological processes make possible to recognize and imitate the values that are represented. The socializing power of stories lies in their emotional power, in their ability to present our own fears, feelings, and internal conflicts. The experiences conveyed by books allow us to live other lives, to identify with other persons or reject them, to know different scenarios and times, to face multiple conflicts, to explore our relationships against them, and to take certain criteria or stands.

Some authors such as Iser (1978) and Rosenblatt (1977) dealt with the power of poetic language and literary texts to build reality, identifying the linguistic sign as an element of aesthetical stimulus. Texts intend to stimulate the interpreter's personal reality in a specific way, so that he/she conveys a deep response about the world around him/her from his/her inner self. The metaphorical power of words and their permanent distancing effect provide readers with a renewed, vigilant view of reality, making him/her question himself/herself critically and efficiently about the existence of real things.

On the basis of Reception Theories of Iser (1978) and Jauss (1982) as well as from Rosenblatt's Transactional Theory (1977), the meaning of texts lies in the reader, who creates the meaning through the text's guidance and his/her own expe-

---

[1] Jauss (1982) also has a scheme for describing identification on five levels of response to the hero. This response may be: (1) *associative* when the audience assumes a role in the closed, imaginary world of a play action; (2) *admiring* when the model has a perfection beyond tragic or comic; (3) *sympathetic*, when the audience projects itself into an alien self and eliminates distance in favor of solidarity with the suffering hero; (4) *cathartic*, when the audience is freed from the real interests and entanglements of its world and finds liberation through tragic emotion or comic relief; and (5) *ironic* when the identification is offered to the audience only to be subsequently refused by the destruction of illusion.

riences. To the highest extent, this interaction or transaction, as Rosenblatt prefers to call it, is an experience where cognitive rational things are subject to aesthetical transactional things. The result of this interdependence enshrines in the reader's response, in his/her own aesthetical creation. The act of reading then becomes a vital event, not just a means to collect information. In this sense, Rosenblatt points out the existence of two kinds of reading, two different ways to interpret the words of a text: nonliterary reading or efferent reading and literary reading or aesthetic reading. These theories lie in the affective dimension of literary reading, especially in the first approach to the text and in the importance of the reader's contribution, whose prior life experience—affective and emotional—shall make dialog and transaction with the text possible. Based on these theories, we should understand that literary texts are not construed unidirectionally but following multiple interpretations. Understanding the text shall be subject to the reader's prior knowledge and to the fact said knowledge is up to date during the reading process (Short 1989).

Without calling into question the educational role played by reading, we should keep in mind that perceptive differentiation by the different readers is the key to the process. This way, each reader shall make his/her own perceptive choice from the contents of the text itself, which shall basically be based on his/her experiences, on what he/she learnt, and on all those values and beliefs assimilated throughout his/her socialization process.

Literary texts should also be created on the basis of pictures, empty spaces, or open structures that allow readers create their own meaning, making interpretative cooperation with them possible. Literary texts that are conceived that way are, no doubt, books that are "open" to a certain extent. Readers are aware that each sentence and picture are open to a multiform series of meanings that they should discover; they may even chose the most exemplary key to reading and use the meaning they wish depending on their mood (Eco 1962, 1979). If readers are provided with the whole story and cannot do anything, their imagination would never come into play, possibly resulting in boredom. Nevertheless, reading becomes active and creative when texts gear imagination (Iser 1978).

Guided by these theories, one's experiences influence one's reading, understanding, and thinking about texts. Reading also influences one's understandings about current situations, new scenarios, and future dilemmas (Pytash 2013). This idea that literature can modify people's beliefs and attitudes has been present in bibliography for a long time. For example, Fisher (1968) presents the results obtained on the basis of reading to modify the beliefs of Native Americans, Koeller (1977) describes an experience from which prejudices towards the Mexican community in America decrease, and Liebkind and McAlister (1999) work on tolerance towards immigrant communities. Many recent studies also show how reading offers possibilities to help the youngest with specific personal and social issues and conflicts: night terrors (Lewis et al. 2015), mental diseases such as anxiety or depression (Harvey 2010), mourning when a family member is lost (Heath and Cole 2012), suicide (Kaywell 1993), domestic violence (Wang et al. 2013), and sexual abuse (Kaywell 2004; Malo-Juvera 2014). Literary reading has also been successfully used to promote integration of students with a disability within the classroom (Cameron and

Rutland 2006), with different sexual orientations (Mitchell 2009), and to reduce aggressive behavior in children (Jones 1991; Shechtman 1999, 2000, 2006).

In this sense, it is noteworthy to point out the increasing number of studies that deal with bullying and cyberbullying through reading and children's and young people's literature, including, among others, the studies of Beane (2005), Flanagan et al. (2013), Freeman (2010, 2014), Henkin (2005), Kriedler (1996), McNamara and McNamara (1997), Pytash, (2013), and Ross (1996). Despite these studies showing good results by using literature in the classroom, further research is needed to establish whether its use can result in measurable changes in the children's and young people's attitudes or not.

13.2   Dealing with Bullying and Cyberbullying in Children's and Young People's Literature

School violence is nothing new in children's literature. For many years, bullying was a reality that affected the main characters of many stories from children's and young people's books. Violent situations were anecdotic many times. Nevertheless, with the changes undergone in children's literature in recent years, bullying has become a central issue, mainly due to the serious consequences suffered by the victims. As some authors point out (Hunt 1990a, 1990b; Cart 2010), this change is mainly due to two reasons: because of the force of the realistic movement in children's and young people's literature today, which pits the reader with daily problems enabling him/her to discover himself/herself and the environment with books that are very close to psycho-literature. On the other hand, it is due to the special use of these books in the field of literary communication because these books that often focus on realistic, current problems are used to prevent and modify certain behaviors.

There is a wide range of resources provided by some publications in which selections of children's literature books are offered to prevent bullying, such as *The Bully-Free Classroom* by Beane, which includes a selection of more than 50 books for children and strategies to keep the classroom free from bullying. Also, *Confronting Bullying: Literacy as a Tool for Character Education* by de Henkin and *Keys to Dealing with Bullies* by McNamara and McNamara. Likewise, some websites such as *Anti-Bullying Alliance* or *Best Children's Books* promote reading children's literature books as an instrument to prevent and stop bullying. In Spanish-speaking countries, it is noteworthy the publication *Pasa página al acoso escolar,* published by Fundación Caja Navarra, which offers a selection of literary books by age together with other resources for parents and teachers. Other lists of children's literature books that can be taken on board are especially those published by the "National School Safety Center," including *Bullying in Schools: Fighting the Bully Battle* (Quiroz et al. 2006), a guide that identifies strategies to diminish the incidence of bullying, among other resources.

Regarding the approach to bullying in children's and young people's literature, there are differences regarding the focalization of the subject, the characterization and the ages of the characters, as well as the description of the harassment and the kind of solution proposed.

Children's literature stories usually present the subject from the victim's point of view to create empathy, sorrow, or mercy, while there are few examples in which the bully is the main character of the story. As described by Borgia and Myers (2010), there are many books dealing with bullying in comparison to cyberbullying in fiction stories for the moment, although there are children under 14 who use the social media without their parent's approval. According to a study by *EU Kids Online* (Pérez-Barco 2013), 11.9 % of children aged 9 and 10 have a profile on a social network, a percentage that reaches 43 % among those aged 11 and 12. In this sense, there are books like *The Berenstain Bears Lost in Cyberspace* (Berenstain and Berenstain 1999), *Destroying Avalon* (McCaffrey 2006), *Abash and the Cyber-Bully* (Casper and Dorsey 2008), *Beacon Street Girls: Just Kidding* (Bryant 2009), *Twisted* (Anderson 2007), *The Secret Life of Girls* (Daughtery 2006), and *Chrissa Stands Strong* (Casanova 2009).

There are many children's literature books that star humanized animals, especially those for younger kids. A few examples of these simple stories presenting situations especially linked to verbal harassment and exclusion to younger kids are picture books such as *Chrysanthemum* (Henkes 1991), *Chester's Way* (Henkes 1988), *The Berenstain Bears and the Bully* (Berenstain and Berenstain 1993), *Henry and the Bully* (Carlson 2010), and *Hazel's Amazing Mother* (Wells 1992).

As far as gender is concerned, bullies are presented generally as male, while victims are presented as both male and female (Entenmen et al. 2005). Verbal and relational bullying is portrayed more often, followed by physical bullying. Violent behaviors usually take place at school and at home, that is, situations where small kids interact with peers. Likewise, many books emphasize elements that lead to victimization, the most common being physical appearance, behavior, some kind of disability, personality, being a newcomer, having strange interests or hobbies, academic success or failure, or growing up in a "different" household.

As described by Oliver et al. (1994), there are books on bullying where revenge is the strategy sought by their main characters to solve harassment situations. Those books published in the 1980s often present characters that are victims of bullying and believe that violence is the only answer to the harassment situation suffered by them. Books such as *Hang on, Harvey!* (Hopper 1984), *The Revenge of the Incredible Dr. Rancid and His Youthful Assistant, Jeffrey* (Conford 1980), *The Once in a While Hero* (Adler 1982), *Wilted* (Kropp 1982), *Rafa's Dog* (Griffiths 1983), *Bundle of Sticks* (Mauser 1987), and *The Boy Who Lost His Face* (Sachar 1991) are noteworthy.

It is important to choose books where the answer to these situations emerges from strategies that focus on institutional support and dialog when it comes to use literature as a sensitization and prevention tool. Oliver et al. (1994) categorized the books surveyed in order of coping and problem-solving strategies that are represented. They were subsequently classified in terms of whether they described more short-term coping strategies or more long-term problem resolution strategies. It is noteworthy that only three of the books included in this chapter dealt with coping or resolution strategies or skills for bullying behavior: *Blubber* (Blume 1983), *Turkey-legs Thompson* (McCord 1979), and *There's a Boy in the Girls' Bathroom* (Sachar 1987). In the first book, *Blubber*, the story revolves around Jill, who goes along with most of the others in her fifth-grade class in tormenting an overweight classmate derisively named Blubber. It is only when the class turns on Jill as the next victim of harassment that she finds out what it is like to become a target of bullying.

Many of these examples include observers who propose very different answers, from helping and defending victims to encouraging to attack. Many books present an adult who offers his/her help or intervention and, despite the solution to the problem was different as the case may be, most bullies were punished for their attack. The subject is generally dealt with in a sweetened, trivial way. The solutions offered are generally naïve and witty, like ignoring the problem, racing the aggressor, or becoming his/her friend; these solutions usually tend to make the problem even worse (Kochenderfer-Ladd 2004; Sandstrom 2004). For example, although some authors have warned about the fact that physical confrontation is usually counterproductive (Kochenderfer-Ladd 2004; Sandstrom 2004), the study conducted by Oliver et al. (1994), in which they analyzed 22 books for children aged between 9 and 12 years, identified that many of these books show characters that respond to bullying with violence.

When coping through difficult issues, many people want to identify with others who are coping with similar problems. Writers seek the identification of the reader with the main character of the story and, therefore, the characters are similarly aged as the reader in most cases. The fact that characters are of the same age as readers and that they are involved in realistic situations shall contribute to the children's and young people's identification with the story (Sridhar and Vaughn 2000). If a child is able to identify with the main character and relate to events that unfold in the book, he or she is likely to become emotionally involved in the story. When children are emotionally involved, they develop meaningful ties to the main character, and in doing so the literature facilitates a release of pent-up emotions. After the child has identified with the story and experienced a catharsis of emotions, he/she develops awareness that his/her problems might be solved in a manner similar to the characters in the book (Gregory and Vessey 2004). Indeed, fiction books allow speaking about a content that is emotionally tough with a certain security distance.

Certainly, literature helps students to have vicarious experiences through the book's characters, helping them to empathize with situations just like if they were the main characters (Tompkins 2007). Many times, the characters become role models that do not only have an expressive and representative function within the text but also a modeling function. In certain situations, the character's attitudes and behaviors show the reader his/her position before the conflicts presented and his/her place in the story. The models shown in stories, literature, and movies contain moral principles and values and encourage transferring some of these moral identity features to the recipient. The rewards and punishments received by the characters as a consequence of their behavior in the story help the reader to take a stand before those behaviors described.

Likewise, in children's literature, many of these books use the picture book as a vehicle, appealing to the reader's feelings in a more powerful way. It is easier to make the reader identify himself/herself with the events told by using pictures, infringing certain conventions such as the storyteller's point of view, for example. This way, in some stories that are written in first person, the fact that pictures show the story from outsider make the reader participate in two kinds of visual information and three stories at the same time: one story is told by the text, one is reflected in the pictures, and another one emerges by combining both of them. Genette (1972, p. 241) distinguishes between the person who is speaking (who is telling the story) and the person who is watching (through whose point of view the story is presented). In many picture books, "the person who speaks" is not "the person who watches": the text is written in first person, but the pictures seem to be in third person. The opposite also happens in those stories that are written in third person where pictures place the reader in the place of the main character to apprehend his/her feelings, thoughts, fears, and ideas, bearing in mind that he/she is suffering from bullying.

In the case of young people's stories, we find some changes regarding the approach to this subject, in comparison to those for children. In books for young people, we find more examples that deal with cyberbullying, where the problem is approached from the aggressor's point of view. In these stories, the main character has generally suffered from violence or harassment and uses the social media to seek revenge from his/her aggressor, showing that some victims in turn become aggressors sometimes (Craig 1998; DuRant et al. 2000; DuRant et al. 1999; Vossekuil et al. 2000). These books present problems for those therapists who use them in bibliotherapy because their texts tend to justify bullying when it turns into revenge. The main characters struggle between what they are doing is right or wrong, but they move forward to solve "yet greater evil."

Similarly, these stories for youngsters,[2] mostly commercial, usually present only one storyteller with an ideological perspective who tells the reader what is right and what is wrong in a Manichean way (vid. Lluch 2012). Normally, bullies themselves justify their behavior. Similarly, these storytellers show their most intimate thoughts and feelings trying to establish empathic relationships with the reader. Finally, the narrative structure of these stories is usually presented according to Adam's quinary model (1985, pp. 57–63), but it is often combined with the folk tale's structure. This way, the hero, upon overcoming several setbacks, emerges victorious with the help of secondary characters and magical objects. In this sense, the stories usually present secondary characters who perpetrate harassment in his/her name or the network turns into the magical object that redeems the hero.

Indeed, it can be noticed that these stories try to induce the identification of the reader over and over again. For example, these books flatter those people and the world around them. The stories take place in scenarios that are easily identifiable by them: high school, discotheques, the neighborhood, etc. In these books, experiences are also shared, the story being placed at present. We must not forget that they are

---

[2] We should include "impulse readings" (Lluch, 2012: 42) as well as other more validated readings that are approved by critics and literary prizes.

often presented as "bildungsroman" or "learning novels" where the main character finally becomes an adult by going through a more or less traumatic adventure. In this sense, bullying turns into a tool allowing them to become "grown-ups."

Examples of this can be found in books for young people that focus on cyber-bullying, such as *El-juego.com* (Algar) by Gemma Lluch and *E-boy* (Penguin) by Kevin Brooks. In *El-juego.com,* there is a game that consists of a bullying situation perpetrated by the main character to seek revenge from her ex-boyfriend. In short, it is about revenge, although it is embellished with the game, as assured by the main character herself:

> You hate someone a lot and start imagining the misfortunes you would like him to go through, anything. You imagine what you want him to go through, what you want him to feel, without limits, do you know? Without fears, without such thing as moral, without punishment [...] you know someone will make them happen for you. It is not you. You only imagine... [...] that was not OK. Now I know. Although it was a game, you just cannot wish all that bad to anyone (Lluch 2004, p. 134).

In *E-boy,* the trigger is a violent aggression against Lucy, the girl, the main charac-ter, is in love with, perpetrated by "The Crow Town kids" gang. The Crows also call E-Boy a nickname to mock of his wounds and his haircut. E-Boy's way of acting is an act of bravery: He tries to protect Lucy and other people from the neighborhood against further aggressions. The gang sexually assaulted Lucy and also perpetrated some bullying acts, such as insulting her or spraying her house's door ["the Word SLAG had been sprayed across the door in bright red aerosol paint"] (Brooks 2010, p. 47), that makes E-Boy very angry, who wishes to "hit someone, to really hurt someone...I wanted to find out who'd done it and throw them off the tower..." (Brooks 2010, p. 47). Tom Harvey, with the help of E-Boy's powers, avenges Lucy, although she refuses thereto: "You said you wanted to hurt them, to kill them...you wanted them to suffer" (Brooks 2010, p. 119).

Indeed, E-Boy is the enforcement arm of revenge using Tom's body. The author even includes an opening statement dealing with unrest, the "fugue state" whereby the individual's life is dissociated, even creating a new identity. This turns E-Boy into a relentless robot that does not wonder why street kids behave like that because they are not persons but things to him. This way, E-Boy embarks in seeking revenge from the Crows:

> ...timeless hours spent working on the computer in my head: sending false texts and pho-toshopped pictures, posting videos on YouTube, spreading malicious lies in chat rooms and blogs. Lies become rumors, rumors become facts: Nathan Craig's a grass; Big and Little Jones are terrorists; De Wayne Firman has posted a Facebook message calling Howard Ell-man a queer.... (Brooks 2010, p. 167)

In *El-juego.com,* the character's virtual alter-egos create a game whereby they originally try to get away from their problems as if the game was a new universe. Llum—the main character—later realizes that the game is not as naïve and unreal because the acts performed on the net have an impact in real life. Dirty tricks are played on her, infecting her computer with a virus that eliminates all information from the hard drive; she receives threatening e-mails; her e-mail is jammed up, she is not getting any information for few days, and she, therefore, loses customers because several companies unsubscribed from her server. Her telephone and electricity supplies are cut off, besides other commodities. Charges are made on her credit card; her computer turns on playing very loud music in the middle of the night. All these actions aim at destroying the victim's life.

These stories are built up on the basis of the guidelines of folktales (Lluch) and the hero's signs are recognized. The characters have suffered injuries and the Internet, the social media, and cyberbullying are presented as magical objects that they will use to restore justice, overcome a series of tests, and beat the aggressor. These stories end up with the victory of the main characters and, in the case of book for young people, let us not forget, are the characters who perpetrate the aggression. We then see that aggressors in these books become "heroes" that seek revenge due to an offence, damage, or tort. As we can see, it is about facing violent situations by using more violence. It is about seeking revenge with their own hands by using the possibilities offered by the Internet, which does not seem very appropriate.

13.3   Main Sensitization and Intervention Strategies

13.3.1   Selecting the Books

One of the aspects to take into account when working on the reading is the importance of selecting the books that are going to be used. Which book, for which reader, and when are the keys to success for this kind of actions. Caution must be taken because some books contain flawed strategies for responding to bullies, such as retaliating, ganging up and fighting the bully, or embarrassing the bully. As suggested earlier, it is wise to read potential books before selecting and sharing stories with children. Henkin (2005) similarly warns that many bullying books are overly simplistic and unrealistic, thus of limited utility. It is advisable that the bullying situation in the book be resolved in a prosocial and realistic manner. Prior to selecting bully-themed books, adults must consider the core message in each book and determine if this message aligns with desirable behaviors they intend to promote.

As described by Heath and Cole (2012), it is important to consider the following guidelines when selecting books to share with students:

(a) Select books that align with desired classroom behavior.
(b) Select books with a clear and direct core message focusing on positive rather than negative behaviors.
(c) Select age-appropriate books sensitive to students' social and emotional maturity, attention span, interests, and unique characteristics (e.g., gender, cultural, ethnic, and religious beliefs).
(d) Prior to sharing books with the classroom, it is important to carefully read, screen, and select the books. Care should be taken to ensure content is appropriate in text and illustration and supports school values and rules.

As pointed out by Morris et al. (2000), it is also important to take into account that there is no need to make all readings focus on stories that deal with this subject explicitly when dealing with bullying and cyberbullying in the classroom but working with other readings that present strategies of positive problem-solving and conflict-resolving skills. Using the categories of skill of the peaceful classroom suggested by Smith (1993), we can suggest readings linked to the development of friendship, compassion, cooperation, and kindness.

13.3.2   The Educator's Role

The ideological function or the transmission of values in narrative texts should not be magnified nor thinking of the immediate or mechanical transfer effects between the models presented and the readers. Reading is a complex cognitive activity, and it may then lead to a process whereby the values presented by the author initially and selected as appropriate by the educator himself/herself are not perceived by the target readers, if not all, at least by those whose vital and contextual features make them have different perceptions. As stated by Mendoza Fillola (2003) and Sánchez-García and Yubero (2013), the meaning of a book is perceived differently depending on the historical, social, and cultural context of each reader because every literary creation can transmit new suggestions and valuations from the perspective it is read or analyzed. "The author's intentions never exhaust the meaning of a literary book. As the book passes from one context into another, whether cultural or historical, new meanings that may have never been foreseen by the author or the target public at the time can be extracted" (Eagleton 1988, p. 91).

Mediators are essential when educating in values through reading, since he/she shall develop different strategies aimed at recognizing and analyzing the values contained, whether direct or indirectly, in the texts. To that end, the fact that stories provide with reflection and valuation material on the characters of the text, their actions and emotions, should be taken into account.

The role played by the mediator should not consist in imposing one single, officially validated reading or in avoiding relativism when construing the text to guide the reader to identify certain values. Using literary books shall, on the contrary, promote dialog between the reader and the text, helping the reader to think about the vicissitudes of the characters, to value or reject their acts, and to link the behaviors presented in the texts with his/her own experiences and values. The role played by the mediator/educator shall consist on accompanying when reading, introducing subjects to help children to form their own opinions and create their own meanings.

As described by King (2001), there is also a danger of aiming these readings at developing other knowledge. The teaching of reading and literature has traditionally focused on engaging kids in stove-piped "reading" exercises where aspects as grammatical constructions and lexicon were prioritized. Texts were in short used to extract other kinds of learning. These practices are necessary for curricular learning but are very far from the real aesthetic nature of reading.

Reading must be put in the first place in this kind of actions. Rosenblatt (1977) emphasizes the idea that we must focus on the affective dimension of literary reading, especially in the first approach to the text and in the importance of the reader's contribution, whose prior life experience—affective and emotional—shall make dialog and transaction with the text possible.

13.3.3   Main Strategies and Activities

The educator must have the knowledge, handle the strategies, and use the necessary instruments to perform an efficient action through reading. Reading, discussion, and writing are the main weapons in this kind of actions.

Reading is an essential aspect that should be taken into account. Oliver et al. (1994) and Heath and Cole (2012), among others, emphasize the importance of reading aloud. Reading the story aloud is preferable because the activity becomes a shared experience and does not place slower readers at a disadvantage. When reading aloud, to increase students' interest, the reader should inject feeling, matching his/her expression to realistically reflect characters and situations. When reading from picture books, Sipe (2008) suggested the book's pictures be large enough for children to see from a distance.

In general, the activities linked to selected readings are structured as follows: pre-, during-, and post-reading strategies (Hillsberg and Spak 2006).

(1) *Pre-reading activities* aim at advancing the conflict dealt with in the story somehow, as well as creating some expectations in the reader (Freeman 2014; Heath and Cole 2012). Activities before reading are designed to activate prior knowledge and build background knowledge with the purpose of assisting students' comprehension of text (Quinn et al. 2003). When introducing the book, heighten students' interest by asking a few carefully posed questions, showing the cover of the book, and possibly giving a short background of the author or illustrator. A few points should be considered for classroom discussion. The teacher could ask one or two questions to help the children think about the book's message. In general terms, all pre-reading activities must focus on connecting prior knowledge with the text and encouraging students to make predictions about the content.

(2) *During-reading activities* mainly aim at making text comprehension easier, as well as promoting dialog and debate about the conflicts described in the story. The activities proposed are directly linked to character education (Freeman 2014). Regarding the strategies more frequently used, the studies analyzed agree on proposing *literature circles,* discussion, and interaction groups for students of all ages. The advantages of *literature circles* lie in the development of significant interactions between the readers and the text (King 2001). Pooling readings in small groups promotes expressivity because the students are able to articulate affective responses between the texts and their own experiences. In

literature circles, participants play different roles (Daniels 2001) that may vary aiming at providing different views to the group:

(a) *Connector:* This student is responsible for finding connections between the text and the outside world. For example, the student can connect to his or her own life, happenings at school or in the community, similar events at other times and places, other books or stories, other writings on the same topic, or other writings by the same author.

(b) *Questioner:* This student's job is to write down three questions about the reading selection. Students should explain why they have this question and why they think this question is important.

(c) *Passage master:* This student's job is to locate key sentences that the group should review. The idea is to help others notice important parts of the text. The student should explain why the passage was selected.

(d) *Vocabulary enricher:* This student is responsible for finding especially important vocabulary in the story. Vocabulary selected should focus on words that are unfamiliar, interesting, important, repetitive, puzzling, or descriptive or those used in an unusual way.

(e) *Researcher:* This student's job is to share background information on topics related to the story. This information should help the group better understand the text.

They act as experts in their areas of focus and share the information with a larger group for open discussion (Quinn et al 2003). Students may rotate roles for each meeting (Burns 1998).

Some authors like Pytash (2013) and Day and Kroon (2010) support the instruction possibilities of *online literature circles*. These groups, which use a dynamics similar to the traditional structure of these groups, transfer conversations to the website, enabling asynchronous conversations with the same possibilities and results as the in-person sessions but in which the students work the search of information on the subjects.

As it has been mentioned previously, the dialogical nature of the reading process and the fact that the reader confers a meaning upon the texts makes the reader's own experiences help him/her to advance, make hypotheses design, compare, and evaluate. It is also likely that all the readers of the same book do not agree on what is reflecting in the text. Reading and discussion on the reading enable the students recognizing what they would do as readers and why, besides learning the other student's opinions and valuations.

Nystrand and Gamoran (1991) emphasized the importance of dialog as an educational tool. Dialogical readings allow children:

(a) To link the story with their own experience.

(b) To evaluate the characters' behavior and justifying his/her opinions.

(c) To develope an active attitude towards reading: seeking answers, advancing events, empathizing with the characters and imaging events that are described.

(d) To contribute constructively to sharing discussions on literature, answering, and contributing to form other students' opinions.

Nystrand et al. (1997) and Nystrand and Gamoran (1991) support the importance of dialogic instruction, as dialogic classroom discourse, such as open discussion, with monologic discourse, in which the teacher controls the content and direction of the talk. Dialogic instruction provides students with the ability to learn to talk, invites discussion that allows students to interact with each other using their own languages and dialects, includes scaffolding to help students become adept at discussion, and often incorporates controversies and divergent points of view (Caughlan et al. 2013; Juzwik et al. 2013). Many of these studies show that dialogic instruction has been correlated with increased academic performance in different studies (Applebee et al. 2003; Nystrand et al. 1997; Nystrand and Gamoran 1991).

(3) *Post-reading activities:* Once the text is read in its entirety, students should be offered opportunities to extend and personalize the meaning of the story. These activities should encourage students to analyze, evaluate, and judge the text on a personal, emotional, and literal level (Atwell 1998; Rasinski and Padak 2000). The post-reading activities that are more frequently used are role-playing and different participative techniques such as dialogs, discussions, presentations in public, and decision-making before a moral dilemma (Oliver et al. 1994; Quinn et al. 2003; Freeman 2014). Some authors suggest the use of role-playing strategies because they believe there is a reverse effect between empathy and aggressive behaviors (Eron 1987). Therefore, making bullies put in the place of victims is beneficial.

We can see how the bibliography used recently is especially focused on the past years of primary education and secondary education above all. In spite of this trend of focusing action plans on teenagers and youngsters, Freeman (2010, 2014) and Vladchou et al. (2011) justify the importance of dealing with bullying from childhood. In this sense, there is a remarkable series of picture books that deal with bullying and even cyberbullying. Titles such as *Stand Tall, Molly Lou Melon* (Lovell 2001), *Henry and the Bully* (Carlson 2010), *The Bully Blockers Club* (Bateman 2004), *Bye-Bye, Big Bad Bullybug!* (Emberley 2007), *Chrysanthemum* (Henkes 1991), *Chester's Way* (Henkes 1988), *Trouble in the Barkers' Class* (DePaola 2003), *Bootsie Barker Bites* (Bottner 1997), and *The Little Bully* (Bracken 2012), present, mainly by means of personified animals, attitudes related to bullying and its different representations: physical, verbal, social exclusion, rumors, and emotional (Monks et al. 2005).

As far as the way of working on reading with younger kids, Freeman (2014) emphasizes the possibilities offered by pictures and the need to address activities mainly towards character education. It is important that younger kids learn to value aspects that make cohabitation inside the classroom easier: the importance of being kind to others, helping someone in need, sharing, being honest, daring to protect someone who is being intimidated, and using positive language in difficult situations. Bergen (2002) emphasizes playing and cognitive strategies to enhance problem-solving and understanding.

In short, communication and dialog are the cornerstones of most of these projects. It is about dealing with bullying through reading, living examples, and discussing on strategies that will help children to be ready for situations they may be facing in the future.

13.4   Outcome

In the studies analyzed, we can see that using literature as awareness and prevention resource at schools is having some remarkable results. In the course of the actions carried out by preschool children and by children from the first years of primary education, Freeman's (2014) describes some improvements in terms of identifying situations and defense strategies by the students. This study, implemented with children aged between 4 and 6, took place one summer over a 12-week period at three child development centers. After the literature readings and lessons to build positive character based on the picture books about bullying, the children were categorized as having a "good" understanding of a bully and as having an "excellent" understanding of a bully. Also, all participants could give at least two positive strategies found as themes in the literature, for what to do if a bully is mean to them (tell an adult; try to be friends with the bully; stand up to the bully with words or body language; ignore or walk away from the bully; stick with a group of friends).

If we keep in mind that bullying is widespread among youngsters and teenagers, actions aimed at children aged between 9 and 16 are more numerous. In this sense, the studies of Holmgrem et al. (2011), Gregory and Vessey (2004), Quinn et al. (2003), Hillsberg and Spak (2006), and Borgia and Myers (2010) are noteworthy, among others. In general, all these studies yield very similar results. The teachers emphasize that they have been able to build a sense of purpose, belonging, identity, and security that created a safe environment for students to express themselves. Moreover, students felt free to unveil their insecurities. They could identify with the various situations of bullying within the book, and they became willing to address the issue. The children began to think, talk, listen, inquire, and learn. They were empowered to feel a part of the solution.

Anti-bullying and suicide awareness programs encourage teenagers to turn to teachers if they are bullied or they are contemplating suicide. However, teachers are sometimes unsure about how they should intervene with a student (Freedenthal and Breslin (2010). Considering that educators should know how to handle these situations, Pytash (2013) carried out an intervention with undergraduate preservice teachers (PSTs) by reading the novels *Thirteen Reasons Why* (Asher 2011) and *Hate List* (Brown 2009). After reading these books, participants shared their thoughts about the books and their own personal experiences with bullying in an online literature circle. According to the information gathered in the online literature circle discussions and in focus group interviews, the study concluded that PSTs shifted from reflecting on their personal experiences to imagining their future lives as teachers. Readings gave PSTs insight into the lives of young adults while providing opportunities for them to understand that, as teachers, they might be able to help teenagers who are considering suicide. Reading also provided PSTs with opportunities to imagine how they would handle similar situations. In this sense, young literature books provide an opportunity for PSTs to picture themselves in the role model in whom a troubled teenager confides.

In short, all these studies allow us to understand how literature provides readers with the opportunity to feel more generous and confidence. Readers could also perceive more deeply the personal and social implications of the reading experience.

13.5   Final Reflection

In this section, we would like to emphasize that despite being aware of the advantages of literature as consciousness and prevention tools, it is essential to instruct teachers not only in strategies to work on reading but so that they can find available fiction books that deal with these issues (Borgia and Myers 2010). Likewise, in order to work on these issues by using children's and young people's literature successfully, it is necessary that both the students and the educators be interested in reading (Oliver et al. 1994). In addition, this kind of actions linking education in values and the use of literature cannot be ad hoc experiments, but they should be part of the activities carried out throughout the entire school year and continue being an important part of the course of study for subsequent years (Freeman 2014).

Carrying out activities, reading books dealing with bullying and ongoing discussions on this issue are very suitable to alleviate intimidating behaviors in children, both in the younger and the elderly. If teachers, educators, and parents are proactive and educate children by carrying out activities of education in values, the problem can diminish before it starts or can be under control at primary and secondary education.

If students connect to the literature, identify with the main character, and relate the theme to their own experiences, they will achieve a higher level of comprehension (Keene and Zimmerman 1997). This increased understanding of the text can lead to changes in effect and behavior. If literature deals with the terrible consequences of bullying, it could help the victim and the bully. The victim may derive comfort or coping strategies from reading about another in a similar situation. In addition, the bully might begin to identify with a fictional victim, leading to empathy and the possibility for change (Pikas 1989). Finally, we want to emphasize the idea that anti-bullying programs are not only for the victims and the bullies but also for most students who are passive and who stand by and watch it occur (Hillberg and Spak 2006).

References

Adam, J. M. (1985). *Le texte narratif*. París: Natham.

Applebee, A. N., Langer, J. A., Nystrand, M., & Gamoran, A. (2003). Discussion-based approaches to developing understanding: Classroom instruction and student performance in middle and high school English. *American Educational Research Journal, 40*(3), 685–730. doi:10.3102/00028312040003685.

Atwell, N. (1998). *In the middle*. Portsmouth: Heinemann.

Beach, R. (1993). *Reader response theories*. Urbana: National Council of Teacher of English.

Beane, A. L. (2005). *The bully free classroom: Over 100 tips and strategies for teachers K-8*. Minneapolis: Free Spirit.

Bergen, D. (2002). The role of pretend play in children's cognitive development. *Early Childhood Research and Practice, 4*(1), 12–25.

Borgia, L. G., & Myers, J. J. (2010). Cyber safety and children's literatue: A good match for creating classroom communities. *Illinois Reading Council Journal, 38*(3), 29–34.

Burns, B. (1998). Changing the classroom climate with literature circles. *Journal of Adolescent & Adult Literacy, 42*(2), 124–129.

Cameron, L., & Rutland, A. (2006). Extended contact through story reading in school: Reducing children's prejudice toward the disabled. *Journal of Social Issues, 62*(3), 469–488. doi:10.1111/j.1540-4560.2006.00469.x.

Caughlan, S., Juzwik, M. M., Borsheim-Black, C., Kelly, S., & Fine, J. G. (2013). English teacher candidates developing dialogically organized instructional practices. *Research in the Teaching of English, 47*, 213–246.

Cart, M. (2010). *Young adult literature: From romance to realism*. Chicago: American Library Association.

Craig, W. M. (1998). The relationship among bullying, victimization, depression, anxiety, and aggression in elementary school children. *Personality and Individual Differences, 24*, 123–130. doi:10.1016/S0191-8869(97)00145-1.

Daniels, H. (2001). *Literature circles: Voice and choice in bookclubs and reading groups*. Portland: Stenhouse.

Day, D., & Kroon, S. (2010). Online literature circles rock! *Middle School Journal, 42*(2), 18–28.

DuRant, R. H., Kreiter, S., Sinal, S. H., & Woods, C. R. (1999). Weapon carrying on school property among middle school students. *Archives of Pediatrics and Adolescent Medicine, 153*, 21–26. doi:10.1001/archpedi.153.1.21.

DuRant, R. H., Altman, D., Wolfson, M., Barkin, S., Kreiter, S., & Krowchuck, D. (2000). Exposure to violence and victimization, depression, substance abuse, and the use of violence by young adolescence. *Journal of Pediatrics, 137*, 707–713. doi:10.1067/mpd.2000.109146.

Eagleton, T. (1988). *Una introducción a la teoría literaria*. México: Fondo de Cultura Económica.

Eco, U. (1962). *Opera aperta. Forma e indeterminazione nelle poetiche contemporanee*. Milano. Bompiani.

Eco, U. (1979). *Lector in fabula. La cooperazione interpretativa nei testi narrativi*. Milano: Bompiani.

Entenmen, J., Murnen, T. J., & Hendricks, C. (2005). Victims, bullies, and bystanders in K-3 literature. *The Reading Teacher, 59*(4), 352–364. doi:10.1598/RT.59.4.5.

Eron, L. D. (1987). Aggression through the ages. *School Safety (National School Safety Center) News Journal, Fall*, 12–16.

Flanagan, K. S., Vanden Hoek, K. K., Shelton, A., Kelly, S. L., Morrison, C. M., & Young, A. M. (2013). Coping with bullying: What answers does children's literature provide? *School Psychology International, 34*(6), 691–706. doi:0.1177/0143034313479691.

Fisher, F. L. (1968). Influences of reading and discussion on the attitudes of fifth graders toward American Indians. *The Journal of Educational Research, 62*(3), 130–134. doi:10.1080/00220671.1968.10883788.

Freedenthal, S., & Breslin, L. (2010). High school teachers' experiences with suicidal students: A descriptive study. *Journal of Loss and Trauma, 15*(2), 83–92. doi:10.1080/15325020902928625.

Freeman, G. (2010). Picture books to develop strategies for dealing with bullying situations: A resource list created by and for young children. *Reading Matters, 11*, 6–11.

Freeman, G. (2014). The implementation of character education and children's literature to teach bullying characteristics and prevention strategies to preschool childrens: An Action Research Project. *Early Childhood Educational Journal, 42*, 305–316. doi:10.1007/s10643-013-0614-5.

Genette, G. (1972). *Figures III*. Paris: Editions du Seuil.

Gregory, K. E., & Vessey, J. A. (2004). Bibliotherapy: A strategy to help students with bullying. *The Journal os School Nursing, 30*(3), 127–133. doi:10.1177/10598405040200030201.

Harvey, P. (2010). Bibliotherapy use by welfare teams in secondary colleges. *Australian Journal of Teacher Education, 35*(5), 29–39. doi:10.1177/0143034305060792.

Heath, M. A., & Cole, B. V. (2012). Strengthening classroom emotional support for children following a family memnber's death. *School Psychology International, 33*(3), 243–262. doi:10-177/01430311415800.

Henkin, R. (2005). *Confronting bullying: Literacy as a tool for character education*. Portsmouth: Heinemann.

Hillsberg, C., & Spak, H. (2006). Young adult literature as the centerpiece of an anti-bullying program in middle school. *Middle School Journal, 38*(2), 23–28.

Holmgren, J., Lamb, J., Miller, M., & Werderich, C. (2011). *Decreasing bullying behaviors through discussing Young-adult literatura, role-playing activities and establishing a schoolwide definition of bullying in accordance with a common set of rules in language arts and math*. Degree of Master of Arts in teaching and leadership. Chicago: Saint Xavier University.

Hunt, P. (1990a). *Children's literature: The development of criticism*. London: Routledge.

Hunt, P. (1990b). *Children's literature: An illustrated history*. Oxford: Oxford University Press.

Iser, W. (1978). *The act of reading: A theory of aesthetics response*. Baltimore: Johns Hopkins University Press.

Jauss, H. R. (1982). *Aesthetic experience and literary hermeneutics*. Minneapolis: University of Minnesota Press.

Jones, C. B. (1991). Creative dramatics: A way to modify aggressive behavior. *Early Child Development and Care, 73*, 43–52. doi:10.1080/0300443910730105.

Juzwik, M. M., Borsheim-Black, C., Caughlan, S., & Heintz, A. (2013). *Inspiring dialogue: Talking to learn in the English classroom*. New York: Teachers College Press.

Kaywell, J. F. (1993). *Adolescents at risk: A guide to fiction and nonfiction for young adults, parents, and professionals*. Westport: Greenwood Press.

Kaywell, J. F. (2004). *Using literature to help troubled teenagers cope with abuse issues*. Westport: Greenwood Press.

Keene, E. O., & Zimmermann, S. (1997). *Mosaic of thought*. Portsmouth: Heinemann.

King, C. (2001). "I like group reading because we can share ideas": The role of talk within the Literature Circle. *Reading, 35*(1), 32–36. doi:10.1111/1467-9345.00157.

Kochenderfer-Ladd, B. (2004). Peer victimization: The role of emotions in adaptive and maladaptive coping. *Social Development, 13*(3), 329–349. doi:10.1111/j.1467-9507.2004.00271.x.

Koeller, S. (1977). The effect of listening to excerpts from children's stories about Mexican-Americans on the attitudes of sixth graders. *Journal of Educational Research, 70*(6), 329–334. doi:10.1080/00220671.1977.10885017.

Kriedler, W. (1996). Smart ways to handle kids who pick on others. *Instructor, 106*, 70–77.

Lewis, K. M., Amatya, K., Coffman, M. F., & Ollendick, T. H. (2015). Treating nighttime fears in young children with bibliotherapy: Evaluating anxiety symptoms and monitoring behavior change. *Journal of Anxiety Disorders, 30*(1), 103–112. doi:10.1016/j.janxdis.2014.12.004.

Liebkind, K., & McAlister, A. L. (1999). Extended contact through peer modelling to promote tolerance in Finland. *European Journal of Social Psychology, 29*, 765–780. doi:10.1002/(SICI)1099-0992(199908/09)29:5/6<765::AID-EJSP958>3.0.CO;2-J.

Lluch, G. (2012). La narrativa para los adolescentes del siglo XXI. In B. Roig Rechou, I. Soto López, & M. N. Rodríguez (coords.) (Eds.), *A narrativa xuvenil a debate (2000–2011)* (pp. 39–57). Vigo: Xerais.

Malo-Juvera, V. (2014). Speak: The effect of literary instruction on adolescents' rape myth acceptance. *Research in the Teaching of English, 48*(4), 407–427.

McNamara, B. E., & McNamara, F. J. (1997). *Keys to dealing with bullies*. New York: Barron's Educational Series.

Mendoza Fillola, A. (2003). Los intertextos: del discurso a la recepción. In A. M. Fillola & P. C. Cerrillo (coord.) (Eds.), *Intertextos: Aspectos sobre la recepción del discurso artístico* (pp. 17–60). Cuenca: Ediciones de la Universidad de Castilla-La Mancha.

Mitchell, M. (2009). When consciousness dawns: Confronting homophobia with Turkish high school students. *English Journal, 98*(4), 67–72.

Monks, C. P., Smith, P. K., & Swettenham, J. (2005). Psychological correlates of peer victimisation in preschool: Social cognitive skills, executive function and attachment profiles. *Aggressive Behavior, 31*(1), 571–588. doi:10.1002/ab.20099.

Morris, V. A., Taylor, S. I., & Wilson, J. T. (2000). Using children's stories to promote peace in classrooms. *Early childhood Education Journal, 28*(1), 41–50. doi:1082-3301/00/0900-0041.

Nystrand, M., & Gamoran, A. (1991). Instructional discourse, student engagement, and literature achievement. *Research in the Teaching of English, 25*, 261–290.

Nystrand, M., Gamoran, A., Kachur, R., & Prendergast, C. (1997). *Opening dialogue: Understanding the dynamics of language and learning in the English classroom.* New York: Teachers College Press.

Oliver, R. L., Young, T. A., & LaSalle, S. M. (1994). Early lessons in bullying and victimization: The help and hindrance of children's literature. *The School Counselor, 42*(2), 137–146.

Pérez-Barco, M. J. (2013). ¿Cuál es la edad recomendada para usar las redes sociales? *ABC. es,* June 24th. http://www.abc.es/familia-padres-hijos/20130621/abci-edad-redes-sociales-201306131359.html.

Petit, M. (2008). *El arte de la lectura en tiempos de crisis.* Barcelona: Océano.

Pikas, A. (1989). A pure concept of mobbing gives the best result for treatment. *School Psychology International, 10*, 95–104. doi:10.1177/0143034389102003.

Pytash, K. E. (2013). Using YA Literature to help preservice teachers deal with bullying and suicide. *Journal of Adolescent & Adult Literacy, 56*(6), 470–479. doi:10.1002/JAAL.168.

Quinn, K. B., Barone, B., Kearns, J., Stackhouse, S. A., & Zimmerman, M. E. (2003). Using a novel unit to help understand and prevent bullying in schools. *Journal of Adolescent & Adult Literacy, 46*(7), 582–591.

Quiroz, H. C., Arnette, J. L., & Stephens, R. D. (2006). *Bullying in schools: Fighting the bully battle.* National School Safety Center. http://www.schoolsafety.us/free-resources/bullying-in-schools-fact-sheet-series.

Rasinski, T., & Padak, N. (2000). *Effective reading strategies.* Columbus: Prentice-Hall.

Rosenblatt, L. M. (1977). *The reader, the text, the poem.* Carbondale: Southern Illinois University Press.

Ross, D. M. (1996). *Childhood bullying and teasing: What school personnel, other professionals, and parents can do.* Alexandria: American Counseling Association.

Sanchez-García, S., & Yubero, S. (2013). *La literatura de Fernando Alonso: fantástica realidad.* Cuenca: Universidad de Castilla-La Mancha.

Sandstrom, M. J. (2004). Pitfalls of the peer world: How children cope with common rejection experiences. *Journal of Abnormal Child Psychology, 32*(1), 67–81. doi:10.1023/B:JACP.0000007581.95080.8b.

Shechtman, Z. (1999). Bibliotherapy: An indirect approach to treatment of childhood aggression. *Child Psychiatry & Human Development, 30*(1), 39–53. doi:10.1023/A:1022671009144.

Shechtman, Z. (2000). An innovative intervention for treatment of child and adolescent aggression: An outcome study. *Psychology in the Schools, 37*(2), 157–167. doi:10.1002/(SICI)1520-6807(200003)37:2<157::AID-PITS7>3.0.CO;2-G.

Shechtman, Z. (2006). The contribution of bibliotherapy to the counseling of aggressive boys. *Psychotherapy Research, 16*(5), 631–636. doi:10.1080/10503300600591312.

Short, M. (1989). *Reading, analysing and teaching literature.* New York: Longman.

Sipe, L. R. (2008). *Storytime: Young children's literary understanding in the classroom.* New York: Teachers College Press.

Smith, C. A. (1993). *The peaceful classroom.* Mt. Rainier: Gryphon House.

Sridhar, D., & Vaughn, S. (2000). Bibliotherapy for all: Enhancing reading comprehension, self-concept, and behavior. *Teaching Exceptional Children, 33*(2), 74–82. doi:10.1177/004005990003300210.

Tompkins, G. E. (2007). *Literacy for the 21st century: A balanced approach* (4th ed.). Boston: Allyn & Bacon.

Vladchou, M., Andreou, E., Botsoglou, K., & Didaskalou, E. (2011). Bully/victim problems among preschool children: A review of current research evidence. *Educational Psychology Review, 23*(3), 329–358. doi:10.1007/s10648-011-9153-z.

Vossekuil, B., Reddy, M., Fein, R., Borum, R., & Modzeleski, W. (2000). *U.S.S.S. safe school initiative: An interim report on the prevention of targeted violence in schools*. Washington, DC: U.S. Secret Service, National Threat Assessment Center, U.S. Department of Education, National Institute of Justice.

Wang, C.-H., Lin, Y.-J., Kuo, Y.-C., & Hong, S.-S. (2013). Reading to relieve emotional difficulties. *Journal of Poetry Therapy, 26*(4), 255–267. doi:10.1080/08893675.2013.849045.

Wollheim, R. (1983). Flawed crystals. *New Literary History, 15,* 185–192.

Yubero, S., & Larrañaga, E. (2011). Cazando valores, valorando lectores. In *Leer abre espacios para el diálogo* (pp. 145–150). México: Conaculta.

Yubero, S., & Larrañaga, E. (2014). Textos literarios para la prevención del acoso. *International Journal of Developmental and Educational Psychology, 1*(5), 313–318.

Literary books cited

Adler, C. S. (1982). *The once in a while hero*. New York: Coward, McCann & Geoghegan.

Anderson, L. H. (2007). *TwUted*. New York: Viking.

Asher, J. (2011). *Thirteen reasons why*. New York: Razorbill.

Bateman, T. (2004). *The bully blockers club*. Morton Grove: Albert Whitman & Company.

Berenstain, S., & Berenstain, J. (1993). *The Berenstain bears and the bully*. New York: Random House.

Berenstain, S., & Berenstain, J. (1999). *The Berenstain bears lost in cyberspace*. New York: Random House.

Blume, J. (1983). *Blubber*. New York: Dell.

Bottner, B. (1997). *Bootsie barker bites*. New York: The Putnam & Grosset Group.

Bracken, B. (2012). *The little bully*. North Mankato: Capstone Press.

Brooks, K. (2010). *iBoy*. New York: Penguin Books.

Brown, J. (2009). *Hate list*. New York: Little, Brown.

Bryant, A. (2009). *Beacon street girls: Just kidding*. New York: Aladdin Paperbacks.

Carlson, N. (2010). *Henry and the bully*. New York: Puffin Books.

Casanova, M. (2009). *Chrissa stands strong*. Middleton: American Girl Publishing, Inc.

Casper, M., & Dorsey, T. (2008). *Abash and the cyberbully*. Hong Kong: Evergrow Ltd.

Conford, E. (1980). *The revenge of the incredible Dr. Rancid and his youthful assistant, Jeffrey*. Boston: Little, Brown.

Daughtery, L. (2006). *The secret life of girls*. Woodstock: Dramatic Publishing Co.

DePaola, T. (2003). *Trouble in the Barkers' class*. New York: G. P. Putnam's Sons.

Emberley, E. (2007). *Bye-bye, big bad bullybug!* New York: Little, Brown Books for Young Readers.

Griffiths, H. (1983). *Rafa's dog*. New York: Holiday House.

Henkes, K. (1988). *Chester's way*. New York: Puffin Books.

Henkes, K. (1991). *Chrysanthemum*. New York: HarperTrophy.

Hopper, N. J. (1984). *Hang on, Harvey!* New York: Dell.

Kropp, P. S. (1982). *Wilted*. New York: Dell.

Lovell, P. (2001). *Stand tall, molly Lou Melon*. New York: G. P. Putnam's Sons.

Lluch, G. (2004). *El-juego.com*. Alzira: Algar.

Mauser, P. R. (1987). *A bundle of sticks*. New York: Aladdin Books.

McCaffrey, K. (2006). *Destroying Avalon. North Freemantle*. Australia: Free Mantle Press.

McCord, J. (1979). *Turkeylegs Thompson*. New York: Atheneum.

Sachar, L. (1987). *There's a boy in the girl's bathroom*. New York: Bullseye.

Sachar, L. (1991). *The boy who lost his face*. New York: Knopf.

Wells, R. (1992). *Hazel's amazing mother*. New York: Puffin Books.

ERRATUM

Cyberbullying and Restorative Justice

Susan Hanley Duncan

© Springer International Publishing Switzerland 2016
R. Navarro et al. (eds.), *Cyberbullying Across the Globe*,
DOI 10.1007/978-3-319-25552-1_12

DOI 10.1007//978-3-319-25552-1_14

In chapter 12 titled **"Cyberbullying and Restorative Justice"**, the author name Louis D. Brandeis is removed from all instances where mentioned in the chapter header and opener, Table of Contents, and Contributors list.

The updated original online version of the chapter can be found at
http://dx.doi.org/10.1007/978-3-319-25552-1_12

© Springer International Publishing Switzerland 2017
R. Navarro et al. (eds.), *Cyberbullying Across the Globe*,
DOI 10.1007/978-3-319-25552-1_14

Index

© Springer International Publishing Switzerland 2016
R. Navarro et al. (eds.), *Cyberbullying Across the Globe,*
DOI 10.1007/978-3-319-25552-1

CPSIA information can be obtained
at www.ICGtesting.com
Printed in the USA
LVOW13*1956010418
571881LV00009B/739/P